D1195488

Current Controversies in the Anxiety Disorders

CURRENT CONTROVERSIES IN THE ANXIETY DISORDERS

Edited by
RONALD M. RAPEE
Macquarie University

THE GUILFORD PRESS
New York   London

Happy Birthday Alice

©1996 The Guilford Press
A Division of Guilford Publications, Inc.
72 Spring Street, New York, NY 10012

Printed in the United States of America

This book is printed on acid-free paper.

Last digit is print number: 9   8   7   6   5   4   3   2   1

Library of Congress Cataloging-in-Publication Data

Current controversies in the anxiety disorders / edited by Ronald
  M. Rapee.
       p.   cm.
    Includes bibliographical references and index.
    ISBN 1-57230-023-X
    1. Anxiety.   I. Rapee, Ronald M.
    [DNLM: 1. Anxiety Disorders.   WM 172 C9763 1995]
RC531.C87   1995
616.85′223 — dc20
DNLM/DLC
for Library of Congress   95-24718
                                             CIP

Contributors

GAVIN ANDREWS, M.D., FRCPsych., FRANZCP, Clinical Research Unit for Anxiety Disorders, University of New South Wales at St. Vincent's Hospital, Sydney, New South Wales, Australia

MARTIN M. ANTONY, Ph.D., Department of Psychiatry, Clarke Institute of Psychiatry, Toronto, Ontario, Canada

DAVID H. BARLOW, Ph.D., Center for Stress and Anxiety Disorders and Department of Psychology, University at Albany, State University of New York, Albany, New York

NIGEL W. BOND, Ph.D., School of Psychology, Flinders University of South Australia, Adelaide, South Australia, Australia.

TIMOTHY A. BROWN, Psy.D., Phobia and Anxiety Disorders Clinic, Center for Stress and Anxiety Disorders, The University at Albany, State University of New York, Albany, New York

BRUCE F. CHORPITA, B.A., Center for Stress and Anxiety Disorders, The University at Albany, State University of New York, Albany, New York

SIMON J. ENRIGHT, Ph.D., Department of Clinical Psychology, West Berkshire Priority Care Trust, Fair Mile Hospital, Wallingford, Oxfordshire, United Kingdom

EDNA B. FOA, Ph.D., Department of Psychiatry, Medical College of Pennsylvania, Philadelphia, Pennsylvania

SCOTT O. LILIENFELD, Ph.D., Department of Psychology, Emory University, Atlanta, Georgia

RICHARD J. MCNALLY, Ph.D., Department of Psychology, Harvard University, Cambridge, Massachusetts

KAREN R. MYERS, M.D., Department of Internal Medicine, Georgetown University Medical School, Washington, D.C.

ARNE ÖHMAN, Ph.D., Department of Clinical Neuroscience, Section of Psychology, Karolinska Institute and Hospital, Stockholm, Sweden

TERESA A. PIGOTT, M.D., Clinical Therapeutic Research Program and Psychopharmacology Clinic, and Department of Psychiatry and Behavioral Sciences Medical Branch at Galveston, University of Texas, Galveston, Texas

RONALD M. RAPEE, Ph.D., School of Behavioural Sciences, Macquarie University, Sydney, New South Wales, Australia

PAUL M. SALKOVSKIS, Ph.D., Department of Psychiatry, Warneford Hospital, University of Oxford, Oxford, United Kingdom

DAVID A. T. SIDDLE, Ph.D., Department of Psychology, University of Queensland, Brisbane, Queensland, Australia

DAVID A. WILLIAMS, Ph.D., Department of Psychiatry, Georgetown University Medical School, Washington, D.C.

S. LLOYD WILLIAMS, Ph.D., Department of Psychology, Lehigh University, Bethlehem, Pennsylvania

Preface

THE ANXIETY DISORDERS have been some of the most widely studied forms of psychopathology throughout the 1980's and 1990's and will, no doubt, continue to fascinate researchers well into the 21st Century. While dramatic advances in our knowledge of these disorders have occurred over the past decade, a wealth of unsolved mysteries still remains. In order to unravel some of the remaining puzzles of anxiety, we will need to rely on carefully developed theories and hypotheses to guide us. Undoubtedly, many theories will be discarded along the way and almost none will survive without modification. However, it is only through discussion, argument, and empirical validation that advances in our understanding of the nature and modification of the anxiety disorders will continue.

In the literature on anxiety, it is often found that opposing views, and even relevant empirical evidence, are published in diverse and independent journals. As a result, the average reader is hard pressed to clearly understand all sides of an issue. In some cases, even the experts in an area do not clearly see the real differences and similarities between positions because of the lack of simple summaries. The purpose of this book, therefore, is to focus on controversial issues or unresolved debates within the anxiety disorders field and to draw together the most outspoken and expert proponents of particular perspectives to present their respective cases.

I have tried to select issues which represent long term and salient sources of disagreement on a variety of aspects of the anxiety disorders. The rules of the game were simple. Authors were asked to write a brief, clear exposition of their position on a particular issue, with ample support, where possible, from empirical evidence. Chapters were minimally edited by me in order to preserve the author's original intent. Once all authors on an issue had submitted their chapters, the manuscripts were given to the other authors for a brief reply. No alterations to the original chapters were permitted.

It seems to me that the original purpose of this book has been abundantly realized. The basic chapters are clear, definitive statements of each author's position. As a reader I have found myself discovering some of the finer points of many arguments for the first time. In turn, the rejoinders provide a revealing insight to each author's reaction to the other chapters in their set. In some cases, authors have discovered marked similarities between apparently diverse positions, whereas in other cases authors have reaffirmed differences and clarified their arguments.

Probably the main value of this type of book is the hope that, by setting out disparate positions side-by-side, it will lead to further refinements of theory. More importantly, such comparison should help to clarify empirical studies which can test differential predictions of various positions. It is my hope that publication of this book will help to stimulate a range of empirical studies aimed at testing many of the controversial issues highlighted.

Contents

PART III. TREATMENT

I

Classification

1

Comorbidity in Neurotic Disorders: The Similarities Are More Important Than the Differences

GAVIN ANDREWS

IN THIS CHAPTER I argue that even though the anxiety and depressive disorders are defined in both the ICD and DSM systems of classification so that overlap between diagnoses is minimal, these disorders are part of a general class of disorders that share common etiological factors. Furthermore, I argue that the strength of these common factors is more important than the strength of etiological factors specific to each disorder. Much of this argument has been made before (Andrews, Stewart, Morris-Yates, Holt, & Henderson, 1990; Andrews, 1991), and most of the present text has appeared in Andrews (in press).

The DSM-IV criteria and the ICD-10 Diagnostic Criteria for Research (World Health Organization [WHO], 1993a) show remarkable similarity in the criteria used to define the major anxiety disorders. Panic Disorder is described in both classifications as consisting of recurrent, abrupt, unexpected, or unpredictable attacks of fear or discomfort, peaking in minutes and accompanied by symptoms of the flight-or-fight response and outcome fears of physical illness. The criteria for Panic Disorder with Agoraphobia, though different in detail, are likely to prove functionally equivalent. ICD-10 follows the traditional description of excessive or unreasonable fear or avoidance of crowds, public places, traveling alone, or being away from home, accompanied by anxiety symptoms when in or thinking about the situation. DSM-IV is less operationalized but encapsulates the key features of the disorder better: First, the panic attacks lead to avoidance or endurance with marked distress of situations from which escape might be difficult or help unavailable; and, second, the panic attacks themselves must worry or handicap the individual.

Social Phobia is defined as excessive and unreasonable fear and avoidance of scrutiny, or fear of being the focus of attention in social situations in case one acts in a way that will result in humiliation or embarrassment. ICD-10 requires that specific symptoms be present, whereas in DSM-IV a level of handicap is required. Obsessive–Compulsive Disorder is defined as consisting of obsessions (one's own thoughts are intrusive) or compulsions; both are repetitive, cannot be resisted, are excessive and inappropriate, and distress or handicap the individual by occupying time. DSM-IV also requires compulsions to be experienced as repetitive behaviors or mental acts designed to neutralize, while ICD-10 requires a minimum duration of symptoms of 2 weeks. Again, the two sets of criteria will probably be functionally equivalent. Generalized Anxiety Disorder is defined as more than 6 months of tension or anxiety and worry over everyday events and problems, accompanied by somatic symptoms of anxiety. ICD-10 requires more anxiety symptoms than DSM-IV, while DSM-IV requires that the worry handicaps and cannot be controlled. Once again, the two difinitions should be comparable in operation.

The criteria for each disorder, whatever the classification used, are sufficiently distinct that the syndrome can be reliably distinguished on clinical interview and more importantly, distinguished by computerized structured diagnostic interviews such as the Composite International Diagnostic Interview — or the CIDI-Auto (WHO, 1993b). Both classifications reaffirm that patients are very much aware of the salient and distinguishing features of their major disorders.

Advances in science commonly follow the introduction of new measurement techniques. The advent of structured diagnostic interviews such as the CIDI has also drawn attention to the excessive frequency with which patients report having experienced more than one disorder in their lifetimes to date. The importance of this excessive comorbidity is that etiological theories must either postulate that a number of separate causative factors have aggregated in one individual at a rate much greater than chance would allow, or else concede that some general factor has made each person vulnerable to a range of disorders.

Patients with anxiety or depressive disorders are often in no doubt about their vulnerability to multiple disorders and attribute their recurrent episodes to some underlying personality sensitivity. "I have a nervous nature that handles stress badly," they claim. This sensitivity to anxiety and failure to cope used to be defined as Asthenic Personality Disorder (ICD-8), but we (Andrews, Kiloh, & Kehoe, 1978) were able to relate this diagnosis to dimensional measures of trait anxiety and coping. Trait concepts, such as trait anxiety (e.g., neuroticism—Eysenck & Eysenck, 1975) and coping (e.g., locus of control—Craig, Franklin, & Andrews, 1984; defense style—Andrews, Singh, & Bond, 1993), are better descriptions of the dimensional or trait nature of the concept (see also Ormel, 1983; Bolger, 1990; Andrews, 1991). In this chapter, I argue the importance of high trait anxiety and poor coping as components of an important etiological factor in the common anxiety and depressive disorders—the common neurotic disorders.

Trait anxiety has been shown to be an important, clinically relevant concept in the etiology of some disorders. For example, in a longitudinal study of depression, we (Kiloh, Andrews, Neilson, & Bianchi, 1972) identified patients who were admitted to a university teaching hospital complaining of depression, and followed them for 15 years. On the basis of a structured diagnostic interview, treatment response, and other ancillary information from the index admission, the patients were divided into three diagnostic groups: endogenous depression; neurotic depression; and other neuroses but complaining of depression. At the 15-year follow-up, information about 193 of the 212 patients was obtained to construct four measures of outcome (global outcome, percentage of time ill, time in hospital, work incapacity). Using a structural-equation modeling approach, we asked which characteristics evident at time of first admission predicted the course of illness. Neither diagnosis, initial severity, nor life event stressors were good predictors of outcome. Personality vulnerability to anxiety (measured by Eysenck's neuroticism scale and related measures) was the best predictor of outcome in both neurotic groups (neurotic depression and other neuroses), explaining 20% of the variance in long-term outcome. These variables, however, did not account for significant variations in outcome in endogenous depression. These findings were held to be consistent with much previous literature (Andrews, Neilson, Hunt, Stewart, & Kiloh, 1990).

In thinking about the adverse life events as causes of anxiety and depression, it is useful to have a schematic model of mediating personality variables, such as trait anxiety and reality- and emotion-focused coping. In the model we espouse (Andrews, 1991), adversity is regarded as a trigger stimulus for symptoms; trait anxiety as a powerful variable moderating the extent of arousal produced by the arousal produced by the adversity; and reality-focused and emotion-focused coping as trait-like attributes that the person uses to focus attention on resolving the adversity or on preventing the anxiety from becoming debilitating should the adversity persist. Measures of life events and of symptoms are common. In this chapter we use neuroticism as a proxy for trait anxiety, and locus of control and defense style as proxies for reality-focused and emotion-focused coping. When present to a pathological degree, these traits are regarded as constituting a vulnerability factor that can render persons liable to anxiety and depressive symptoms and disorders.

This chapter is also about comorbidity—the observation that persons with mental disorders are at great risk of having other disorders during their lifetimes. There are a number of mechanisms that may explain comorbidity; three are illustrated here. First, a single factor may make people vulnerable to a number of disorders, and as a corollary the patterns of comorbidity will not be specific to any disorder. Second, different factors may render people vulnerable to different groups of disorders; the corollary of this is that comorbid disorders should occur in distinguishable clusters. Third, the stress of one disorder may cause other disorders, in which case the comorbidity will be sequential. These mechanisms can coexist. For example, persons with high trait anxiety who develop generalized anxiety disorder may then develop a major depressive episode, both because of the load of the worrying and because of being made vulnerable to any neurotic disorder by the high level of trait anxiety.

VULNERABILITY TO ANXIETY AND DEPRESSIVE SYMPTOMS: COMMUNITY STUDIES

Are vulnerability factors important in the genesis of anxiety and depressive symptoms that occur in the general population? Duncan-Jones (1987) studied the variation in symptoms of two cohorts in the population; contrary to the ideas of the day, he concluded that short-term stressors were of little import and that long-term vulnerability factors dominated the etiology of neurotic illness, accounting for 70–76% of the variance in symptoms. He later concluded that neuroticism accounted for the majority of this effect. Ormel and Wohlfarth (1991) studied the causal relationships among neuroticism, long-term difficulties, life situation change, and psychological distress in a 7-year, three-wave study in a general population. They concluded that temperament was more powerful than environment; that neuroticism and, to a lesser extent, long-term difficulties were powerful predictors of symptom occurrence over protracted periods of time; and that a substantial proportion of the correlations among long-term difficulties, life change scores, and symptoms could be attributed to the confounding effects of neuroticism on aspects of these variables. From the epidemiological perspective, therefore, personality vulnerability is a necessary and nearly sufficient cause of anxiety and depressive symptoms occuring in the general population.

Jardine, Martin, and Henderson (1984) obtained measures of the neuroticism trait, and of anxiety and depressive symptoms, in 3,810 twin pairs. First, they calculated that 60–67% of the variation in symptom scores was related to stable genetic or environmental factors (a finding resembling that of Duncan-Jones), with the remainder of the variance being related to fluctuating environmental influences or attributable to measurement error. Genetic factors accounted for 50% of the variation in neuroticism, 38% of the variation in anxiety symptoms, and 36% of the variation in depressive symptoms. They conducted a multivariate genetic anaylsis and concluded that "genetic variation in the symptoms of anxiety and depression is largely dependent on the effects of the same genes which determine variation in the trait of neuroticism" (p. 89). In fact, the genes shared with neuroticism accounted for 92% and 83%, respectively, of the genetic influence on anxiety and depressive symptoms.

Kendler, Heath, Martin, and Eaves (1986, 1987) reanalyzed these symptom questions from the Australian twin data and concluded that the "same" genes act in a largely nonspecific way to influence the overall level of psychiatric symptoms. At the time there was considerable interest in the heritability of panic; accordingly, we (Martin, Jardine, Andrews, & Heath, 1988) reanalyzed the two possible "panic symptoms" from the same data set. We found that the additive and dominant genetic effects of the factor shared with neuroticism were more important than the specific genetic determinants of the individual symptoms. Thus both epidemiological and genetic modeling of the variation of symptoms in the general population have supported the importance of trait measures of personality vulnerability (e.g., neuroticism) as an important single factor that determines symptoms. At least in terms of average symptom level, people are very much the victims of their temperaments.

VULNERABILITY TO ANXIETY AND DEPRESSIVE DISORDERS: COMMUNITY STUDIES

The preceding section has discussed vulnerability to symptoms of anxiety and depression. Having symptoms, however, may not be the same as having the particular cluster of symptoms required to meet DSM or ICD criteria for a diagnosis. We (Andrews, Stewart, Allen, & Henderson, 1990) therefore interviewed a quasi-population sample of adult twins (104 monozygotic female pairs, 84 monozygotic male pairs, 86 dizyotic female pairs, 71 dizygotic male pairs, and 103 dizygotic male–female pairs), using trait anxiety and coping measures; measures of anxiety and depressive symptoms; and a draft version of the CIDI to generate DSM-III diagnoses. Were the twins representative? We demonstrated that the twin type correlations for neuroticism and for anxiety and depressive symptoms were comparable to the data reported by Jardine et al. (1984) (i.e., about a third of the variation in symptoms was accounted for by genetic factors, and most of this was shared with neuroticism). Furthermore, the lifetime prevalences of the six common anxiety and depressive disorders (depression, dysthymia, panic disorder with or without agoraphobia, social phobia, obsessive–compulsive disorder, and generalized anxiety disorder) were within the range of age- and sex-controlled site variation figures found in the U.S Epidemiologic Catchment Area study. Thus, the data from the twins in our study seemed to correspond with the data in two of the larger studies in the literature.

Comorbidity was considerable. Multiple diagnoses were four times more common than would be expected on the basis of prevalence alone, while single diagnoses were correspondingly rarer. This study was originally designed to illuminate genetic relationships. It was frustrating that the small numbers of twin pairs concordant for any particular neurosis precluded any stable genetic estimates. Even though 243 subjects met criteria for one or more diagnoses, only 1 pair was concordant for depression, 4 pairs for dysthymia, 2 pairs for panic disorder with or without agoraphobia, 1 pair for social phobia, and 17 pairs for generalized anxiety disorder. No pairs were concordant for obsessive–compulsive disorder. The impact of comorbidity becomes clear if the concordance table is reviewed (see Table 1.1, and also Andrews, Stewart, Allen, & Henderson, 1990). We therefore asked what could be generating such a clustering of diagnoses. The data for the complete sample, now treated as individuals and not twins, are shown in Table 1.2 (adapted from Andrews, Stewart, Morris-Yates, et al., 1990). These data are the lifetime-to-date comorbidities among the six diagnoses mentioned above. Table 1.2 is not a crosstabulation in any usual sense; the probability of having another diagnosis depends of the prevalence of that diagnosis in this sample and not on patterns of comorbidity associated with particular disorders. Thus, when the tetrachoric correlations for the risk of comorbidity were calculated, a first general factor fitted the data well and accounted for 57% of the variance. Nether two- nor three-factor solutions improved the goodness of fit.

Even if there was a common factor underlying the pattern of comorbid diagnoses, it could be possible that each diagnosis was related in a special way to known vulnerability measures. When these relationships were tabulated, there was no indication of significant variation in scores of neuroticism or locus of control among the five major diagnoses, although people with a diagnosis of DSM-III generalized anxiety disorder (a lower-threshold diagnosis) did show lower scores on these vulnerability measures. When people were ranked by the number of these six diagnoses they had experienced, which we took to be a proxy for a general

TABLE 1.1. Concordance of Lifetime Diagnoses by Twin Type: Specific Diagnoses of Twins Concordant for Neurotic Illness

MZF Twin A:Twin B	MZM Twin A:Twin B	DZF Twin A:Twin B	DZM Twin A:Twin B
G:G	YOPG:DYSPG	OG:G	G:G
DYPG:G	G:G	P:G	S:DG
G:YP	G:G	D:P	DYOS:S
YG:DYOG	G:G	DYG:DY	
G:Y	G:G	G:O	
DYOG:G	G:D	P:G	
G:YG	DYG:G	DY:YOSPG	
PG:DYO	YG:G	G:DYOP	
SG:DP		G:DYOSPG	
D:DYPG		PG:DYPG	
DYS:G			

Note. MZF, monozygotic females; MZM, monozygotic males; DZF, dizygotic females; DZM, dizygotic males; D, depression; Y, dysthymia; G, generalized anxiety disorder; P, panic disorder with or without agoraphobia; O, obsessive–compulsive disorder; S, social phobia. In each case, the diagnoses of Twin A are displayed to left of colon and those of Twin B to right. Adapted from Andrews, Stewart, Allen, & Henderson (1990). Copyright 1990 by Journal of Affective Disorders. Adapted by permission.

TABLE 1.2. The Lifetime Co-Occurrence of Six Neurotic Diagnoses in the Twin Sample (*n* = 243)

Diagnosis	*n* cases	Co-occurring diagnoses: Percentage of cases with row diagnosis					
		DEP	DYS	OCD	SOC	PAG	GAD
DEP	65	16[a]	43	23	17	20	66
DYS	52	54	17[a]	29	23	31	58
OCD	48	31	31	33[a]	27	17	35
SOC	33	33	36	39	27[a]	21	42
PAG	34	38	42	24	21	24[a]	56
GAD	168	26	18	10	8	11	60[a]

Note. DEP, depression; DYS, dysthymia; OCD, obsessive–compulsive disorder; SOC, social phobia; PAG, panic disorder with or without agoraphobia; GAD, generalized anxiety disorder. This is not a cross-tabulation, but six overlapping rows of data. For example, of 65 persons (first row) who had met criteria for depression in their lifetimes, 16% had had no other illness but 43% had also met criteria for dysthymia, 23% for obsessive–compulsive disorder, and so on. The 43% who had also met criteria for dysthymia are relisted in the second row, which represents the illness experience of the 52 persons who met criteria for dysthymia. Persons with more than one diagnosis are represented repeatedly, the one person who gave symptoms consistent with all six diagnoses being included in all off-diagonal cells. Persons listed on the diagonal had one diagnosis only. Adapted from Andrews, Stewart, Morris-Yates, Holt, & Henderson (1990). Copyright 1990 by British Journal of Psychiatry. Adapted by permission.

[a]Criteria met for that diagnosis only.

factor there was a strong association ($p < .001$) with neuroticism and locus of control measures (see Andrews, Stewart, Morris-Yates, et al., 1990, for details). It was concluded that the concept of a general neurotic syndrome depends in part on the presence of personality vulnerability factors measured by neuroticism and locus of control.

Exploring the genesis of such a personality vulnerability factor (in the whole study measured by neuroticism, locus of control, and defense style), we showed that although each measure was substantially influenced by genetic factors (neuroticism more than the other two measures), the same genes were implicated in all three measures, as signified by loadings on a common genetic factor (i.e., proportion of variance explained by heredity). These loadings were as follows: neuroticism, 53% (proportion specific to neuroticism 19%, proportion common to all three measures 34%); locus of control, 46% (specific 12%, common factor 34%); and defense style, 37% (specific 18%, common factor 19%) (Andrews, 1991). Questionnaires are imprecise surface markers of the latent traits. It may well be that persons who inherit the latent trait of emotionality arouse quickly and inhibit slowly; as a consequence, they may find it difficult to conceive of the world either as a controllable world in the sense that an internal locus of control would suggest, or as a world in which the mature defenses of suppression, anticipation, sublimation, and humor can be readily employed. It is therefore not surprising that neuroticism, locus of control, and defense style are correlated and determined by a common genetic factor that influences temperament.

Using a structural-equation model, I then showed that once these genetic effects of neuroticism and locus of control on vulnerability had been controlled, there was little evidence of additional genetic effects on illness or symptoms in this population sample (Andrews, 1991). In this sense, the findings of epidemiologists (Duncan-Jones, 1987) and geneticists (Jardine et al., 1984) were supported. Eysenck had always proposed that his neuroticism scale was a proxy for some constitutional trait of emotionality. Roberson, Martin, and Candy (1978) showed that Maudsley reactive rats (bred to be analogues of high-neuroticism humans) had decreased benzodiazepine binding sites in the hippocampus, taken as presumptive evidence of decreased functional gamma-aminobutyric acid (GABA) inhibitory receptor density. If this were found to be applicable to humans, people with high neuroticism scores would, when stimulated, arouse more quickly and inhibit more slowly than persons with low neuroticism scores because of this functional lack of inhibitory GABA interneuron pathways. Using saccadic eye movement peak velocity slowing with a standard dose of benzodiazepine, I have obtained some preliminary data that would support this idea (Andrews, 1991). Whether this biological marker will parallel the genetic basis for neuroticism remains to be demonstrated.

Ormel and Wohlfarth (1991) noted that a substantial proportion of the correlation between chronic life stressors and symptoms can be attributed to the confounding effects of neurotcism. Minimizing any possibility of contamination between measures, we concluded that in this twin sample interpersonal events, but not chance events, occurred more frequently (relative risk = 1.68) in persons with neuroticism scores above the median (Poulton & Andrews, 1992). With David Fergusson, I completed a structural-equation model of these data, and estimated that 12% of all life events could be attributed to a latent trait related to neuroticism (unpublished results, 1991). Given the influence of this general vulnerability factor on life events, symptoms, and illness, it would seem prudent to control for such factors before seeking either the specific environmental or genetic determinants of the individual disorders.

Kendler and colleagues at the Medical College of Virginia are completing a painstaking study of the environmental and genetic determinants of neurosis. They have used structured diagnostic interviews and life events, traits, and coping measures with a volunteer population of 1,033 monozygotic and dizygotic pairs of female twins. This fivefold increase in sample size over our study has allowed the genetics of the individual disorders to be explored. Kendler, Kessler, Heath, Neale, and Eaves (1991) found that two of their three coping measures had a heritability of 30% and concluded, as we have, that genes may affect the vulnerability to psychiatric disorders by influencing coping behavior. In generalized anxiety disorder, Kendler, Neale, Kessler, Heath, and Eaves (1992a) found that the heritability was 30%, and that the genes responsible for major depression and generalized anxiety disorder were likely to be the same (Kendler et al., 1992b). In phobias, Kendler et al. (1992c) estimated the heritability of agoraphobia and social phobia to be 39% and 30%, respectively; however, the correlations between those genes and the genes influencing major depression were more modest (.38, .30) (Kendler, Neale, Kesller, Heath, & Eaves, 1993a). In panic disorder with and without agoraphobia, the heritability of liability again ranged from 32% to 46%, depending on the diagnostic approach used (Kendler et al., 1993b).

Analyzing data on depression from two waves of interviewing 1 year apart, Kendler et al. (1993c) showed that the genetic factors (which accounted for 43% of the variance at each time point) were stable, whereas the environmental factors were occasion-specific. Using the two-wave design to estimate and eliminate the effect of the measurement error that occurs from one estimate alone, they argued that estimates of the heritability of the liability to a lifetime history of major depression were increased substantially over that derived from a single measurement occasion. Exploring the relation between a restricted measure of neuroticism (measured on two occasions and only using 12 of the 23 items) and major depression, Kendler et al. (1993d) found that more than half of the genetic liability of major depression was shared with neuroticism, the remainder being unique to depression. As they considered that the genes influencing generalized anxiety disorder are identicial, neuroticism must be equally important in that disorder.

Kendler and colleagues' studies will dominate the literature for many years to come. They represent profound scholarship, best exemplified by Kendler's (1993) tutorial. Importantly, the results of three different research programs (Jardine et al.'s, my own and colleagues', and Kendler et al.'s) employing twin studies of population samples have, using biometrical genetic modeling techniques, all come to congruent conclusions: that genetic factors contribute between 30% and 42% of the variation in symptoms of anxiety and symptoms of depression, and of the diagnoses of panic disorder, agoraphobia, social phobia, generalized anxiety disorder, and major depression; that many of the symptoms or disorders seem to share the same genes in whole or in part; and that an antecedent construct related to trait anxiety and coping is itself under substantial genetic influence (50% in the case of neuroticism) and may be more than any specific genetic effects on symptoms. This antecedent vulnerability factor may well account for the majority of the variation in both the genetic and environmental determinants of these symptoms and disorders, and hence for the observed comorbidity.

VULNERABILITY TO ANXIETY AND DEPRESSIVE DISORDERS: CLINIC STUDIES

Disorders seen in the general population may not have the same relationship to etiological factors as do the more severe disorders seen in specialist practice. Torgersen (1983) has drawn attention to the effects of sampling variation on observed risks. For example, in his data, genetic factors in neurosis were only significant in an extreme group—males admitted to mental hospitals. Our findings on a clinical population have, however, been largely consistent with the results of the population surveys. We began with a pedigree study of panic disorder with or without agoraphobia, which showed that the risk among first-degree relatives was increased threefold; the data, we felt, were more consistent with the inheritance of neuroticism than with any specific genetic influence (Moran & Andrews, 1985). We then looked at comorbidity and risk factors among 165 patients treated for panic disorder with or without agoraphobia, and found that the comorbidity was similar to the twin study sample; that the neuroticism scores and locus of control scores were 1.5 *SD* units above the population means; and that these scores were correlated with the number of other prior diagnoses identified (Andrews, Stewart, Morris-Yates, et al., 1990). We have previously argued that all these factors are evidence for the importance of a general personality vulnerability in the genesis of disorders, and in addition are associated with treatment seeking.

For many years, we have administered the CIDI to all patients presenting for treatment at our specialized anxiety disorders clinic. We had noted that patients treated for panic disorder with or without agoraphobia or social phobia had lower than expected rates of comorbid obsessive–compulsive disorder, and vice versa (Crino & Andrews, in press); we felt that at this extreme of the range, causative factors other than the general vulnerability factor were becoming evident. Crino and I therefore reviewed the results from 367 patients who completed the CIDI-Auto Version 1.0 (WHO, 1993b). At first glance, the comorbidity matrix resembles that previously published from the twin study, but the clinic sample are clearly more severe (Table 1.3). For example, the scores of the clinic patients on the three vulnerability measures expressed in *SD* units were more extreme, whatever the diagnosis being considered, than those of persons with corresponding diagnoses in the twin sample. The difference from the population mean for neuroticism was 2.1 *SD* in the clinic sample versus 1.0 *SD* in the twin sample; for locus of control, 1.5 *SD* versus 0.6 *SD;* and for defense style, 0.8 *SD* versus 0.5 *SD.* This elevation in vulnerability scores is consistent with an enhanced general vulnerability to neurosis in the clinic patients over that seen in diagnosis-positive persons derived from a population sample.

As would be expected in a clinic-ascertained sample, the number of comorbid diagnoses was increased from an average of 0.6 in the twin study to 1.1 additional diagnoses in the clinic sample. As in the twin sample, there was a significant linear trend among all the vulnerability measures for scores to increase as patients met criteria for increasing numbers of diagnoses (Table 1.4). The concept of a general vulnerability to all six neuroses studied was supported. However, when the probability of comorbid diagnoses was standardized by row and column prevalences, and the odds ratios were calculated (Table 1.3), it was clear that patients who endorsed symptoms that met criteria for generalized anxiety disorder or dysthymia had significantly increased exposure odds ratios for the other four disorders. Patients with the other four disorders did not; the point of rarity in comorbidity between the phobias and obsessive–compulsive disorder noted previously was evident, but did not reach significance. If a point of rarity in comorbidity is detected, it could indicate the operation of additional etiological factors other than the general vulnerability factor that has been the focus of this chapter.

If comorbidity is so ubiquitous and so driving by the vulnerability factor, why do patients mostly complain of only one disorder when, on average, they have had 2.1 comorbid disorders in their lifetimes to date?

TABLE 1.3. Comorbidity in Clinic Patients: Percentage of Patients Comorbid for Other Disorders (CIDI-Auto Version 1.0) with Odds Ratios in Which $p < .05$

	DEP	DYS	OCD	SOC	PAG	GAD
DEP	—	35%	24%	65%	70%	25%
(n = 204)		4.9	n.s	n.s.	n.s.	1.9
DYS	82%	—	29%	72%	68%	33%
(n = 87)	4.9		1.8	1.9	n.s.	2.6
OCD	64%	33%	—	61%	61%	30%
(n = 77)	n.s	1.8		n.s.	n.s.	2.0
SOC	58%	28%	21%	—	73%	25%
(n = 227)	n.s.	1.9	n.s.		1.8	2.2
PAG	57%	24%	19%	67%	—	23%
(n = 74)	n.s.	n.s.	n.s.	1.8		2.0
GAD	68%	39%	31%	76%	78%	—
(n = 74)	1.9	2.6	2.0	2.2	2.0	

Note. DEP, depression; DYS, dysthymia; OCD, obsessive–compulsive disorder; SOC, social phobia; PAG, panic disorder with or without agoraphobia; GAD, generalized anxiety disorder. This is not a cross-tabulation, but six overlapping rows of data. For example, of 65 persons (first row) who had met criteria for depression in their lifetimes, 16% had had no other illness but 43% had also met criteria for dysthymia, 23% for obsessive–compulsive disorder, and so on. The 43% who had also met criteria for dysthymia are relisted in the second row, which represents the illness experience of the 52 persons who met criteria for dysthymia. Persons with more than one diagnosis are represented repeatedly, the one person who gave symptoms consistent with all six diagnoses being included in all off-diagonal cells. Persons listed on the diagonal had one diagnosis only. Adapted from Andrews, Stewart, Morris-Yates, Holt, & Henderson (1990). Copyright 1990 by British Journal of Psychiatry. Adapted by permission.

We have developed a semistructured interview in which the results of the CIDI are reviewed with each patient, and the time course of each episode is dated against life chart markers (Hunt & Andrews, in press). When there are two or more disorders, we ask whether the later disorders are considered to be consequences of the earlier disorder. Hunt and I studied 100 consecutive patients. In 19 patients, the presenting diagnosis was the only diagnosis. In 55, there was a history of more than one diagnosis, but all subsequent diagnoses were judged by the patients to be secondary to their primary diagnosis, and were often seen as an expected and nautral consequence of the stress of the primary disorder. Twenty-six patients identified one or more of their comorbid diagnoses as being independent of the primary diagnosis, and usually related it to other intercurrent stressors. We concluded that both secondary and independent comorbidity could be explained in terms of the impact of stress (of being ill, or of being stressed while ill) on a vulnerable personality structure.

   In summary, therefore, all the studies reviewed have pointed to the

TABLE 1.4. Relation between Number of Lifetime Diagnoses and Vulnerability Factors

No. of diagnoses	Twin sample[a]			Clinic sample			
	n of cases	N ES	LCB ES	n of cases	N ES	LCB ES	DS(I) ES
1	152	0.16	0.06	68	1.4	1.0	0.4
2	54	0.78	0.07	90	1.9	1.4	0.8
3	16	1.31	0.63	79	2.1	1.3	0.7
4	14	1.33	0.87	44	2.3	1.6	1.0
5 or 6	7	1.29	1.04	26	2.3	1.7	1.2
		$p < .001$	$p < .001$		$p < .001$	$p < .005$	$p < .001$

Note. Vulnerability factors measured by neuroticism (N), locus of control (LCB), and defense style (DS) (I, immature factor). Effect size differences from population means (ES). [a]Twin sample retabulated from Andrews, Stewart, Morris-Yates, Holt, & Henderson (1990). Copyright 1990 by British Journal of Psychiatry. Retabulated by permission.

presence of an important single vulnerability factor related to trait anxiety and coping that accounts for the major part of the variation in symptoms and illness. Sequential effects are evident, with the stress of illness acting as a precipitant of additional morbidity in vulnerable persons. Specific environmental and genetic factors have been described, but none have been shown to be more important than the single common factor responsible for the common anxiety and depressive disorders.

VULNERABILITY: IMPLICATIONS FOR TREATMENT AND PREVENTION

What, then, are the implications of these findings? Medicine is about the prevention and treatment of disease. If a common vulnerability factor is a major cause of liability to anxiety and depression, then treatment programs must not only reduce symptoms and disability, but should also reduce this risk factor if relapse is to be prevented. In a similar vein, prevention will mean that such vulnerability factors must be reduced to within the normal range—that is, to within 1 SD of the population mean. Jorm (1989) conducted a meta-analytic review of treatments that had resulted in reductions of trait anxiety. He reported that the cognitive therapies were the only treatments to result in levels of change exceeding those attributable to placebo.

Two studies from our clinic have also demonstrated that changes in vulnerability measures can follow cognitve-behavior therapy. In a 1-year follow-up of patients treated with cognitive-behavior therapy for agoraphobia, we showed that there was a 1-SD improvement in neuroticism and locus of control that became evident in the first few months after treatment had concluded. From regression analyses, we calculated that this drop in vulnerability scores at 6 months accounted for 30% of the patients' well-being 6 months later (Andrew & Moran, 1988). Hunt and I are currently completing a 2-year follow-up of some 200 patients treated for panic disorder with or without agoraphobia or social phobia. There was a marked fall in symptoms and disability with the intensive cognitive-behavior therapy program. The improvement was stable over the 2 years after treatment had ended. There was evidence that scores on neuroticism, locus of control, and defense style normalized with treatment and remained normal during the follow-up period. Thus, identifying risk factors and checking to see whether these risk factors have been reduced by treatment can improve treatment efficacy.

Prevention is always better than cure. There are cognitive-behavior packages available for the treatment of adolescents with anxiety disorders (Kendall, Howard, & Epps, 1988), and these have been modified for use with highly anxious children who have not as yet developed an anxiety disorder. If these programs are successful, the prospect of prevention among those at risk is very real. We conducted a natural experiment with students who were about to spend 12 months in a foreign country. Matching them on relevant personality variables with peers who stayed at home, we showed that the controlled but stressful experience of living abroad resulted in a ninefold increase in personality maturity over that expected from the maturing effect of time alone (Andrews, Page, & Neilson, 1993). We argued that this gain in personality maturity was a reduction in risk and would result in a threefold reduction in incidence of the neurotic disorders defined above. Medicine has always made the largest advances not through improvements in direct treatment, but by reducing the risk of illness among the well. The identification and amelioration of risk factors for the common anxiety and depressive disorders will hasten this process.

CONCLUSION

Personality—in particular, the constitutional part of personality known as temperament—has been shown to be important in the genesis of the common anxiety and depressive disorders. Trait anxiety and habitual coping strategies, whether related to symptoms in the general population, disorders in the general population, or disorders in patients presenting for treatment, account for the majority of the observed comorbidity. In patients presenting for treatment, it is clear that other factors, as yet unspecified, account for some further variation in the patterns of observed comorbidity. In the clinic sample, and perhaps in all samples, the stress of having one disorder interacts with the primary vulnerability factors to render persons liable to additional disorders. As these vulnerability factors can be measured, treatment programs should ensure that they are reduced if relapse is to be inhibited. Prevention programs aimed at persons with high levels of this vulnerability, which increases their risk of developing the anxiety and depressive disorders, would appear to be practical and are likely to prove to be a cost-effective strategy in reducing the incidence of (and considerable disability associated with) these disorders.

The observation that persons who have an anxiety or depressive disorder also have an increased likelihood of having had other anxiety or depressive disorders in their lifetimes to date means either that the specific causes of these disorders have aggregated much more than chance would allow, or that some general vulnerability factor has made each person liable to each and all the disorders they report. Future studies of the etiology of individual anxiety and depressive disorders will therefore need to be more sophisticated than has been usual. Claims that a certain factor is specific to a particular disorder will need to demonstrate (1) that the factor is not typical of a normal nonpatient population matched for age and sex to show that the phenomenon of interest could be associated with the disorder; (2) that the factor is not present in a control group that is high in trait anxiety but nonsymptomatic to show that the phenomenon is not primarily a proxy measure for vulnerability factors such as trait anxiety and coping; and finally (3) that the factor does not occur in patients with other anxiety or depressive disorders, and hence may be specific to the disorder being studied.

In the last 10 years, there has been an explosive growth in knowledge about the anxiety disorders. Diagnostic criteria are agreed upon, diagnostic instruments are reliable and valid (Peters and Andrews, in press), treatments are effective, and information as to causes (both general and specific) is emerging. At the editor's request (and to my own relief, for the effort of reviewing the specific factors would have been considerable), this chapter has focused on the general factors. Nevertheless, it now behooves researchers, as they seek to identify specific factors important in each disorder, to remember that personality vulnerability makes a major contribution to all these disorders and to distinguish such general effects from the effects specific to each disorder. The way ahead is not by lumping or splitting (Andrews, 1990), but by lumping and splitting alternatively—first asking whether this finding could be specific to a particular disorder, and then asking whether this finding could be evidence of a general effect—until we have developed a full understanding of the general and specific characteristics, determinants, and treatment responses of the anxiety and depressive disorders.

REFERENCES

American Psychiatric Association. (1994). *Diagnostic and statistical manual of mental disorders* (4th ed.). Washingtonn, DC: Author.

Andrews, G. (1990). Classification of neurotic disorders. *Journal of the Royal Society of Medicine, 83,* 606–607.

Andrews, G. (1991). Anxiety, personality and anxiety disorders. *International Review of Psychiatry, 3,* 293–302.

Andrews, G. (in press). Comorbidity and the general neurotic syndrome. *British Journal of Psychiatry.*

Andrews, G., Kiloh, L. G., & Kehoe, L. (1978). Asthenic personality: Myth or reality? *Australian and New Zealand Journal of Psychiatry, 12,* 95–98.

Andrews, G., & Moran, C. (1988). Exposure treatment of agoraphobia with panic attacks: Are drugs essential? In I. Hand & H.-U. Wittchen (Eds.), *Panic and phobias II: Treatments and variables affecting course and outcome* (pp. 89–99). Heidelberg: Springer-Verlag.

Andrews, G., Neilson, M. D., Hunt, C., Stewart, G. W., & Kiloh, L. G. (1990). Diagnosis, personality and the long-term outcome of depression. *British Journal of Psychiatry, 157,* 13–18.

Andrews, G., Page, A. C., & Neilson, M. D. (1993). Sending your teenagers away: Controlled stress decreases neurotic vulnerability. *Archives of General Psychiatry, 50,* 585–589.

Andrews, G., Singh, M., & Bond, M. (1993). The Defense Style Questionnaire. *Journal of Nervous and Mental Disease, 181,* 246–256.

Andrews, G., Stewart, G. W., Allen, R., & Henderson, A. S. (1990). The genetics of six neurotic disorders: A twin study. *Journal of Affective Disorders, 19,* 23–29.

Andrews, G., Stewart, G. W., Morris-Yates, A., Holt, P. E., & Henderson, A. S. (1990). Evidence for a general neurotic syndrom. *British Journal of Psychiatry, 157,* 6–12.

Bolger, N. (1990). Coping as a personality process: A prospective study. *Journal of Personality and Social Psychology, 59,* 525–537.

Craig, A., Franklin, J., & Andrews, G. (1984). A scale to measure locus of control of behaivor. *British Journal of Medical Psychology, 57,* 173–180.

Crino, R. D., & Andrews, G. (in press). Obsessive compulsive disorder and Axis I co-morbidity. *Journal of Anxiety Disorders.*

Duncan-Jones, P. (1987). Modelling the aetiology of neurosis: Long-term and short-term factors. In B. Cooper (Ed.), *Psychiatric epidemiology: Progress and prospects* (pp. 178–191). London: Croom Helm.

Eysenck, H. J., & Eysenck, S. B. G. (1975). *Personality Questionnaire (Junior and Adult).* Sevenoaks: Hodder & Stoughton.

Hunt, C., & Andrews, G. (in press). Unravelling comorbidity: The life chart approach. *Journal of Psychiatric Research.*

Jardine, R., Martin, N. G., & Henderson, A. S. (1984). Genetic covariation between neuroticism and the symptoms of anxiety and depression. *Genetics Epidemiology, 1,* 89–107.

Jorm, A. F. (1989). Modifiability of trait anxiety and neuroticism: A meta-analysis of the literature. *Australian and New Zealand Journal of Psychiatry, 23,* 21–29.

Kendall, P. C., Howard, B. L., & Epps, J. (1988). The anxious child: Cognitive behavioral treatment strategies. *Behavior Modification, 12,* 281–310.

Kendler, K. S. (1993). Twin studies of psychiatric illness: Current status and future directions. *Archives of General Psychiatry, 50,* 905–915.

Kendler, K. S., Heath, A., Martin, N. G., & Eaves, L. J. (1986). Symptoms of anxiety and depression in a volunteer twin population. *Archives of General Psychiatry, 43,* 213–221.

Kendler, K. S., Heath, A., Martin, N. G., & Eaves, L. J. (1987). Symptoms of anxiety and symptoms of depression: Same genes, different environments? *Archives of General Psychiatry, 44,* 451–457.

Kendler, K. S., Kessler, R. C., Heath, A. C., Neale, M. C., & Eaves, L. J. (1991). Coping: A genetic epidemiological investigation. *Psychological Medicine, 21,* 337–346.

Kendler, K. S., Neale, M. C., Kessler, R. C., Heath, A. C., & Eaves, L. J. (1992a). Generalized anxiety disorder in women: A population-based twin study. *Archives of General Psychiatry, 49,* 267–272.

Kendler, K. S., Neale, M. C., Kessler, R. C., Heath, A. C., & Eaves, L. J. (1992b). Major depression and generalized anxiety disorder: Same genes, (partly) different environments) *Archives of General Psychiatry, 49,* 716–722.

Kendler, K. S., Neale, M. C., Kessler, R. C., Heath, A. C., & Eaves, L. J. (1992c). The genetic epidemiology of phobias in women: The interrelationship of agoraphobia, social phobia, situational phobia, and simple phobia. *Archives of General Psychiatry, 49,* 273–281.

Kendler, K. S., Neale, M. C., Kessler, R. C., Heath, A. C., & Eaves, L. J. (1993a). Major depression and phobias: The genetic environmental sources of comorbidity. *Psychological Medicine, 23,* 361–371.

Kendler, K. S., Neale, M. C., Kessler, R. C., Heath, A. C., & Eaves, L. J. (1993b). Panic disorder in women: A population-based twin study. *Psychological Medicine, 23,* 397–406.

Kendler, K. S., Neale, M. C., Kessler, R. C., Heath, A. C., & Eaves, L. J. (1993c). A longitudinal twin study of 1-year prevalence of major depression in women. *Archives of General Psychiatry, 50,* 843–852.

Kendler, K. S., Neale, M. C., Kessler, R. C., Heath, A. C., & Eaves, L. J. (1993d). A longitudinal twin study of personality and major depression in women. *Archives of General Psychiatry, 50,* 853–862.

Kiloh, L. G., Andrews, G., Neilson, M., & Bianchi, G. N., (1972). The relationship of the syndromes called endogenous and neurotic depression. *British Journal of Psychiatry, 121,* 183–196.

Martin, N. G., Jardine, R., Andrews, G., & Heath, A. C. (1988). Anxiety disorders: Are there genetic factors specific to panic? *Acta Psychiatrica Scandinavica, 77,* 698–706.

Moran, C., & Andrews, G. (1985). The familial occurrence of agoraphobia. *British Journal of Psychiatry, 146,* 262–267.

Ormel, J. (1983). Neuroticism and well-being inventories: Measuring traits or states? *Psychological Medicine, 13,* 165–176.

Ormel, J., & Wohlfarth, T. (1991). How neuroticism, long-term difficulties, and life situations change influence psychological distress: A longitudinal model. *Journal of Personality and Social Psychology, 60,* 744–755.

Peters, L., & Andrews, G. (in press). A procedural validity study of the CIDI-Auto. *Psychological Medicine.*

Poulton, R., & Andrews, G. (1992). Personality as a cause of adverse life events. *Acta Psychiatrica Scandinavica, 85,* 35–38.

Robertson, H. A., Martin, I. L., & Candy, J. M. (1978). Differences in benzodiazepine receptor binding in Maudsley reactive and Maudsley nonreactive rats. *European Journal of Pharmacology, 50,* 455–457.

Torgersen, S. (1983). Genetics of neurosis: The effects of sampling variation upon the twin concordance ration. *British Journal of Psychiatry, 142,* 126–132.

World Health Organization (WHO). (1993a). *The ICD-10 Classification of Mental and Behavioural Disorders: Diagnostic Criteria for Research.* Geneva: WHO.

World Health Organization (WHO). (1993b). *CIDI-Auto Version 1.0: Administrator's Guide and Reference.* Sydney: Training and Reference Centre for WHO-CIDI.

2

Validity of the DSM-III-R and DSM-IV Classification Systems for Anxiety Disorders

TIMOTHY A. BROWN

RELATIVE TO OTHER FIELDS of science, the classification of emotional disorders is in its infancy, having changed rapidly over the past 40 years. Examination of the DSM classification system across time reveals a marked increase in the number of diagnostic categories with each revision. Indeed, in the case of the anxiety disorders, only three categories existed in DSM-II (American Psychiatric Association [APA], 1968): phobic neurosis, anxiety neurosis, and obsessive–compulsive neurosis. With the publication of DSM-IV (APA, 1994), fully 12 anxiety disorder categories for adults exist in the nomenclature.[1] This rise in the number of diagnoses has been accompanied by a greater incidence in the "subtyping" of these categories. For example, when assigning a diagnosis of specific phobia under the DSM-IV system (named "simple phobia" in DSM-III-R), clinicians are required to specify the "type" of phobia from a list of five (e.g., animal, natural environment, situational).

This state of affairs might imply that researchers have attained greater precision and consensus in the organization and understanding of the parameters of human psychopathology. Although this may be true to some extent, considerable controversy has surrounded each step in the evolution of the DSM system. Among the foci of these debates have been such issues as how to differentiate "normal" and "pathological" behavior, what constitute the "boundaries" among the various disorders, and even whether such classification should be attempted at all (see Barlow, 1988). Whereas DSM-III-R and DSM-IV represent substantial advances to our clinical science (particularly with regard to their heuristic value), for these and other reasons to be articulated later, most researchers would concede that these systems represent more of a beginning than a "final word" on the nature of psychological disorders (see Barlow, 1988, 1991a; Maser, Kaelber, & Weise, 1991).

In the study of emotional disorders, as in any science, classification is of paramount importance. Beyond the practical implication of communication among investigators, classification should assist in the understanding of the nature and treatment of the phenomena it is designed to organize. Needless to say, the endeavor to organize, in a clinically meaningful manner, the seemingly endless and diverse array of features that could be subsumed under the emotional disorders represents a tremendously large and challenging enterprise. As is the case with any form of measurement, the utility of the classification system can be gauged to a large extent by its reliability and validity. Accordingly, *reliability* can be evaluated in part by the extent to which independent observers (diagnosticians) agree on the presence of domains in the classification system. In the case of human psychopathology, such "domains" could entail both the diagnostic categories (i.e., DSM disorders) and the features (dimensions) comprising these categories (e.g., diagnostic criteria). The *validity* of the classification system may be gauged by the extent to which the identification of the disorders (or features comprising the disorders) has value. In the DSM system, this utility could be indicated by whether the establishment of a diagnosis provides information about likely associated features (e.g., coexisting symptoms or syndromes), the course of the disorder, parameters of its onset (e.g., age and nature of onset), and, ideally, selection of treatment and prognosis.

Although the DSM system has been lauded for its atheoretical and descriptive nature, perhaps the most substantial criticism that has been levied against it is the fact that this system represents a *categorical* approach to classification. An implicit assumption of the approach adopted in the DSM system is that the disorders comprising the taxonomy represent distinct, nonoverlapping entities that are qualitatively different from one another (and from nonpathological behavior). Conversely, *dimensional* approaches to classification have been proposed to accommodate the alternative position that the features comprising the DSM criteria for the various disorders are quantitative and continuous in nature (see Blashfield, 1990; Frances, Widiger, & Fyer, 1990; Moras & Barlow, 1992). In other words, inherent in this approach is the assumption that individuals assigned a DSM-IV diagnosis differ from "normal" persons only in the frequency and/or severity with which they experience the features that form the diagnostic criteria. In this chapter and elsewhere (e.g., Barlow, 1988; Brown & Barlow, 1992a; Moras & Barlow, 1992), my colleagues and I have adopted a somewhat intermediary position—one that acknowledges the value (validity) of the DSM system, but champions the utility of incorporating dimensional elements, particularly in the recording of co-occurring key and common features (often at the subthreshold level) that may have a substantial impact on the course of the "principal" disorder and its treatment. This proposal does not imply that the current nosological system is invalid. Instead, this approach is viewed as a method of providing a greater amount of clinically useful information than can be generated from a purely categorical approach. For instance, whereas the majority of patients with panic disorder do not present with comorbid hypochondriasis, a large number do evidence features of this disorder (e.g., fear that the symptoms of panic and anxiety reflect an undetected cardiac problem). Just as overvalued ideation may be a predictor of treatment response in obsessive–compulsive disorder (Foa & Kozak, 1989), the extent of belief conviction on the part of panic disorder patients' perceptions of panic symptomatology may be associated with outcome and longitudinal course of the disorder as well. Adding these dimensional elements to the classification system would allow for such an analysis.

Thus, a central thesis offered in this chapter is that although the DSM-III-R and DSM-IV anxiety disorders possess many overlapping and common features, and indeed may share a common diathesis (e.g., biopsychosocial vulnerability), they can be differentiated on certain key features. This differentiation has important clinical ramifications (e.g., selection of treatment, course of disorder). Nevertheless, although inherent to the process of differentiation is the incorporation of categorical classification, the addition of dimensional elements is viewed as an important adjunct to the classificatory system in order to record additional features that may exert a powerful influence on the expression of the principal disorder and its treatment.

RELIABILITY AND COMORBIDITY AMONG ANXIETY DISORDERS

As noted above, one indicator of the merit of the DSM classificatory system would be the degree of interrater reliability of its constituent diagnoses. As we have articulated in detail elsewhere (Brown & Barlow, 1992a), comorbidity rates (i.e., the co-occurrence of two or more disorders in the same individual) may potentially provide another important index of the utility of the classification system. For example, extremely high rates of comorbidity could indicate poor discriminant validity among the diagnostic categories; in other words, the system may be erroneously distinguishing phenomena that actually reflect variations in symptom manifestations of a larger, underlying syndrome (Blashfield, 1990). Moreover, extensive overlap or co-occurrence of symptoms would potentially have an adverse effect on diagnostic reliability as well. Accordingly, it could be argued that partial support for the distinction among the DSM-III R (APA, 1987) anxiety disorders would be provided by (1) favorable rates of diagnostic agreement, and (2) reasonable (i.e., not excessively high) rates of comorbidity among disorders.

Reliability

As shown in Table 2.1, evidence for the reliability of the DSM-III-R anxiety disorders is provided by a large-scale study ($n = 267$) recently conducted at our center (Di Nardo, Moras, Barlow, Rapee, & Brown, 1993). Kappas were calculated on the basis of diagnoses assigned during two independent administrations of the Anxiety Disorders Interview Schedule—Revised (ADIS-R; Di Nardo & Barlow, 1988). Excellent reliability was obtained for principal diagnoses of simple phobia, social phobia, and obsessive–compulsive disorder (OCD); good reliability was obtained for panic disorder with mild and moderate agoraphobia (PDA [mild and moderate]); and fair reliability was obtained for generalized anxiety disorder (GAD),

TABLE 2.1. Interrater Reliability of DSM-III-R Anxiety Disorder Diagnoses Using the ADIS-R ($n = 267$)

Principal diagnosis	n	kappa
PD	38	.43
PDA (mild)	89	.60
PDA (moderate)	50	.71
PDA (severe)	7	.44
GAD	38	.57
Simple phobia	21	.82
Social phobia	45	.79
OCD	19	.80
PSD	3	.46
PDA (all levels)	131	.72
PD and PDA (all levels)	152	.79

Note. See text for abbreviations. n indicates the number of cases in which the diagnosis was assigned by either or both raters. Brown & Barlow (1992a). Copyright 1992 by the American Psychological Association. Reprinted by permission.

panic disorder without agoraphobia (PD), panic disorder with severe agoraphobia (PDA [severe]), and posttraumatic stress disorder (PTSD), although the kappas for PTSD and PDA (severe) were not that meaningful, given the small sample sizes for these categories.

These results are particularly encouraging when one considers the stringency of the methods used to calculate interrater agreement (e.g., use of independent diagnostic interviews). Moreover, in order for a case to be considered an agreement, diagnosticians were required to concur, when two or more diagnoses were present, on which disorder represented the "principal" diagnosis (i.e., the disorder associated with the highest degree of distress or life interference). It is also interesting to note how the categorical nature of DSM-III-R affected the diagnostic agreement for some disorders. For instance, as shown in Table 2.1, the reliability of PDA was "good" when all levels of agoraphobic avoidance were pooled. Indeed, we (Di Nardo et al., 1993) reported a correlation of .81 between the two interviewers' ADIS-R avoidance ratings assigned to patients with PD and PDA (summation of a series of 0–4 ratings of a variety of commonly avoided situations). Thus, we concluded that it was possible to rate the severity of agoraphobic avoidance reliably; however, this concordance faltered when we attempted to apply the DSM-III-R descriptors of agoraphobia severity. Partly because of these data, DSM-IV no longer requires the differentiation of levels of agoraphobia (or levels of panic severity).

Comorbidity

As discussed earlier, comorbidity rates may provide an important indicator of the discriminant validity of disorders that constitute the diagnostic system. For purposes of discussion, cross-sectional comorbidity data from a study recently completed at our center are presented in Figure 2.1 (Brown & Barlow, 1992a; Moras, Di Nardo, Brown, & Barlow, 1994). These data were derived from a large sample ($n = 468$) of carefully diagnosed patients who presented for evaluation and/or treatment to our anxiety disorders clinic. The ADIS-R was used for establishing diagnoses. This instrument was designed to evaluate comprehensively the anxiety, mood, and somatoform disorders (and to screen for the presence of other disorders—e.g., psychotic). Thus, patterns of comorbidity were largely confined to these classes of disorders.

Consistent with previous findings (e.g., de Ruiter, Rijken, Garssen, van Schaik, & Kraaimaat, 1989; Sanderson, Di Nardo, Rapee, & Barlow, 1990), rates of comorbidity were high. Indeed, 50% of patients with a principal anxiety disorder had at least one additional clinically significant anxiety or depressive disorder. The principal diagnoses of GAD and PDA (severe) were the categories associated with the highest comorbidity rates (82% and 72%, respectively); individuals with a principal diagnosis of

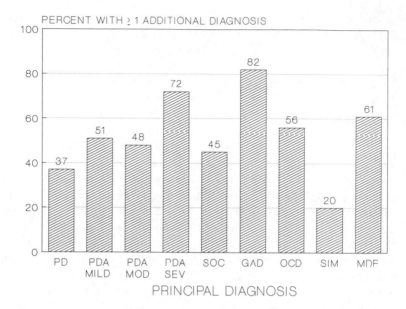

FIGURE 2.1. Cross-sectional comorbidity rates for principal DSM-III-R diagnoses (percentage of cases with at least one additional diagnosis). PD, panic disorder; PDA, panic disorder with agoraphobia; SOC, social phobia; GAD, generalized anxiety disorder; OCD, obsessive–compulsive disorder; SIM, simple phobia; MDE, major depression.

simple phobia were the least likely to be assigned an additional diagnosis (20%). Although not shown in Figure 2.1, GAD was the most frequently assigned additional diagnosis (23%), followed by social phobia (14%). The latter finding is consistent with data indicating that GAD and social phobia were the most frequently assigned additional diagnoses in a study examining patients with a principal disorder of major depression or dysthymia (Sanderson, Beck, & Beck, 1990).

Discussion of Reliability and Comorbidity Findings

Overall, good to excellent diagnostic reliability has been obtained for the DSM-III-R anxiety disorders. These findings are noteworthy, not only because of the stringent methods employed in the Di Nardo et al. (1993) study for calculating interrater agreement, but because high rates of comorbidity were found for some disorders. Some anxiety disorder categories (e.g., simple phobia) were found to evidence excellent reliability and low rates of comorbidity. However, other categories were associated with no more than fair reliability and/or higher comorbidity rates (e.g., GAD, PD).

In addition to the parameters discussed above, another factor that appeared to influence rates of interrater agreement (and perhaps comorbidity) was the extent to which the disorder possessed an outstanding key feature that facilitated differential diagnosis. For example, the categories with the highest reliability in the Di Nardo et al. (1993) study were OCD, simple phobia, and social phobia, each containing some form of overt marker (e.g., compulsions, circumscribed avoidance). Moreover, it is interesting to note that another study found that when diagnostic agreements involving the principal diagnosis of OCD occurred, the majority of these disagreements involved OCD patients without overt behavioral compulsions (Brown, Moras, Zinbarg, & Barlow, 1993). This factor may have contributed in part to the lower reliability of GAD and PD without avoidance. But as we have asserted previously (Brown & Barlow, 1992a), a more salient factor contributing to the reliability and perhaps comorbidity of these diagnoses may be that the core features of PD and GAD (i.e., panic, anxious apprehension) represent characteristics that are present to some extent in all of the anxiety disorders. Because this could be taken as evidence in support of the position claiming poor differentiation among the DSM-III-R and DSM-IV anxiety disorders, particular attention will be paid to GAD and PD in a later section of this chapter.

DIMENSIONS OF THE DSM-III-R AND DSM-IV ANXIETY DISORDERS

Many diverse phenomena (e.g., somatic manifestations of panic, intrusive thoughts, fear of social evaluation, agoraphobic avoidance) are subsumed under the broad heading of anxiety disorders in DSM-III-R and DSM-IV. Although reliability and comorbidity data may speak to some degree to the merit of these nosologies, much more needs to be learned about the nature and phenomenology of these problems before they can be categorized and dimensionalized with the most validity and parsimony. For example, one important research direction is the initiation of longitudinal studies in which the patterns and relationships among syndromes (and, more importantly, constituent symptoms) are examined across time. Another useful endeavor would be to conduct treatment studies to examine what influence the treatment of one disorder has on the course of its co-occurring disorders and symptoms. Although these strategies have many practical limitations (e.g., large sample sizes, multiple measures), greater emphasis should be placed on model-fitting statistical procedures than on analyses that are essentially descriptive in nature, as has been common practice to date.

In a study that has a bearing on the issue of the DSM-III-R anxiety disorders' construct validity, Zinbarg and Barlow (1995) measured key features of anxiety and related affects—including panic, sensitivity to social evaluation, anxiety sensitivity, depression, worry, obsessions, compulsions, and specific fears—among 432 patients and 32 normal controls. These features were measured by two methods: (1) the ADIS-R, and (2) a wide variety of questionnaires. First, a series of item-level factor analyses of the questionnaires was performed for data reduction. The questionnaire items were grouped into subscales on the basis of these preliminary factor analyses, as well as previously available psychometric data and item content. In all, the items from the entire questionnaire battery were grouped into 23 subscales. The scores of all subjects on the 23 subscales were entered into a factor analysis to examine the dimensionality of the anxiety symptom domain. The range of numbers of factors to be rotated was determined by a scree test and Kaiser's criterion (i.e., the number of eigenvalues greater than 1). A solution with six first-order factors was judged to be most acceptable structurally and substantively. These first-order factors were identifiable as relating to social anxiety, generalized anxiety, agoraphobia, panic (fear of fear), obsessions and compulsions, and simple (or specific) fears. Structural equation modeling (LISREL) indicated that a higher-order model consisting of one higher-order factor (loaded on by each of the six first-order factors) provided a significantly better fit than a model in which the six first-order factors were constrained to be orthogonal. Following Tellegen (1985), this higher-order factor was labeled "Negative Affect."

Next, factor score estimates were computed for the higher-order factor of Negative Affect and each of the six first-order factors for each subject. These factor scores were used to examine the extent to which the different DSM-III-R principal diagnostic groups (determined by the ADIS-R) displayed characteristic factor score profiles (group membership was defined by DSM-III-R principal diagnoses, established using the ADIS-R). A discriminant-function analysis yielded five functions that were statistically significant in differentiating the diagnostic groups; a sixth function approached significance. One function, defined primarily by the higher-order factor of Negative Affect, discriminated each of the patient groups from the normal controls, with the social phobic and simple phobic groups significantly lower than all other patient groups that did not differ from each other. The second function, defined primarily by the Panic (fear of fear) factor, discriminated patients with a principal diagnosis of PD or PDA from each of the other groups. The third function, defined primarily by the Agoraphobia factor, discriminated PDA patients from each of the other groups. The fourth function, defined primarily by the Social Anxiety factor, discriminated social phobics from the other groups. The fifth function, defined primarily by the Obsessions and Compulsions factor, discriminated patients with OCD from the other groups. The sixth function, defined primarily by the Generalized Anxiety factor, discriminated simple phobics and normal controls from each of the other groups. Figure 2.2 presents the multivariate profiles for seven principal diagnoses, plotting each group's mean elevation above the normal control group, on each of the six discriminant functions. For most clinical groups, the profiles are plotted twice—the first including the entire sample, the second including patients with no other diagnoses other than their principal diagnosis (the second profile was not plotted for patients with principal diagnoses of GAD, OCD, or major depression/dysthymia, because of low sample sizes when comorbid cases were excluded).

Thus, Zinbarg and Barlow (1995) concluded that the results indicated a reasonably good match between the discriminant-function classification and the established DSM-III-R anxiety disorder diagnoses. The results of the factor analyses and the discriminant function analyses provided empirical evidence for the construct validity of the DSM-III-R groupings. The emergence of the higher-order factor and its corresponding discriminant function indicated that the various DSM-III-R anxiety disorders are related and belong in a common family or group of disorders (i.e., the classification has convergent validity). Indeed, while acknowledging some limitations in the study design (e.g., lack of measures of trait anxiety or neuroticism), Zinbarg and Barlow (1995) concluded that their findings were consistent with conceptual models positing a trait vulnerability factor that is common to all anxiety disorders (Barlow, 1988). Nevertheless, whereas this general higher-order factor accounted for a large proportion of the variance, the first-order factors and their corresponding discriminant functions indicated that it was possible to differentiate reliably among the members of this family.

ANXIETY DISORDERS WITH "UBIQUITOUS" KEY FEATURES

It is beyond the scope of this chapter to discuss extensively the extant literature attesting to the validity of each of the DSM-III-R and DSM-IV anxiety disorders, although the findings of Zinbarg and Barlow (1995) speak to this issues to some degree. Therefore, this section focuses on the discussion of GAD and PD. Arguably, these diagnoses could be considered to have the most diffuse boundaries among the anxiety and mood disorders, given that their key features (anxious apprehension, panic attacks) are present in the other disorders. This may have been reflected to some extent by the diagnostic reliability and comorbidity findings discussed earlier.

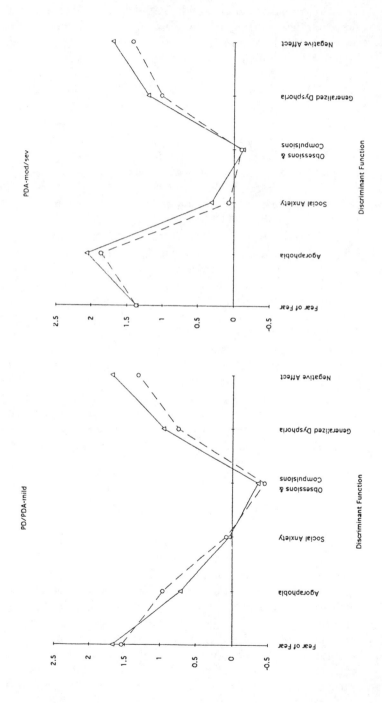

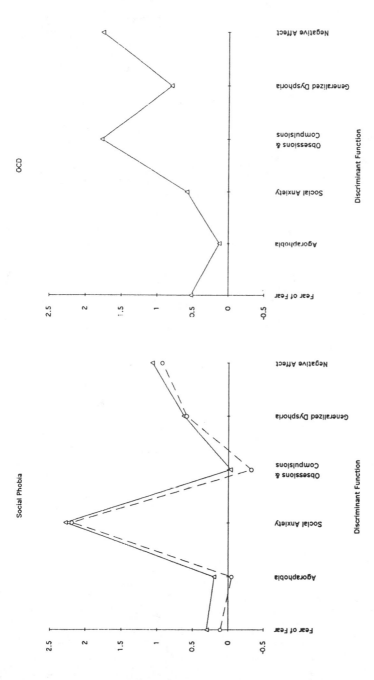

FIGURE 2.2. Discriminant-function profiles of principal DSM-III-R anxiety and mood disorders categories (Zimbarg & Barlow, 1995), using the total sample (triangles, solid lines) and excluding patients with comorbid diagnoses (circles, dashed lines). PD/PDA-mild, panic disorder with no more than mild agoraphobia; PDA-mod/sev, panic disorder with moderate or severe agoraphobia. OCD, obsessive–compulsive disorder.

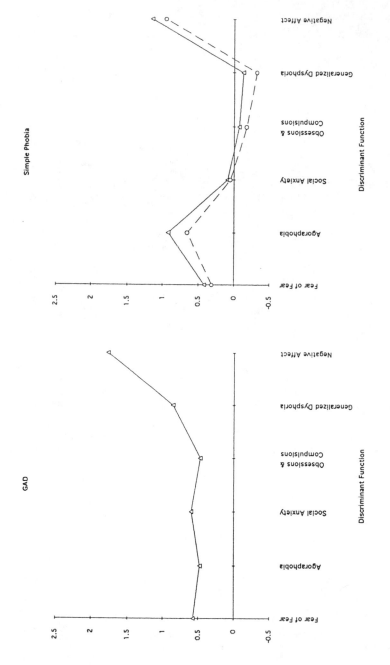

FIGURE 2.2. (*continued*) GAD, generalized anxiety disorder.

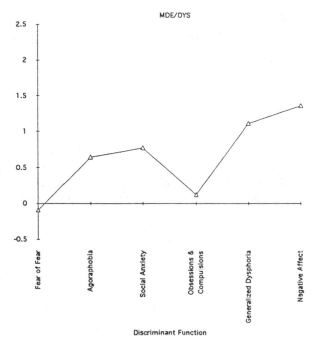

MDE/DYS

FIGURE 2.2. (*continued*) MDE/DYS, major depression or dysthymia.

Empirical Basis for Generalized Anxiety Disorder

Advocates of the notion of poor discriminant validity among anxiety and mood disorders would be wise to focus their arguments on GAD. GAD was the focus of considerable debate and controversy during the process of evaluating and revising the diagnoses and diagnostic criteria for DSM-IV. Indeed, many researchers involved in the development of DSM-IV argued for the elimination of GAD or moved to place this category in the appendix of disorders in need of further study. This proposition was largely based on the findings briefly reviewed above pertaining to the reliability and comorbidity of GAD. Thus, a principal argument against the retention of GAD was that in light of its lower interrater reliability in the context of other anxiety disorders and high rate of comorbidity, GAD should be subsumed under the diagnoses with which it co-occurs. This argument was based on the principle (noted earlier in the chapter) that low reliability and high comorbidity may be indicative of poor discriminant validity among categories in the classification system (i.e., the system is distinguishing phenomena that would be more parsimonious if combined).

Some of the factors that may have contributed to lowering the diagnostic reliability of GAD have been discussed earlier (e.g., ubiquity of anxious apprehension/worry across disorders, lack of an overt behavioral marker, high comorbidity rate). Moreover, additional findings from the Zinbarg and Barlow (1995) study bear on the issues of the reliability and distinctiveness of GAD. These authors found that patients with GAD, while having higher factor scores than normal controls on all six factors (listed earlier), were not differentiated from the other anxiety disorder groups on any one factor. Nevertheless, profile analyses revealed significant differentiation between patients with GAD and the other groups, indicating that these patients had a characteristic factor score profile. Thus, these data suggest that whereas patients with GAD could not be differentiated on the basis of any specific dimension assessed in this study (attesting to a proposed source of lower diagnostic reliability), their presentation was unique with regard to their profile of scores on a variety of dimensions of anxiety.

Elsewhere (Brown, Barlow, & Liebowitz, 1994), we have articulated a number of other features of GAD that support its validity and distinguishability. For example, GAD can be readily distinguished from OCD (Brown, Moras, et al., 1993). This is noteworthy because OCD could be considered the closest "neighbor" to GAD, given that its essential features are quite similar to the features of GAD (e.g., obsessions vs. excessive worry; compulsions vs. worry behavior). Moreover, GAD seems to be differentiated by its age and manner of onset. A consistent finding in the literature is that, on the whole, GAD is associated with an earlier (e.g., since childhood) and more gradual onset than most other anxiety disorders (e.g., Anderson, Noyes, & Crowe, 1984; Barlow, Blanchard, Vermilyea, Vermilyea, & Di Nardo, 1986; Cameron, Thyer, Nesse, & Curtis, 1986; Noyes et al., 1992; Sanderson & Barlow, 1990). Data from family and twin studies have provided data indicating a familial aggregation of GAD (Kendler, Neale, Kessler, Heath, & Eaves, 1992; Noyes, Clarkson, Crowe, Yates, & McChesney, 1987; Noyes et al., 1992), although nonsignificant findings exist in the literature (Cloninger, Martin, Clayton, & Guze, 1981; Torgersen, 1983).

In addition, patients with GAD can be differentiated from other anxiety disorder groups on dimensions of worry and associated symptomatology (Brown et al., 1994). For instance, patients with GAD can be differentiated from other anxiety disorder groups and normal controls on indices reflecting the parameters of controllability and pervasiveness of the worry process, as indicated by differences on responses to structured interviews (e.g., Borkovec, Shadick, & Hopkins, 1991; Brown, Moras, et al., 1993; Craske, Rapee, Jackel, & Barlow, 1989; Sanderson & Barlow, 1990) and by scores on psychometrically established questionnaires (e.g., Brown, Antony, & Barlow, 1992; Brown, Moras, et al., 1993; Meyer, Miller, Metzger, & Borkovec, 1990).

Another rather recent finding that has been obtained consistently is that GAD is associated with a set of somatic symptoms different from those associated with other anxiety disorders (e.g., Brown, Marten, & Barlow, 1995; Hoehn-Saric, McLeod, & Zimmerli, 1989; Marten et al., 1993). These symptoms do not involve any of those generally believed to be associated with autonomic arousal (e.g., accelerated heart rate, shortness of breath); rather, they are symptoms that were formally found in the motor tension and vigilance-and-scanning clusters of the DSM-III-R associated symptom criterion for GAD (e.g., irritability, muscle tension, feeling keyed up or on edge). Initial studies indicate that the presence of these symptoms differentiates patients with GAD from other anxiety disorder groups and from normal controls (e.g., Brown, Antony, & Barlow, 1992; Brown et al., 1995). Accordingly, the associated symptom criterion for GAD has been revised considerably in DSM-IV to incorporate these findings (see Brown et al., 1994).

We have also argued that the motion among some researchers in DSM-IV to subsume GAD under the disorders with which it co-occurs may be flawed on a number of accounts (Brown et al., 1994). For example, an examination of patterns of comorbidity reveals that the clinical features of several of the diagnoses that most frequently co-occur with GAD possess little ostensible overlap with the features of GAD. For example, in the Brown and Barlow (1992a) study, the most commonly occurring additional diagnosis in GAD patients was social phobia (29%) — a diagnosis where chronic anxiety and worry are infrequently present, except in severe "generalized" social phobics. In the Noyes et al. (1992) study, the most frequent additional diagnosis was simple phobia. On the other hand, comorbidity findings indicate that GAD is not highly comorbid with diagnoses associated with potentially overlapping features (e.g., OCD, mood disorders). Indeed, several studies indicate that OCD and GAD co-occur infrequently (e.g., Brown, Moras, et al., 1993; Moras et al., 1993). Moras et al. (1993) noted that 18% and 11% of patients with GAD had an additional diagnosis of dysthymia and major depression, respectively. Thus, the majority (71%) of GAD patients in the Moras et al. (1993) study had symptoms that could not be subsumed under a mood disorder. On a practical level, omission of the GAD diagnosis would result in a loss of coverage for the fairly large percentage of patients (20% or more) currently receiving the diagnosis in the absence of additional diagnoses.

Another difficulty with the position that GAD could be subsumed under other diagnoses is the fact that this argument discounts findings pertaining to temporal sequence and the fact that GAD is quite often associated with an earlier onset than many of the disorders with which it frequently co-occurs (e.g., PD). Accordingly, findings of high comorbidity could be interpreted to support recent conceptual models (e.g., Sanderson & Wetzler, 1991) that the features of GAD may act as vulnerability factors to the subsequent development of these co-occurring conditions. However, the question of whether the specific features of GAD act as vulnerability factors independent of more general constructs of vulnerability (e.g., trait anxiety, neuroticism) awaits future research.

Empirical Basis for Panic Disorder

A now widely accepted finding is that panic attacks are not unique to PD, but occur in all of the anxiety disorders and the mood disorders as well (Barlow, Brown, & Craske, 1994; Barlow et al., 1985). Consistent with these data, a revision introduced in DSM-IV is the presentation of the criteria for panic attacks (see Table 2.2) at the beginning of the chapter on anxiety disorders, prior to listing the criteria for the anxiety disorders themselves. In DSM-IV, it is stated explicitly that "Panic Attacks occur in the context of several different Anxiety Disorders" (APA, 1994, p. 394). Thus, the ubiquity of panic attacks across these diagnoses could be cited as evidence for poor discriminability among the anxiety disorder categories.

Data similar to those presented in the discussion of GAD could be offered here in support of PD as a distinct category (e.g., familial aggregation; see Noyes et al., 1987; Torgersen, 1983). However, this section focuses on changes to the diagnostic criteria in DSM-IV that provide the major boundary between PD and other anxiety disorders. In DSM-IV, it is asserted that "in determining the differential diagnostic significance of a Panic Attack, it is important to consider the context in which the Panic Attack occurs" (p. 394). Thus, three types of panic attacks are defined in DSM-IV, characterized by the prototypical relationships between the onset of the attacks and situational triggers: (1) unexpected (uncued); (2) situationally bound (cued); and (3) situationally predisposed (see APA, 1994, pp. 394–395).

In DSM-IV, the first part of Criterion A of PD reads: "recurrent unexpected Panic Attacks" (APA, 1994, p. 402). A key aspect of this criterion is the word "recurrent." For example, it would be problematic to place diagnostic significance on a patient's initial panic attack, given that (1) unexpected panic attacks mark the onset of the disorders for many persons with phobic disorders (McNally & Steketee, 1985; Munjack, 1984); and (2) many individuals with PD report an unfavorable experience with drugs (e.g., marijuana, cocaine, anesthesia) as the setting event for their first panic attack (Aronson & Craig, 1986; Last, Barlow, & O'Brien, 1984). Thus, the nature of the initial panic attack does not appear to be helpful in establishing the boundary between PD and other disorders, given that (1) initial panics would be experienced as "unexpected" or "out of the blue" by most patients, regardless of the anxiety disorder to which they are subsequently assigned; and (2) both patients with PD and pa-

TABLE 2.2. DSM-IV Panic Attack Criteria and Types of Panic

A discrete period of intense fear or discomfort, in which four (or more) of the following symptoms developed abruptly and reached a peak within 10 minutes:

(1) palpitations, pounding heart, or accelerated heart rate
(2) sweating
(3) trembling or shaking
(4) sensations of shortness of breath or smothering
(5) feeling of choking
(6) chest pain or discomfort
(7) nausea or abdominal distress
(8) feeling dizzy, unsteady, lightheaded, or faint
(9) derealization (feelings of unreality) or depersonalization (being detached from oneself)
(10) fear of losing control or going crazy
(11) fear of dying
(12) paresthesias (numbing or tingling sensations)
(13) chills or hot flushes

Types of DSM-IV panic:

(1) *Unexpected (uncued):* the onset of the panic attack is not associated with a situational trigger (i.e., occurring spontaneously "out of the blue").
(2) *Situationally bound (cued):* the panic attack almost invariably occurs immediately on exposure to, or in anticipation of, the situational cue or trigger (e.g., seeing a snake or dog always triggers an immediate panic attack).
(3) *Situationally predisposed:* the panic attacks are more likely to occur on exposure to the situational cue or trigger, but are not invariably associated with the cue and do not necessarily occur immediately after the exposure (e.g., attacks are more likely to occur while driving, but there are times when the individual drives and does not have a panic attack or times when the panic attack occurs after driving for a half hour).

Note. Reprinted with permission from the *Diagnostic and Statistical Manual of Mental Disorders,* Fourth Edition (p. 395). Copyright 1994 by American Psychiatric Association.

tients with phobic disorders report initial panic attacks that are (and are not) associated with situational cues.

As we have articulated in detail elsewhere (Barlow et al., 1994), a salient feature setting the boundary between PD and the phobic disorders is that patients with PD continue to experience unexpected (uncued) attacks, whereas patients with phobic disorders can always identify the cue and almost always experience the panic immediately upon confronting the situation. Even in patients with PDA, who may in the later stages of the disturbance report that virtually all of their panics are situational (e.g., occur in shopping malls), expectancy (predictability) of panic is quite useful in distinguishing PD from the phobic disorders. For example, Craske (1989) examined the timing of the panic attack in relation to exposure

to the phobic cue in patients with PDA, social phobia, and specific phobia. Whereas 15% and 30% of specific phobics and social phobics, respectively, reported that the timing of their panics was typically delayed, fully
92% of patients with PDA reported that they had no clear idea when to
expect the panic, despite being exposed to a situation that was identified
in their minds as a reliable panic "cue."

Thus, the key aspect distinguishing the panic attacks experienced by
patients with PD or PDA is that the patient at some time (but not necessarily initially) reports several unexpected (uncued) panic attacks (or temporal discontinuity between the cue and the attack). Moreover, a
substantial literature indicates that the phenomenon of "recurrent unexpected" panic attacks is associated with other important parameters that
foster the distinction of PD from other disorders. A major distinguishing
feature found in individuals with PD is marked anxiety over the possibility of experiencing additional panic attacks. This feature mediates a number of other parameters that have been shown to differentiate PD from
other anxiety disorders (e.g., response to biological challenge, increased
awareness of and sensitivity to somatic cues; Rapee, Brown, Antony, &
Barlow, 1992; Ehlers & Breuer, 1992; Ehlers, Margraf, Roth, Taylor,
& Birbaumer, 1988). Accordingly, these data (see Barlow et al., 1994,
for an extensive review) are reflected in the second part of Criterion A
for DSM-IV PD:

> (2) at least one of the attacks has been followed by 1 month (or more) of
>   one (or more) of the following:
>   (a) persistent concern about having additional attacks;
>   (b) worry about the implications of the attacks or its consequences (e.g.,
>   losing control, having a heart attack, "going crazy")
>   (c) a significant change in behavior related to the attacks (p. 402)

CLASSIFICATION OF ANXIETY DISORDERS: TREATMENT IMPLICATIONS

Whereas most of the data reviewed thus far pertain to the concurrent validity of the anxiety disorders (i.e., convergent and discriminant validity),
I have noted earlier that another important index of the utility of a system for classification is the extent to which it possesses predictive validity. In this section, one important parameter of predictive validity is briefly
discussed: treatment prescription.

Among the sequelae to the increased discrimination of anxiety disorders in the DSM system has been the development of specific treatments
targeting each disorder. For virtually all anxiety disorders, there now

exist controlled studies illustrating the effectiveness of cognitive-behavioral treatments compared with no treatment or some well-construed alternative psychosocial intervention. Although these treatments for anxiety disorders contain some overlapping elements (e.g., exposure to anxiety-provoking cues, cognitive restructuring), the specificity of cognitive-behavioral treatments for anxiety disorders in many ways outstrips the specificity of pharmacological treatments (Brown, Hertz, & Barlow, 1992).

Although there are difficulties inherent in the attempt to validate a diagnostic category on the basis of its treatment response, it is fair to say that considerable advances have been achieved in the therapeutic management of anxiety disorders via the tailoring of new treatments to key features of the disorder. Perhaps nowhere is this more true than in the development of cognitive-behavioral treatments for PD. Whereas situational exposure elements have long been in place for the treatment of agoraphobic avoidance, nonpharmacological approaches that directly target unexpected (uncued) panic attacks have only recently been available. Guided by recent empirical developments, these treatments contain components specifically targeting the most salient parameters of panic (e.g., cognitive restructuring of misattributions concerning the consequences of panic; interoceptive exposure to ameliorate marked sensitivity to a variety of somatic cues). In addition to being markedly effective in comparison to waiting-list control conditions, these cognitive-behavioral treatments for panic have been compared with leading drug treatments and have been found to be of equal or greater effectiveness, particularly over long-term follow-up (Brown & Barlow, 1992b). Thus, an implication of these findings is that the differential diagnosis of PD may have important ramifications for the selection of a treatment uniquely tailored to target the key features of the disorder.

It is interesting to note that in comparison to the treatment of PD, cognitive-behavioral treatments of GAD have produced modest results (e.g., Barlow, Rapee, & Brown, 1992). Consequently, Barlow (1988) has asserted that whereas the process of anxious apprehension (worry) is found in all anxiety disorders, when this process is the primary focus (as in GAD) "it is in many ways the most difficult of all anxiety disorders to treat" (p. 355). In addition, we (Brown et al., 1994) have speculated that the modest outcome findings may in part be attributable to the fact that most of the treatments examined to date have contained components that are relatively nonspecific to essential features of GAD (e.g., relaxation training, cognitive restructuring). Although highly specialized treatments have been developed that target the key features of GAD (e.g., excessive and uncontrollable worry), the question of whether these treatments produce more substantial gains awaits future study (Brown, O'Leary, & Barlow, 1993).

Also germane to the issue of treatment prescription is the utility of "subtyping" of disorders, which has become increasingly prevalent with each revision of the DSM. In DSM-IV, subtyping occurs for the majority of anxiety disorders (e.g., for PD, with or without agoraphobia; for specific phobia, animal, natural environment, blood–injection–injury, situational, other; for social phobia, generalized; for OCD, with poor insight; for PTSD, acute, chronic, with delayed onset). In some instances, the subtype of disorder may have substantial treatment implications. For example, the blood–injection–injury subtype of specific phobia is typically associated with a physiological reaction (hypotension, fainting) that is entirely different from that of other specific phobics, dictating a quite different approach to treatment (e.g., applied tension; Öst, Sterner, & Fellenius, 1989). Research has also shown that persons with the situational subtype of specific phobia (e.g., driving phobics, claustrophobics) often possess characteristics that place them on a continuum closer to PD (e.g., presence of situationally predisposed panic attacks, sensitivity to somatic cues). This finding may likewise have important implications for treatment (e.g., incorporation of panic control treatment elements such as interoceptive exposure; Zarate, Craske, Rapee, & Barlow, 1988). The provision of subtypes may potentially provide important information on treatment selection and response for social phobia as well (Heimberg et al., 1990).

Preliminary evidence from studies examining panic control treatments for PD and PDA suggests that when agoraphobia is present even in its mildest form, then this feature should represent a specific target of treatment. For example, we (Craske, Brown, & Barlow, 1991) reported that whereas the majority (81%) of PD patients (with no more than mild agoraphobia) receiving panic control treatment (consisting of cognitive restructuring and interoceptive exposure, but no situational exposure) were panic-free 2 years after treatment, only 50% met criteria for high-endstate status. This finding seemed to be attributable in part to continued mild agoraphobic avoidance in some patients, suggesting that the elimination of panic may not alone result in the amelioration of agoraphobic avoidance. Thus, situational exposure may be essential to the treatment of PD when the presence of agoraphobia is identified.

CONCLUSION

To return to the issue discussed at the beginning of the chapter, a fundamental issue in the nosology of emotional disorders is whether classification should be categorical (as in the DSM system) or dimensional. Given evidence attesting to marked overlap in symptomatology (high rates of symptom and syndrome comorbidity), it would seem that a purely dimensional approach to the assessment of anxiety disorders would be optimal. Although this point has not been given wide attention in this chapter, extensive overlap can be found in relation to the mood disorders, particularly for some anxiety disorders (GAD, OCD). Indeed, recent theories have conceptualized anxiety and depression to be constructs sharing a common vulnerability but falling at different points on a helplessness–hopelessness continuum (Alloy, Kelly, Mineka, & Clements, 1990; Barlow, 1988, 1991b). A dimensional approach to classification is more consistent with the principles held by cognitive-behavioral researchers and therapists.

However, as the evidence reviewed above has hopefully indicated, there appears to be considerable value to the identification of the clusters of symptoms specified by the DSM-III-R and DSM-IV anxiety disorder categories. Nevertheless, these categories should be viewed with caution, so as not to imply the presence of "real" or "distinct" entities that possess orthogonal parameters of etiology and psychopathology. The disorders contained in DSM-IV should be heralded for their heuristic value, which will foster future research on such important issues as the impact of coexisting symptoms and syndromes on treatment outcome and the expression of the principal disorder across time. This line of inquiry will probably point to the incorporation of some dimensional scaling into the nosology as the optimal approach to assessment and treatment planning (Barlow, 1988; Brown & Barlow, 1992a).

NOTE

1. Diagnoses under the heading of "Anxiety Disorders" in DSM-IV include panic disorder without agoraphobia, panic disorder with agoraphobia without history of panic disorder, specific phobia, social phobia, obsessive–compulsive disorder, posttraumatic stress disorder, acute stress disorder, generalized anxiety disorder, anxiety disorder due to a general medical condition, substance-induced anxiety disorder, and anxiety disorder not otherwise specified.

REFERENCES

Alloy, L. B., Kelly, K. A., Mineka, S., & Clements, C. M. (1990). Comorbidity of anxiety and depressive disorders: A helplessness–hopelessness perspective. In J. D. Maser & C. R. Cloninger (Eds.), *Comorbidity of mood and anxiety disorders* (pp. 499–543). Washington, DC: American Psychiatric Press.

American Psychiatric Association. (1968). *Diagnostic and statistical manual of mental disorders* (2nd ed.). Washington, DC: Author.

American Psychiatric Association. (1987). *Diagnostic and statistical manual of mental disorders* (3rd ed., rev.). Washington, DC: Author.

American Psychiatric Association. (1994). *Diagnostic and statistical manual of mental disorders* (4th ed.). Washington, DC: Author.

Anderson, D. J., Noyes, R., & Crowe, R. R. (1984). A comparison of panic disorder and generalized anxiety disorder. *American Journal of Psychiatry, 141,* 572–575.

Aronson, T. A., & Craig, T. J. (1986). Cocaine precipitation of panic disorder. *American Journal of Psychiatry, 143,* 643–645.

Barlow, D. H. (1988). *Anxiety and its disorders: The nature and treatment of anxiety and panic.* New York: Guilford Press.

Barlow, D. H. (1991a). Introduction to the special issue on diagnosis, dimensions, and DSM-IV: The science of classification. *Journal of Abnormal Psychology, 100,* 243–244.

Barlow, D. H. (1991b). The nature of anxiety: Anxiety, depression, and emotional disorders. In R. M. Rapee & D. H. Barlow (Eds.), *Chronic anxiety: Generalized anxiety disorder and mixed anxiety–depression* (pp. 1–28). New York: Guilford Press.

Barlow, D. H., Blanchard, E. B., Vermilyea, J. A., Vermilyea, B. B., & Di Nardo, P. A. (1986). Generalized anxiety and generalized anxiety disorder: Description and reconceptualization. *American Journal of Psychiatry, 143,* 40–44.

Barlow, D. H., Brown, T. A., & Craske, M. G. (1994). Definitions of panic attacks and panic disorder in DSM-IV: Implications for research. *Journal of Abnormal Psychology, 103,* 553–564.

Barlow, D. H., Rapee, R. M., & Brown, T. A. (1992). Behavioral treatment of generalized anxiety disorder. *Behavior Therapy, 23,* 551–570.

Barlow, D. H., Vermilyea, J. A., Blanchard, E. B., Vermilyea, B. B., Di Nardo, P. A., & Cerny, J. A. (1985). The phenomenon of panic. *Journal of Abnormal Psychology, 94,* 320–328.

Blashfield, R. K. (1990). Comorbidity and classification. In J. D. Maser & C. R. Cloninger (Eds.), *Comorbidity of mood and anxiety disorders* (pp. 61–82). Washington, DC: American Psychiatric Press.

Borkovec, T. D., Shadick, R., & Hopkins, M. (1991). The nature of normal and pathological worry. In R. M. Rapee & D. H. Barlow (Eds.), *Chronic anxiety: Generalized anxiety disorder and mixed anxiety–depression* (pp. 29–51). New York: Guilford Press.

Brown, T. A., Antony, M. M., & Barlow, D. H. (1992). Psychometric properties of the Penn State Worry Questionnaire in a clinical anxiety disorders sample. *Behaviour Research and Therapy, 30,* 33–37.

Brown, T. A., & Barlow, D. H. (1992a). Comorbidity among anxiety disorders: Implications for treatment and DSM-IV. *Journal of Consulting and Clinical Psychology, 60,* 835–844.

Brown, T. A., & Barlow, D. H. (1992b). Long-term clinical outcome following cognitive-behavioral treatment of panic disorder and panic disorder with agoraphobia. In P. H. Wilson (Ed.), *Principles and practice of relapse prevention* (pp. 191–212). New York: Guilford Press.

Brown, T. A., Barlow, D. H., & Liebowitz, M. R. (1994). The empirical basis of generalized anxiety disorder. *American Journal of Psychiatry, 151,* 1272–1280.

Brown, T. A., Hertz, R. M., & Barlow, D. H. (1992). New developments in cognitive-behavioral treatment of anxiety disorders. In A. Tasman (Ed.), *American Psychiatric Press review of psychiatry* (Vol. 11, pp. 285–306). Washington, DC: American Psychiatric Press.

Brown, T. A., Marten, P. A., & Barlow, D. H. (1995). Discriminant validity of the symptoms constituting the DSM-III-R and DSM-IV associated symptom criterion of generalized anxiety disorder. *Journal of Anxiety Disorders, 9,* 317–328.

Brown, T. A., Moras, K., Zinbarg, R. E., & Barlow, D. H. (1993). Diagnostic and symptom distinguishability of generalized anxiety disorder and obsessive–compulsive disorder. *Behavior Therapy, 24,* 227–240.

Brown, T. A., O'Leary, T. A., & Barlow, D. H. (1993). Generalized anxiety disorder. In D. H. Barlow (Ed.), *Clinical handbook of psychological disorders: A step-by-step treatment manual* (2nd ed., pp. 137–188). New York: Guilford Press.

Cameron, O. G., Thyer, B. A., Nesse, R. M., & Curtis, G. C. (1986). Symptom profiles of patients with DSM-III anxiety disorders. *American Journal of Psychiatry, 143,* 1132–1137.

Cloninger, C. R., Martin, R. L., Clayton, P., & Guze, S. B. (1981). A blind follow-up and family study of anxiety neurosis: Preliminary analysis of the St. Louis 500. In D. F. Klein & J. G. Rabkin (Eds.), *Anxiety: New research and changing concepts* (pp. 137–148). New York: Raven Press.

Craske, M. G. (1989). *The boundary between simple phobia and panic disorder* (Report to the DSM-IV Anxiety Disorders Workgroup). Albany: Center for Stress and Anxiety Disorders, The University at Albany, State University of New York.

Craske, M. G., Brown, T. A., & Barlow, D. H. (1991). Behavioral treatment of panic disorder: A two-year follow-up. *Behavior Therapy, 22,* 289–304.

Craske, M. G., Rapee, R. M., Jackel, L., & Barlow, D. H. (1989). Qualitative dimensions of worry in DSM-III-R generalized anxiety disorder subjects and non-anxious controls. *Behaviour Research and Therapy, 27,* 397–402.

de Ruiter, C., Rijken, H., Garssen, B., van Schaik, A., & Kraaimaat, F. (1989). Comorbidity among the anxiety disorders. *Journal of Anxiety Disorders, 3,* 57–68.

Di Nardo, P. A., & Barlow, D. H. (1988). *Anxiety Disorders Interview Schedule— Revised (ADIS-R).* Albany, NY: Graywind.

Di Nardo, P. A., Moras, K., Barlow, D. H., Rapee, R. M., & Brown, T. A. (1993). Reliability of DSM-III-R anxiety disorder categories using the Anxiety Disorders Interview Schedule — Revised (ADIS-R). *Archives of General Psychiatry, 50,* 251–256.

Ehlers, A., & Breuer, P. (1992). Increased cardiac awareness in panic disorder. *Journal of Abnormal Psychology, 101,* 371–382.

Ehlers, A., Margraf, J., Roth, W. T., Taylor, C. B., & Birbaumer, N. (1988). Anxiety induced by false heart rate feedback in patients with panic disorder. *Behaviour Research and Therapy, 26,* 1–11.

Foa, E. B., & Kozak, M. J. (1989). *Obsessions, overvalued ideas, and delusions in obsessive–compulsive disorder* (Report to the DSM-IV Anxiety Disorders Workgroup). Philadelphia: Eastern Pennsylvania Psychiatric Institute at the Medical College of Pennsylvania.

Frances, A., Widiger, T., & Fyer, M. R. (1990). The influence of classification methods on comorbidity. In J. D. Maser & C. R. Cloninger (Eds.), *Comorbidity of mood and anxiety disorders* (pp. 41–59). Washington, DC: American Psychiatric Press.

Heimberg, R. G., Dodge, C. S., Hope, D. A., Kennedy, C. R., Zollo, L. J., & Becker, R. E. (1990). Cognitive behavioral group therapy for social phobia: Comparison with a credible placebo control. *Cognitive Therapy and Research, 14,* 1–23.

Hoehn-Saric, R., McLeod, D. R., & Zimmerli, W. D. (1989). Somatic manifestations in women with generalized anxiety disorder: Psychophysiological responses to psychological stress. *Archives of General Psychiatry, 46,* 1113–1119.

Kendler, K. S., Neale, M. C., Kessler, R. C., Heath, A. C., & Eaves, L. J. (1992). Generalized anxiety disorder in women: A population-based twin study. *Archives of General Psychiatry, 49,* 267–272.

Last, C. G., Barlow, D. H., & O'Brien, G. T. (1984). Precipitants of agoraphobia: Role of stressful life events. *Psychological Reports, 54,* 567–570.

Marten, P. A., Brown, T. A., Barlow, D. H., Borkovec, T. D., Shear, M. K., & Lydiard, M. B. (1993). Evaluation of the ratings comprising the associated symptom criterion of DSM-III-R generalized anxiety disorder. *Journal of Nervous and Mental Disease, 181,* 676–682.

Maser, J. D., Kaelber, C., & Weise, R. E. (1991). International use and attitudes toward DSM-III and DSM-III-R: Growing consensus in psychiatric classification. *Journal of Abnormal Psychology, 100,* 271–279.

McNally, R. J., & Steketee, G. (1985). The etiology and maintenance of severe animal phobias. *Behaviour Research and Therapy, 23,* 431–435.

Meyer, T. J., Miller, M. L., Metzger, R. L., & Borkovec, T. D. (1990). Development and validation of the Penn State Worry Questionnaire. *Behaviour Research and Therapy, 28,* 487–495.

Moras, K., & Barlow, D. H. (1992). Dimensional approaches to diagnosis and the problem of anxiety and depression. In W. Fiegenbaum, A. Ehlers, J. Margraf, & I. Florin (Eds.), *Perspectives and promises of clinical psychology* (pp. 23–37). New York: Plenum Press.

Moras, K., Di Nardo, P. A., Brown, T. A., & Barlow, D. H. (1994). *Comorbidity and depression among the DSM-III-R anxiety disorders.* Manuscript submitted for publication.

Munjack, D. J. (1984). The onset of driving phobias. *Journal of Behavior Therapy and Experimental Psychiatry, 15,* 305–308.

Noyes, R., Clarkson, C., Crowe, R. R., Yates, W. R., & McChesney, C. M. (1987). A family study of generalized anxiety disorder. *American Journal of Psychiatry, 144,* 1019–1024.

Noyes, R., Woodman, C., Garvey, M. J., Cook, B. L., Suelzer, M., Clancy, J., & Anderson, D. J. (1992). Generalized anxiety disorder vs. panic disorder: Distinguishing characteristics and patterns of comorbidity. *Journal of Nervous and Mental Disease, 180,* 369–379.

Öst, L.-G., Sterner, U., & Fellenius, J. (1989). Applied tension, applied relaxation, and the combination in the treatment of blood phobia. *Behaviour Research and Therapy, 27,* 109–121.

Rapee, R. M., Brown, T. A., Antony, M. M., & Barlow, D. H. (1992). Response to hyperventilation and inhalation of 5.5% carbon dioxide-enriched air across the DSM-III-R anxiety disorders. *Journal of Abnormal Psychology, 101,* 538–552.

Sanderson, W. C., & Barlow, D. H. (1990). A description of patients diagnosed with DSM-III-R generalized anxiety disorder. *Journal of Nervous and Mental Disease, 178,* 588–591.

Sanderson, W. C., Beck, A. T., & Beck, J. (1990). Syndrome comorbidity in patients with major depression or dysthymia: Prevalence and temporal relationships. *American Journal of Psychiatry, 147,* 1025–1028.

Sanderson, W. C., Di Nardo, P. A., Rapee, R. M., & Barlow, D. H. (1990). Syndrome comorbidity in patients diagnosed with a DSM-III-R anxiety disorder. *Journal of Abnormal Psychology, 99,* 308–312.

Sanderson, W. C., & Wetzler, S. (1991). Chronic anxiety and generalized anxiety disorder: Issues in comorbidity. In R. M. Rapee & D. H. Barlow (Eds.), *Chronic anxiety: Generalized anxiety disorder, and mixed anxiety-depression* (pp. 119–135). New York: Guilford Press.

Tellegen, A. (1985). Structures of mood and personality and their relevance to assessing anxiety with an emphasis on self-report. In A. H. Tuma & J. D. Maser (Eds.), *Anxiety and the anxiety disorders* (pp. 681–706). Hillsdale, NJ: Erlbaum.

Torgersen, S. (1983). Genetic factors in anxiety disorders. *Archives of General Psychiatry, 40,* 1085–1089.

Zarate, R., Craske, M. G., Rapee, R. M., & Barlow, D. H. (1988, November). *The effectiveness of interoceptive exposure in the treatment of simple phobia.* Paper presented at the meeting of the Association for Advancement of Behavior Therapy, New York.

Zinbarg, R. E., & Barlow, D. H. (1995). *The structure of anxiety and the DSM-III-R anxiety disorders: A hierarchical model.* Manuscript submitted for publication.

It Is the Same Penny: We See the Head and They See the Tail

GAVIN ANDREWS

BOTH BROWN AND MYSELF are blessed with good structured diagnostic interviews. The Anxiety Disorders Interview Schedule—Revised is a highly reliable interview for DSM-III-R anxiety disorders. The CIDI-Auto is a highly reliable, computerized, self-administered interview that covers all the common DSM-III-R and ICD-10 mental disorders. The results of both interviews tell us the same things: that patients tend to have clinical histories of more than one disorder in their lifetimes to date, and that patients with the individual anxiety and depressive disorders can be reliably differentiated. Brown argues in Chapter 2 of this book that this differentiation is of value. We concur, and in fact our recent textbook *Treatment of Anxiety Disorders* (Andrews, Crino, Hunt, Lampe, & Page, 1994) is organized by disorder, demonstrating the characteristics that are unique to each disorder and demonstrating the different treatment approaches that work best with each disorder. In effect, Brown's chapter, like our book, represents the tail of the penny—the observable consequence of a sequence of processes that is recognized as disorder.

I have described the head of the penny in Chapter 1 of the present book. In it I have sought to explain why the common anxiety and depressive illnesses may occur in the first place, and then co-occur more than chance would dictate. Beginning with two longitudinal studies that showed how antecedent neuroticism measures could predict the occurrence of symptoms or disorder, I have reviewed community studies of symptoms, community studies of disorders, and finally clinic studies of disorders, before concluding that personality vulnerability is a necessary and nearly sufficient cause for the six common anxiety and depressive disorders studied.

Disproving this claim is simple. It merely requires two things. First, a cohort of persons who meet criteria for the six diagnoses studied must be shown to have scores on measures of trait anxiety and coping that are not elevated; second, it must be shown that persons who do not meet criteria for these diagnoses and yet who have high scores on these measures are not vulnerable to these diagnoses if followed through the years of risk. The genetic information I have presented in Chapter 1 simply underscores the position that this personality vulnerability is in part inherited and therefore causal in the proper sense, and not simply attributable to the confounding effects of illness on questionnaire completion. One consequence of this position is that treatment should be directed at ameliorating the symptoms of the disorder and at reducing these vulnerability factors if cure is to result. Another consequence is that prevention must result in this vulnerability being reduced, given that cure or successful prevention means that the person thereafter should have only the age- and sex-standardized population risk of developing the disorder.

I apologize to the editor. He had so hoped for a passionate controversy. Instead I claim that both Brown and I are correct, and that together we have begun to illustrate the cause and the manifestation of some of the common anxiety and depressive disorders. Even if this claim is not controversial, it must make for a valuable and complementary pair of chapters.

REFERENCE

Andrews, G., Crino, R., Hunt, C., Lampe, L., & Page, A. (1994). *Treatment of anxiety disorders*. New York: Cambridge University Press.

On the Validity and Comorbidity of the DSM-III-R and DSM-IV Anxiety Disorders

TIMOTHY A. BROWN
BRUCE F. CHORPITA

PRIOR TO RESPONDING SPECIFICALLY to issues raised in Chapter 1 by Andrews, we briefly reiterate a few of the major points conveyed in Chapter 2. First, the chapter states that clinical investigators should regard DSM-III-R and now DSM-IV primarily for their heuristic value rather than as some representation of truth (cf. Maser, Kaelber, & Weise, 1991). Similarly, given the overlap in symptomatology across diagnostic categories and the dimensional nature of symptoms forming the criteria for the various emotional disorders, the chapter argues that a dimensional approach to classification (or a combination of a dimensional approach and the categorical approach that prevails in DSM-IV) would be optimal. Finally, drawing on our conceptual model of emotional disorders (see Barlow, 1988; Brown, Antony, & Barlow, 1995) and on recent data from our clinic (e.g., Zinbarg & Barlow, 1995), the chapter asserts that anxiety and mood disorders share common diatheses (e.g., biological vulnerabilities) but differ on important dimensions (e.g., focus of attention, degree of psychological vulnerability), to the extent that increased differentiation of these pathological phenomena is warranted (e.g., has implications for treatment). Consequently, identification of clusters of symptoms as specified by the DSM-IV appears to have considerable value (rather than "lumping" these symptoms into one larger syndrome).

Since Chapter 2 was written, Brown et al. (1995) have completed a study that we believe has a bearing on the last point. This study examined the impact and course of comorbid diagnoses associated with cognitive-behavioral treatment of panic disorder (PD). Although space limitations preclude a full elaboration of these findings, an observation relevant to this reply was that treatment for PD resulted in a significant decline in comorbidity at posttreatment. Indeed, whereas 40% of patients had at least one additional diagnosis at pretreatment, this rate declined to 17% at posttreatment. However, by 24-month follow-up the rate of comorbidity increased to a level (30%) that was no longer significantly different from the pretreatment level, despite the fact that patients continued to improve upon their treatment gains for PD symptomatology over this period. This finding suggests a considerable degree of independence between panic symptomatology and comorbid syndromes. Brown et al. also suggested that this finding can be taken to support the position that although treatment was successful in eliminating the specific, maintaining processes of PD, a shared diathesis remained that had etiological significance in the emergence or resilience of other disorders. (This may also be supportive of Andrews's assertion of the importance of focusing on common vulnerability as the target of treatment and prevention.) Nevertheless, whereas these data provide many interesting hints about the nature of psychopathology and its organization, this study (like most research conducted to date) raises more questions than it answers, for the reasons discussed below.

In Chapter 1, Andrews provides a thoughtful integration and discussion of the literature germane to issues pertaining to classification and the distinctiveness of anxiety and mood disorders as specified by the DSM and ICD classification systems. Although Brown has placed greater emphasis on the value of differentiating various emotional phenomena in Chapter 2, both chapters appear to converge on the existence and importance of a shared diathesis among the anxiety and mood disorders. Indeed, to borrow from Andrews's chapter title, a comparison of the positions taken in the two chapters suggest that the similarities appear to be more important than the differences. However, because this book is about controversy, we would like to make a few points to caution readers against placing too much emphasis on the role of general vulnerability in the emotional disorders, at least at this stage in our knowledge about the nature of these disorders.

In building the case for the position that the anxiety and mood disorders share a common vulnerability, Andrews and others have relied a great deal on studies pertaining to the comorbidity among diagnostic syndromes. As has been noted elsewhere (e.g., Blashfield, 1990; Frances,

Widiger, & Fyer, 1990), when two disorders are observed to co-occur on a descriptive level, it is difficult to ascertain which interpretation is the most relevant: (1) Disorders X and Y are both influenced by another underlying or causal factor Z (i.e., they share the same diathesis); (2) disorder X predisposes or causes disorder Y (or vice versa); (3) disorders X and Y co-occur because of chance factors; (4) disorders X and Y are associated because they share overlapping definitional criteria; or (5) disorders X and Y should not be considered comorbid, because they are best subsumed into one larger category that has been artificially split into separate parts. Thus, whereas we and presumably Andrews would predict that comorbidity is attributable primarily to the first explanation, the extant literature (much of which is reviewed by Andrews) is not sufficient to support any particular interpretation (or multiple interpretations such as the combination of underlying vulnerability plus the stress of a preexisting disorder, as suggested by Andrews).

Given this state of affairs, it is far too early to center our thinking around any one explanation. One hindrance to the advancement of our knowledge in this area is the preponderance of research that has examined these issues at the level of diagnosis rather than at the level of symptoms. Although studies conducted at the syndrome level may provide useful information about the degree and possible meaning of comorbidity, they are restricted by their adherence to the disorders defined by the diagnostic system (indeed, by using diagnoses as the units of analysis, researchers are in a sense implicitly accepting the validity of the classification system they are evaluating). Hence, studies of this nature do not provide basic information pertaining to the extent to which the syndromes defined by ICD and DSM are empirically valid in terms of symptom covariance or clustering. Indeed, as noted by Andrews, it is quite plausible that a general factor may influence *a priori* syndrome definitions. However, it is of equal concern whether the definitions themselves reflect the true patterns in nature.

To effectively address the question of how the anxiety and mood disorders are best conceptualized and classified, it is important to consider more closely the nature of the processes in question. Although much of the evidence reviewed by Andrews is compelling, it often fails to operate at the multiple levels of analysis necessary. Namely, it seems that a cogent examination of the anxiety and mood disorders must involve analysis of both general and specific factors, longitudinal influences, measurement theory (e.g., reliability), symptom as well as syndrome covariance, and the dimensional rather than the categorical nature of psychopathology.

Information emanating from studies examining comorbidity among the anxiety and mood disorders may be misleading because the validity of the disorders themselves has yet to be firmly established. For example, if a high comorbidity rate between PD and specific phobia were observed, this could be an artifact of there being completely overlapping clusters of symptoms (i.e., one syndrome). Alternatively, the interpretation of high rates of co-occurrence between PD and specific phobia would be misleading if specific phobia had been erroneously classified as a single syndrome when, in fact, it empirically clustered into two distinct syndromes.

In addition, most analyses of comorbidity (and analyses of the influence of genetics or familial aggregation) rely on data that do not reflect the dimensional nature of psychopathology. There are a number of limitations associated with this approach to analysis. As a rule, any categorization of dimensional variables will forfeit meaningful information by artificially collapsing variability above and below an arbitrary threshold. For example, dichotomous classification of the symptomatology forming a DSM-IV diagnostic category ignores the wide range of variability in symptomatology above and below the threshold that is used to define what is a disorder and what is not. On the other hand, if the assessment of these phenomena were to be performed at the dimensional level, this would allow the researcher to evaluate more accurately the interrelationships among symptoms and syndromes, and their relative loading onto a general, higher-order factor. Thus, although the notion of a diagnostic threshold may be useful for some applications (e.g., defining inclusion criteria in treatment outcome studies), it is likely to create conceptual and statistical limitations for the researcher studying the nature and classification of psychopathological phenomena.

Thus, future studies should place greater emphasis on the dimensional assessment of the multitude of symptoms forming the anxiety and mood disorder constructs and associated vulnerability variables. With the advances in statistical modeling procedures, it is possible to examine the interrelationship of measurement issues, dimensional elements, multiple-level factor structures, and longitudinal phenomena associated with anxiety and depression. Using these techniques, researchers can directly compare the various and often opposing conceptual models pertaining to the structure of psychopathology in the anxiety and related disorders. Studies that examine the relative contribution of a variety of explanations for these phenomena will lead to substantially greater advances in our understanding of the nature and organization of psychopathology than will studies attempting to validate a unitary position.

REFERENCES

Barlow, D. H. (1988). *Anxiety and its disorders: The nature and treatment of anxiety and panic.* New York: Guilford Press.

Blashfield, R. K. (1990). Comorbidity and classification. In J. D. Maser & C. R. Cloninger (Eds.), *Comorbidity of mood and anxiety disorders* (pp. 61–82). Washington, DC: American Psychiatric Press.

Brown, T. A., Antony, M. M., & Barlow, D. H. (1995). Diagnostic comorbidity in panic disorder: Effect on treatment outcome and course of comorbid diagnoses following treatment. *Journal of Consulting and Clinical Psychology, 63,* 408–418.

Frances, A., Widiger, T., & Fyer, M. R. (1990). The influence of classification methods on comorbidity. In J. D. Maser & C. R. Cloninger (Eds.), *Comorbidity of mood and anxiety disorders* (pp. 41–59). Washington, DC: American Psychiatric Press.

Maser, J. D., Kaelber, C., & Weise, R. E. (1991). International use and attitudes toward DSM-III and DSM-III-R: Growing consensus in psychiatric classification. *Journal of Abnormal Psychology, 100,* 271–279.

Zinbarg, R. E., & Barlow, D. H. (1995). *The structure of anxiety and the DSM-III-R anxiety disorders: A hierarchical model.* Manuscript submitted for publication.

II

Etiology

3

Emotion Theory as a Framework for Explaining Panic Attacks and Panic Disorder

MARTIN M. ANTONY
DAVID H. BARLOW

SINCE THE DIAGNOSIS of panic disorder (PD) was introduced in DSM-III (American Psychiatric Association, 1980), a dramatic surge of research activity on the nature and treatment of panic has occurred. In addition, various etiological theories accounting for panic have been published. These models come from a broad range of theoretical perspectives, including those advocating the importance of biological factors (e.g., Gorman, Liebowitz, Fyer, & Stein, 1989; Klein, 1981, 1993; Klein & Gorman, 1987; Nutt, 1989; Nutt & Lawson, 1992), hyperventilation (e.g., Ley, 1987), classical conditioning (e.g., Goldstein & Chambless, 1978; Wolpe & Rowan, 1988), psychodynamic factors (Shear, Cooper, Klerman, Busch, & Shapiro, 1993), evolutionary factors (e.g., Marks, 1987; Nesse, 1987), cognitive factors (e.g., Beck & Emery with Greenberg, 1985; Clark, 1986, 1988; Rapee, 1993), and variations on these approaches (e.g., Ehlers & Margraf, 1989).

As is typically the case early in the study of a particular area, much of the research and thought regarding PD has been driven by theoretical perspectives that might be best described as unidimensional. For example, although biological theorists have acknowledged that psychological factors may be relevant to PD (particularly in the development of agoraphobic avoidance), little attention has been paid to the specific nature of

55

these variables. Similarly, most cognitive and behavioral theorists have tended to de-emphasize the role of biological factors in their models. Furthermore, the majority of clinical theorists have made little reference to theory and data from relevant areas of basic psychological research, including emotion theory and cognitive science. In response to these problems, Barlow (1988) has published a model of panic and PD that incorporates current thinking from emotion theory while attempting to integrate findings from a variety of perspectives, including cognitive, learning, and biological.

This chapter describes PD from an emotion theory perspective, and provides empirical support for the model from relevant research on panic and PD. In addition, we discuss limitations of the model, as well as future research that might test aspects of the theory.

AN EMOTION-BASED MODEL OF PANIC
AND PANIC DISORDER

The Nature of Emotion

Barlow's (1988) model of panic is compatible with the thinking of contemporary emotion researchers such as Peter Lang and other theorists, who have applied an information-processing framework to emotional phenomena and more recently to disorders of emotion such as depression (e.g., Bower, 1981; Lang, 1988; Teasdale, 1993; Watts, 1992). Lang (1988) and others have used the computer as a metaphor for the mind, which is viewed as an organized, logical information-processing system. Emotions are described by Lang as behavioral dispositions that prepare an organism for action. In the case of fear, such dispositions include strong motivation to escape from a dangerous situation.

Following recent models of memory, Lang believes that bits of information about stimuli and responses (including emotional responses) are stored in associative memory, as is the situation or context in which these responses occur. Memory is hypothesized to be organized in associative networks in which concepts are stored and linked to one another with connections of varying strength. For example, the concept "collie" may be more strongly associated with the concept "dog" than with the concept "animal." Emotional reactions occur when stimuli activate particular networks in emotional memory.

Lang (1988) has criticized cognitive appraisal models for relying on conscious rational analysis (or unconscious analysis that resembles conscious thought) to explain panic. While arguing that cognitive processing is important for the experience of emotion, he also suggests that these

processes are different from the rational (or irrational) appraisals hypothesized to occur in most cognitive models of panic (e.g., Clark, 1986, 1988).
This view is consistent with that expressed by Zajonc (1980, 1984), who,
though acknowledging that conscious appraisal may precede emotional
reactions in some situations, has argued that such appraisal is not necessary for emotion to occur.

The Nature of Panic, Fear, and Anxiety

With few exceptions (e.g., Beck et al., 1985), most recent models of panic
disorder fail to define the terms "panic," "anxiety," and "fear" adequately, and also fail to specify how these states may be similar or different.
Like most emotion theorists, Barlow (1988, 1991) views fear and anxiety
as fundamentally different processes and has tried to provide specific definitions for each term.

Barlow shares Lang's view of "fear" as a tightly organized, cohesive
affective structure or what Izard (1977) describes as a distinct, primitive,
basic emotion. Recall that for Lang, an emotion is primarily a behavioral
disposition that prepares an organism to act. Consistent with this view,
fear is an alarm reaction in which there is an intense push to escape from
potential danger and in which the organism is mobilized, both physically
and cognitively, for action. Fear is viewed as a possibly hard-wired, fight-
or-flight response that is present across cultures and species and can vary
in intensity across situations. When fear occurs in the absence of any real
threat, the fear reaction is called a "false alarm" or "panic attack." Thus,
in Barlow's model, "panic" is phenomenologically identical to the emotion of fear.

Consistent with Lang's (1985) view, Barlow (1988) sees "anxiety"
(or "anxious apprehension") as a loosely defined, widespread affective network stored in memory, or what Izard (1977) describes as a blend of emotions. Furthermore, in contrast to basic emotions such as fear, what gets
labeled as anxiety varies across people and situations. Although basic emotions such as fear and sadness are easy to distinguish, affective states such
as anxiety and depression appear to have more in common and are therefore harder to distinguish. This point is supported by the high correlations typically found among measures of anxiety, depression, and other
states characterized by elevated negative affect (Dobson, 1985; Gotlib &
Cane, 1989; Zinbarg & Barlow, 1991).

According to Barlow (1988), anxiety is a future-oriented emotional
state characterized by high negative affect and a sense that upcoming events
are uncontrollable and unpredictable. When one is anxious, one's attentional focus shifts rapidly back and forth between the task at hand and
an internal, self-evaluative focus. This accounts for the difficulty in con-

centrating reported by people who are anxious. This process results in self-preoccupation, worry, and an intensification of the arousal associated with anxiety.

To summarize, panic is an acute reaction to immediate danger, similar to the feeling that occurs when one must veer out of the way of an oncoming car or quickly grab the sides of a ladder to avoid falling after missing a step. The reaction to such events must be immediate to allow appropriate actions to be taken in time to remove oneself from the danger. In contrast, anxiety is future-oriented apprehension over some possible threat. For example, after experiencing an automobile collision, one may be anxious over the possibility of encountering such a situation in the future and may be vigilant for early signs and signals such as driving too fast.

One implication of Barlow's (1988) model is that many episodes of anxious apprehension may be misdiagnosed as panic. According to DSM-III-R (American Psychiatric Association, 1987) and DSM-IV (American Psychiatric Association, 1994), a panic attack must reach a peak within 10 minutes. However, it is difficult to imagine an episode of fear, as defined by Barlow (1988), taking up to 10 minutes to peak and still being able to protect a person from immediate danger. Many people report that their panic attacks peak immediately or within seconds. These attacks are probably most similar to the fight-or-flight responses described by Barlow as panic/fear. Episodes of heightened arousal that take minutes or hours to peak are probably examples of what Barlow calls anxious apprehension, even though they might meet current diagnostic criteria for panic. This issue has been discussed in some detail by Barlow, Brown, and Craske (1994), who have recommended that a shorter "rise time" of 5 minutes be used by PD researchers to define panic attacks.

A Model of Panic Disorder

Barlow's model of PD (see Figure 3.1) may be summarized as follows. The initial panic attack typically occurs following a period of stress in individuals who possess a *biological* vulnerability to experiencing surges of fear in the absence of any specific triggers. According to Barlow, some people are susceptible to developing panic attacks following stress, just as some other individuals develop headaches, hypertension, and other similar problems. These attacks are called "false alarms," because they occur in the absence of any real threat. Following stressful life events, some individuals are assumed to be more vulnerable to having panic attacks than others, just as other people might develop headaches or essential hypertension in response to stress. Presumably, the factors contributing to this vulnerability include a genetically inherited predisposition to experience panic attacks. For many people, the attacks are attributed to some be-

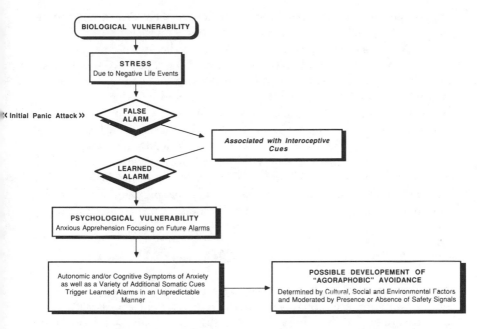

FIGURE 3.1. A model of the etiology of panic disorder. From Barlow (1988, p. 367). Copyright 1988 by The Guilford Press. Reprinted by permission.

nign cause (e.g., something they ate, being anxious, etc.). This would describe a typical attack for a nonclinical panicker (Norton, Dorward, & Cox, 1986).

As illustrated in Figure 3.1, some individuals possess an additional *psychological* vulnerability to developing PD. This vulnerability consists of a sense that events in general and emotions in particular are uncontrollable and unpredictable. The results of this sense of poor control and predictability are an increase in arousal and an inward shift in attention; thus begins the process of anxious apprehension focused on having additional panic attacks. For Barlow (1988), it is this process of anxious apprehension that turns the harmless (although uncomfortable) experience of panic into a disorder characterized by frequent panic attacks, high levels of anxiety between panic attacks, and in some cases agoraphobic avoidance.

For people who develop anxious apprehension over future panic, interoceptive cues become associated (through classical conditioning) with the original false alarm, and the result is what Barlow calls "learned alarms." The occurrence of learned alarms is often triggered by changes in specific bodily sensations. If anxiety develops and becomes focused on future panic, additional somatic and cognitive cues become available to trigger the panic attacks, resulting in the development of PD. Depending on cultural, social, and environmental factors, as well as on the presence of safety signals, agoraphobic avoidance may then develop.

Barlow's (1988) model does not depend on conscious appraisal to account for panic attacks. However, it does specify cognitive processes that may be involved in panic (e.g., memory, perceived control, internal focus of attention). This is consistent with modern theories of Pavlovian conditioning (e.g., Rescorla, 1988), which hypothesize some level of cognitive processing in all animal learning. This model does not rule out the possibility that some attacks may be preceded by a conscious appraisal of danger in response to fluctuations in physical sensations; however, this need not be the case for most attacks. Clearly, people can respond to the environment and behave outside of awareness.

EMPIRICAL EVIDENCE FOR BARLOW'S MODEL

Now that Barlow's (1988) model of panic has been described in some detail, we turn our attention to some of the research that addresses the various components of the theory. Specifically, research on the relationships among panic, anxiety, and fear is discussed, as is the evidence for a biological vulnerability to experiencing panic attacks (false alarms) and for the role of stress in the onset of false alarms. Finally, the literature on factors associated with a psychological vulnerability to developing anxiety (e.g., perceived control, predictability) is reviewed, as well as data on nonclinical panic and its relationship to PD.

The Relationship between Panic and Anxiety

Despite Barlow's assertion that anxiety and panic are fundamentally distinct states, many investigators have disagreed with this view. Several theorists, such as Ley (1987) and Clark (1986, 1988), have implied that panic and anxiety are essentially identical. Theorists who do not distinguish between these states tend to view panic as an intense form of anxiety that increases quickly through a positive feedback loop involving the catastrophic misinterpretation of bodily sensations triggered by hyperventilation (Ley, 1987) or by one of a variety of other benign causes (Clark, 1986, 1988).

Like Clark (1986, 1988) and Ley (1987), Ehlers and Margraf (1989) view panic and anxiety as differing quantitatively but not qualitatively. To support their view, Ehlers and Margraf (1989) have argued that panic attacks occur in anxiety disorders other than PD, as well as in nonclinical populations. In addition, they point out that panic and anxiety share many symptoms, and even suggest that the differences in severity between panic and anxiety may be smaller than previously assumed. Specifically, they argue that the majority of panic attacks are not as intense as patients' retrospective self-reports might suggest. Margraf, Taylor, Ehlers, Roth, and Agras (1987) used panic attack diaries and ambulatory monitoring to measure physiological activity associated with panic; they found that actual attacks tended to be less severe on both measures than in subsequent retrospective reports by the subjects.

Despite these arguments against the distinctiveness of panic and anxiety, there are several reasons to consider them different states. First, the argument that panic attacks occur in disorders other than PD is probably irrelevant to the distinction between panic and anxiety. Those who view panic and anxiety as qualitatively different (e.g., Barlow, 1988) would argue that panic and anxiety are different regardless of the disorder in which they occur. For example, an individual with specific phobia may experience panic under certain circumstances (e.g., when encountering a snake) and anxious apprehension under other circumstances (e.g., when anticipating encountering a snake in the future).

Second, despite the overlap in physical symptoms highlighted by Ehlers and Margraf (1989), some investigators have reported a tendency for symptoms to cluster differently in panic and general anxiety (Borden & Turner, 1989). Furthermore, it could be argued that high symptom overlap in panic and anxiety does not necessarily mean that the two states are the same. For example, a person who is very angry may experience many of the same sensations (e.g., breathlessness, palpitations, etc.) as one who is very excited; yet few would argue that anger and excitement are qualitatively identical.

It seems that at least two criteria may be relevant to the question of whether panic and anxiety are qualitatively different. First, are there different biological mechanisms underlying panic and anxiety? Studies comparing the neurochemical basis, relevant brain structures, genetics, and specific drug responses of panic and anxiety may help to answer this question.

Second, are panic and anxiety experienced differently? This question may best be answered by studies examining the specific symptoms reported by subjects, differences in the abruptness with which each occurs (assessed via both subjective and objective measures), and subjects' ability to distinguish reliably between episodes of panic and anxiety. Furthermore, if panic is different from anxiety but identical to the basic emotion of fear, one might expect the behavioral component of fear (i.e., overwhelming urge to escape) to be present during panic but not during episodes of anxiety (Barlow et al., 1994).

Biological Evidence

Many biological theorists have hypothesized different mechanisms for panic and anxiety, although they have disagreed with respect to the specific brain areas involved. For example, Gorman et al. (1989) have proposed that acute panic attacks are based on abnormal noradrenergic activity in the locus ceruleus, whereas anticipatory anxiety is believed to involve areas of the limbic system, particularly the hippocampus. Gray (1982, 1987) also suggests that anxiety is based in the septo-hippocampal region, in what he calls the "behavioral inhibition system." However, according to Gray, panic attacks are based in the "fight-or-flight system," located primarily in the amygdala, hypothalamus, and midbrain. Gray suggests that these two systems interact, although he sees them as functionally distinct.

Differences in effects of specific drug classes have also been cited in support of the distinction between panic and anxiety (Klein & Gorman, 1987). Early studies suggested that antidepressants such as imipramine might be effective antipanic agents, but might have little effect on anticipatory anxiety (e.g., Klein, 1964; Klein & Fink, 1962). Although the effectiveness of imipramine for blocking panic has been replicated (Cross-National Collaborative Panic Study, Second Phase Investigators, 1992; Mavissakalian & Perel, 1989), imipramine has also been used successfully to treat generalized anxiety (Kahn et al., 1986), despite Klein's original findings. In addition, various benzodiazepines, including high-potency drugs such as alprazolam and low-potency drugs such as diazepam, have been shown to be effective treatments for panic (Ballenger et al., 1988; Dunner, Ishiki, Avery, Wilson, & Hyde, 1986; Pollack & Rosenbaum, 1988; Wilkinson, Balestrieri, Ruggeri, & Bellantuono, 1991), despite their traditional use for managing generalized anxiety. Overall, it seems that similar drugs can be useful for alleviating both anxiety and perhaps panic attacks.

Despite the overlap in drug effects on panic and anxiety, it may be premature to conclude that panic and generalized anxiety are neuroanatomically equivalent. First, medications typically act on more than one part of the brain. Furthermore, activity in one brain area can have significant effects on many other areas of the central nervous system. Therefore, even if medications are not specific to panic or generalized anxiety, the two phenomena may still be qualitatively different and neuroanatomically independent.

Furthermore, anxious apprehension appears to play a large role in the maintenance of PD and the occurrence of learned alarms. It is possible that some classes of drug help PD patients by blocking anxiety, whereas other drugs have a direct effect on panic. Illustrating the point that different drugs can act on different aspects of a disorder, Hoehn-Saric, McLeod, and Zimmerli (1988) found that alprazolam and imipramine were both effective at decreasing symptomatology in generalized anxiety disorder (GAD) patients. However, alprazolam was more effective at decreasing hyperarousal and somatic symptoms, whereas imipramine was more effective at improving dysphoria and negative thinking patterns.

More convincing evidence that panic and anxiety are biologically distinct comes from genetic and epidemiological research. If panic were simply a more severe form of general anxiety, one might expect PD and GAD to aggregate in the same families, but this seems not to be the case (Crowe, Noyes, Pauls, & Slymen, 1983; Harris, Noyes, Crowe, & Chaudhry, 1983; Noyes et al., 1986). Despite evidence that PD and GAD are each familial in nature, PD is no more common in first-degree relatives of GAD patients than in controls. Similarly, GAD is no more common in first-degree relatives of PD patients than in controls.

In addition, Torgersen (1983) studied twin data and concluded that genetic factors contribute to the familial nature of PD but not to that of GAD. However, this finding was not replicated by Kendler, Neale, Kessler, Heath, and Eaves (1992), who studied female twin pairs and found GAD to be a moderately familial disorder with a heritability of about .30.

Overall these data support the independence of PD and GAD (Weissman, 1990). However, it should be emphasized that the extent to which these disorders (i.e., PD, GAD) overlap with the constructs of panic and anxiety is unclear.

The Phenomenology of Panic and Anxiety

Borden and Turner (1989) examined the profiles of symptoms typically occurring in PD, GAD, and obsessive–compulsive patients, and obtained results supporting the assertion that panic and anxiety are distinct states. When overall levels of anxiety were controlled, a panic factor emerged that distinguished PD patients from the other two groups. Furthermore, correlations between specific panic symptoms and state–trait anxiety were generally low.

More recently, Zinbarg and Barlow (1992) factor analyzed scores from 23 subscales of measures completed by over 430 anxiety disorder patients and 32 normal controls. Panic and general anxiety were two of five primary factors that emerged (others included agoraphobia, social anxiety, and obsessions–compulsions) supporting the independence of panic and anxiety.

Also supporting the distinctiveness of panic and anxiety, Noyes et al. (1992) found a number of differences between GAD and PD patients, including different patterns of comorbidity, a different course for each disorder, different family histories, and different symptom profiles. Specifically, GAD patients reported more symptoms of central nervous system hyperarousal (e.g., trouble sleeping, restlessness, muscle tension), whereas PD patients reported more symptoms indicating autonomic hyperarousal (e.g., palpitations, shaking, breathlessness). Despite the differences in the frequency of symptoms reported, there was also much overlap in symptoms. This is not surprising, given the elevated anxiety typically reported by PD patients.

Clinical and research findings suggesting differences in the abruptness of panic and anxiety episodes have been reviewed by Barlow et al. (1994). For example, several studies have shown that measurable abrupt surges in heart rate occur during panic, and that these surges are distinguishable from heart rate patterns occurring during anticipatory anxiety (e.g., Freedman, Ianni, Ettedgui, & Puthezhath, 1985; Taylor et al., 1986).

Finally, patients often report a strong urge to escape during panic attacks, whereas such urges are typically not reported during episodes of anxiety. This clinical observation has yet to be systematically studied; however, to the extent that it is an accurate observation, this finding supports the notion that panic (but not anxiety) is a basic emotion with a clear behavioral component.

The Relationship between Panic and Fear

A few theorists have suggested that panic and fear are different phenomena. For example, in support of his suffocation alarm model of panic, Klein (1993) has argued that uncued panic and fear differ in that panic lacks the hypothalamic–pituitary–adrenal (HPA) activation found in normal fear, stress, and pain responses. He has also argued that panic and fear have different symptom profiles, with dyspnea being a prominent symptom of spontaneous panic but not of fear.

Despite Klein's assertions, several researchers have argued against the distinctiveness of panic and fear. In fact, reviews by Barlow (1988), Craske (1991), and Kathol, Noyes, and Lopez (1988) have all come to the conclusion that spontaneous panic and phobic fear are not physiologically distinct. Kathol et al. (1988) argued that HPA activation is typical of acute *physical* stress (e.g., the period immediately following surgery), but not of acute *psychological* stress (e.g., the period immediately preceding surgery, noise exposure). They concluded that HPA activation is similarly small in PD patients and normals experiencing external, psychological stress. Likewise, Barlow (1988) concluded that HPA activation is weak and inconsistent among both simple (specific) phobics exposed to fear cues (Nesse et al., 1985) and PD patients during panic provocation (Liebowitz et al., 1985; Woods, Charney, Goodman, & Heninger, 1987). Further-more, there is evidence that the slight HPA activation observed in some individuals is more closely related to the novelty of the situation than to the fear itself (Nesse et al., 1985). These conclusions are consistent with the view that panic and fear are similar processes.

With regard to Klein's assertion that spontaneous panic and fear have different symptom profiles, Craske (1991) reviewed a variety of data from retrospective interviews, self-monitoring diaries, and studies of experimen-tally induced fear; she concluded that PD patients and simple phobics report very similar symptom profiles, although PD patients tend to report more symptoms. This finding is not surprising in light of the fact that PD patients tend to report greater anxiety over sensations (Taylor, Koch, & McNally, 1992), and therefore may be more vigilant for these sensations.

Furthermore, despite Klein's (1993) assertion that dyspnea occurs in panic but not fear, studies of mixed simple phobics (Craske, Burton, & Barlow, 1989) and injection phobics (Öst, 1989) both found dyspnea to be a relatively common symptom among individuals with specific fears. Similarly, Rapee, Sanderson, McCauley, and Di Nardo (1992) found that the frequency of dyspnea was not significantly greater during unexpected panic attacks in PD patients (63.3%) than during fear reactions reported by simple phobics, social phobics, and patients with obsessive–compulsive disorder (42.2%).

Still, some other theorists such as Gray (1991) have argued that pan-ic and fear are fundamentally different states. According to Gray (1991), fear is a subtype of anxiety and originates in the behavioral inhibition sys-tem, unlike panic, which is based in the fight-or-flight system. However, as Gray notes, much of the disagreement between his view and that of Barlow (1991) may be in the way terms such as "fear," "anxiety," and "panic" are defined, and not in the nature of the states to which the terms refer. Gray's (1991) critique highlights the need for a common vocabu-lary among anxiety and emotion researchers.

In summary, the data suggest that uncued panic attacks and phobic fear, as defined by Barlow (1988), differ only in their specific triggering cues (internal cues in the case of PD; external cues in the case of phobic disorders) and not in their qualitative natures.

Biological Vulnerabilities

Several areas of research have been used to support the assertion that bio-logical factors are relevant to the onset and maintenance of PD. These include studies demonstrating the efficacy of biological treatments for PD; brain imaging studies showing distinct patterns of cerebral blood flow in PD patients relative to nonpanickers; and studies showing that PD patients are more likely than nonpanickers to panic in response to biological challenges (e.g., sodium lactate infusion, yohimbine, caffeine, hyperventilation, carbon dioxide [CO_2]. Although these studies clearly indicate that biological processes are involved in panic and anxiety, several authors have argued convincingly that they do not necessarily support a unique biological etiology for panic, and that these findings can be explained equally well by psychological models of panic (Antony, Brown, & Barlow, 1992; Clark, 1993; Margraf, Ehlers, & Roth, 1986).

Perhaps the most compelling data supporting Barlow's assertions about the existence of a biological vulnerability to experiencing panic have come from the previously reviewed genetics and family studies. These studies suggest that PD runs in families and has a genetic component (Weissman, 1990), although additional twin studies and studies of genetic linkage are needed before such a conclusion can be made confidently (Judd, Burrows, & Hay, 1987). Interestingly, studies have also shown that panic runs in families of nonclinical panickers (Norton, Cox, & Malan, 1992), although these studies are limited by subjects' possible recall biases.

The Role of Stress in the Onset of Panic Disorder

Consistent with Barlow's model, several studies have found that PD patients with agoraphobia report a greater number of stressful life events prior to the onset of their disorder than do nonanxious controls for a comparable period (Faravelli & Pallanti, 1989; Roy-Byrne, Geraci, & Uhde, 1986). Studies comparing PD patients to patients with other anxiety disorders have found that stressful life events tend to precede the onset of these other disorders as well. For example, Rapee, Litwin, and Barlow (1990) showed that although there were no group differences in the number of stressful events, PD patients and those with other anxiety disorders reported a greater *negative impact* of these events in the period preceding the disorder onset relative to nonanxious controls. The lack of differences between PD patients and those with other anxiety disorders suggests that stress is not a specific cause of PD, but rather a possible trigger for a variety of problems in individuals with specific vulnerabilities. Consistent with this view, de Loof, Zandbergen, Lousberg, Pols, and Griez (1989) found few differences in the frequency of stressful life events preceding the onset of PD and obsessive–compulsive disorder.

One criticism of the hypothesis about stressful life events has been that patients with PD and other forms of psychopathology may be biased toward recalling negative life events (e.g., Rapee et al., 1990). Pollard, Pollard, and Corn (1989) addressed this criticism by using panic patients as their own controls in a within-subject design. In that study, life events were assessed by retrospective self-report for two times in the course of the disorder: (1) the period preceding the first panic attack, and (2) a period 4 years after the initial panic. Panic patients were more likely to report stressful life events immediately preceding the first panic than during the period 4 years later. Of course, it is possible that panic patients are more negatively biased in their recall of events occurring before the first panic. To address this possibility adequately, patients would need to be studied at the time of the first panic attack (e.g., when they report to emergency rooms) and perhaps compared to matched surgical controls. Such a study has yet to be completed.

Psychological Vulnerabilities

According to Barlow (1988), people who are susceptible to experiencing false alarms may develop anxious apprehension and possibly PD if they have the necessary psychological vulnerabilities, which include a sense that events in general and emotions in particular are uncontrollable and unpredictable. One situation in which perceived control and predictability have been examined is that of panic induced in the laboratory. The fact that PD patients tend to panic in response to CO_2 inhalation (and other biological challenges) more often than other groups (e.g., Rapee, Brown, Antony, & Barlow, 1992) has been used as evidence to support noradrenergic or central CO_2 sensitivity models of panic (e.g., Gorman et al., 1989). However, recent data suggest that variables such as perceived control, predictability, and other cognitive factors (e.g., Clark, 1993) may mediate the occurrence of panic during these "biological" challenges.

Sanderson, Rapee, and Barlow (1989) examined the effects of breathing CO_2-enriched air in PD patients who either believed or did not believe they had control over the flow of CO_2. Patients with perceived control reported fewer panic attacks, lower levels of anxiety, and fewer panic symptoms than did subjects who believed they had no control. In a related study, Carter, Hollon, Carson, and Shelton (1995) demonstrated that the presence of a "safe person" (e.g., a spouse) significantly decreased PD patients' response to CO_2 inhalation. Similarly, Telch and Harrington (1992) found that among patients high in anxiety sensitivity (i.e., anxiety over panic sensations), those who expected to feel relaxed were more likely to panic during CO_2 inhalation than those who expected to feel aroused. The one study that failed to show the expected effects of predictability and controllability on panic symptoms during CO_2 inhalation (Van den Bergh, Vandendriessche, De Broeck, & Van de Woestijne, 1993) compared normal subjects high and low on trait anxiety. These subjects were not screened for the presence of PD or for the presence of related symptomatology (e.g., elevated anxiety sensitivity), and therefore would not be expected to respond to CO_2 inhalation in the same way as typical panic patients. Overall, these studies suggest that among panic patients, perception of control and ability to predict the occurrence of panic can have a significant effect on the occurrence of panic during CO_2 inhalation, perhaps because of the mediating role of anxiety.

Several other studies have addressed the roles of perceived control and expectancy in PD patients. Cloitre, Heimberg, Liebowitz, and Gitow (1992) measured locus of control (Levenson, 1973) in PD patients, social phobics, and normals, and found that both clinical groups had a lower sense of internal control than normals. Furthermore, PD patients tended to view events as occurring in a random and uncontrollable fashion, whereas social phobics tended to perceive events as controlled by powerful others.

Lopatka (1989) found that the predictability of exposure to a feared stimulus determined subsequent avoidance of the stimulus. Specifically, snake phobics who were exposed to a snake at unexpected times were subsequently more likely to avoid the snake than those who were exposed an equal number of times at expected intervals. Similarly, Arntz, Van Eck, and De Jong (1991) demonstrated that subjects exposed to unpredictable intensities of pain were subsequently less tolerant of pain than subjects initially exposed to predictable pain levels. To the extent that avoidance behavior in these studies is mediated by anxiety over possible danger, these findings support Barlow's (1988) view regarding the relationship between predictability and the development of anxious apprehension.

Nonclinical Panic

Barlow's (1988) model leads to very specific predictions regarding the nature of nonclinical panic and its relationship to PD. As Barlow sees it, there should exist a group of people who share the biological vulnerability to experiencing false alarms in response to stress, but who do not have the prerequisite psychological vulnerabilities to developing anxious apprehension and PD. That is, they do not experience anxious apprehension over the occurrence of panic; they do not have a decreased sense of the controllability and predictability of events; and they do not experience panic as frequently, because of the relative absence of learned alarms (cued, in part, by symptoms of anxious apprehension).

Data from several researchers suggest that panic attacks occur frequently in the general population. Although some studies (e.g., Norton et al., 1986) have reported past-year prevalence rates of nearly 35% in nonclinical populations, other investigators have criticized these findings on the grounds that the self-report measure used by Norton et al. (1986)

and others to measure panic may lead subjects to confuse panic with generalized anxiety. Using a modified measure, and specifying for the subjects the differences between panic and general anxiety, Brown and Cash (1990) found a past-year panic prevalence of 25.7%. In a follow-up study, using a structured interview assessment of nonclinical panic, Brown and Deagle (1992) obtained similar results (a past-year panic prevalence of 29.2%). However, only 2.3% of Brown and Deagle's subjects reported an uncued panic attack in the past year. Although panic attacks were common, the frequency of uncued panic was low, and not much greater than the prevalence of PD in this population (1.2%).

Other investigators have confirmed the relatively low rate of uncued panic in the population. Telch, Lucas, and Nelson (1989) reported lifetime uncued panic prevalence rates of approximately 12%. Although this number is higher than estimates by Brown and Deagle (1992), the difference may be attributable to the method of data collection, since Telch et al. used a self-report measure of panic. In the study by Telch et al., 2.36% were panicking frequently enough to meet DSM-III-R criteria for PD. Other epidemiological studies using clinical interviews to look at lifetime PD prevalence in random community samples have found rates consistent with these data (Joyce, Bushnell, Oakley-Browne, Wells, & Hornblow, 1989) or slightly lower (Robins et al., 1984). In any case, it seems clear that uncued panic does occur in people without PD. Furthermore, as is the case among PD patients, panic seems to run in families among nonclinical panickers (Norton et al., 1986).

Several studies have examined the specific factors that distinguish between clinical and nonclinical panickers. Telch et al. (1989) showed in a study of college students that anxiety sensitivity was higher among those meeting criteria for PD than among nonclinical panickers and nonpanickers, who did not differ. Furthermore, PD subjects specifically reported greater anxious apprehension than nonclinical subjects over the future occurrence of panic.

In a related study, Cox, Endler, and Swinson (1991) compared clinical and nonclinical panickers on a variety of dimensions, and confirmed a variety of the predictions following from Barlow's (1988) model. First, panic attacks were similar among the two groups (i.e, symptom profiles, rapid onset, etc.). Furthermore, there were no differences in family history of panic, consistent with Barlow's view that there is a common biological predisposition to false alarms in PD patients and nonclinical panickers. Clinical panickers reported more frequent attacks, more agoraphobic avoidance, higher depression, higher anxiety sensitivity, and a higher likelihood of future unpredictable panics. Interestingly, nonclinical panickers were more likely than clinical panickers to report that their attacks were associated with stress. (Cox et al., 1991; Cox, Endler, Swinson, & Norton, 1992). This supports Barlow's view that false alarms occur in the context of stress, whereas learned alarms are less likely to be associated with stress. Finally, Cox et al. (1992) found that nonclinical panickers were more likely to use adaptive strategies to cope with panic (e.g, seeking a friend, relaxation) than were PD patients, who tended to use avoidance and self-medication as their primary coping strategies.

Overall, these findings support Barlow's view that what separates clinical and nonclinical panickers is their anxiety over experiencing false alarms. Nevertheless, there is still a need for systematic replication of these data before any firm conclusions can be made.

CONCLUDING REMARKS

This chapter has provided a summary of Barlow's (1988) model of PD and of some of the relevant research from which the model was derived. Specifically, the literature supports the conclusion that PD develops within a context of multiple etiological factors, including biological variables, learning, cognitive mechanisms, and stress.

Unfortunately, the space restrictions inherent in the present format do not allow for a thorough discussion of all the research relevant to the model, although areas that could not be reviewed herein have been discussed elsewhere. For example, Barlow (1988) has reviewed the research related to his view of anxious apprehension and the role of self-focused attention in anxiety over the experience of panic. In addition, evidence arguing for and against the concept of basic emotions has been reviewed recently by several authors (e.g., Eckman, 1992; Izard, 1992; Oatley & Johnson-Laird, 1987; Ortony & Turner, 1990).

Barlow's model of panic has been criticized by several authors on the grounds that it lacks clarity and precision at certain points. Maser and Cuthbert (1991) believe that Barlow (1991) has been vague in his descriptions of states such as fear, panic, anxiety, and anxious apprehension. We have therefore tried to explain more fully in this chapter how these concepts are similar and different.

Other authors, such as Mineka, Luten, and Pury (1991), have raised questions about the relationship between perceived control and emotional disorders. Specifically, they have argued that the model is unclear about whether the lack of perceived control hypothesized to predispose one to develop PD refers to control over emotions, life events, or other factors. This too has been clarified in this chapter, although much more research needs to be done before this aspect of the model can be supported or refuted with confidence.

Although PD has been a very popular topic of study among anxiety researchers in recent years, this review highlights the need for much more research to tease out exactly how the various factors contributing to the onset of panic and PD interact with one another. Studies examining biological and cognitive correlates of panic in isolation do little to provide insight into the causes of panic and PD.

There is a great need for longitudinal studies of people at risk for developing PD, in order to prospectively examine those factors that lead some people to panic and those that protect others from developing PD. In addition, more studies examining the nature of certain specific types of panic (e.g., nonclinical panic, nonfearful panic, nocturnal panic) may help to answer certain questions about panic among PD patients. These special cases also have implications for certain models of panic, particularly those relying on conscious appraisal to explain panic attacks.

REFERENCES

American Psychiatric Association. (1980). *Diagnostic and statistical manual of mental disorders* (3rd ed.). Washington, DC: Author.

American Psychiatric Association. (1987). *Diagnostic and statistical manual of mental disorders* (3rd ed., rev.). Washington, DC: Author.

American Psychiatric Association. (1994). *Diagnostic and statistical manual of mental disorders* (4th ed.). Washington, DC: Author.

Antony, M. M., Brown, T. A., & Barlow, D. H. (1992). Current perspectives on panic and panic disorder. *Current Directions in Psychological Science, 1,* 79–82.

Arntz, A., Van Eck, M., & De Jong, P. (1991). Avoidance of pain of unpredictable intensity. *Behaviour Research and Therapy, 29,* 197–201.

Ballenger, J. C., Burrows, G. R., DuPont, R. L., Lesser, I. M., Noyes, R., Pecknold, J. C., Rifkin, A., & Swinson, R. P. (1988). Alprazolam in panic disorder and agoraphobia: Results from a multicenter trial. 1. Efficacy in short term treatment. *Archives of General Psychiatry, 45,* 413–422.

Barlow, D. H. (1988). *Anxiety and its disorders: The nature and treatment of anxiety and panic.* New York: Guilford Press.

Barlow, D. H. (1991). Disorders of emotion. *Psychological Inquiry, 2,* 58–71.

Barlow, D. H., Brown, T. A., & Craske, M. G. (1994). Definitions of panic attacks and panic disorder in DSM-IV: Implications for research. *Journal of Abnormal Psychology, 103,* 553–564.

Beck, A. T., & Emery, G., with Greenberg, R. L. (1985). *Anxiety disorders and phobias: A cognitive perspective.* New York: Basic Books.

Borden, J. W., & Turner, S. M. (1989). Is panic a unique emotional experience? *Behaviour Research and Therapy, 27,* 263–268.

Bower, G. H. (1981). Mood and memory. *American Psychologist, 36,* 129–148.

Brown, T. A., & Cash, T. F. (1990). The phenomenon of nonclinical panic: Parameters of panic, fear, and avoidance. *Journal of Anxiety Disorders, 4,* 15–29.

Brown, T. A., & Deagle, E. A. (1992). Structured interview assessment of non-clinical panic. *Behavior Therapy, 23,* 75–85.

Carter, M. M., Hollon, S. D., Carson, R., & Shelton, R. C. (1995). Effects of a safe person on induced distress following a biological challenge in panic disorder with agoraphobia. *Journal of Abnormal Psychology, 104,* 156–163.

Clark, D. M. (1986). A cognitive approach to panic. *Behaviour Research and Therapy, 24,* 461–470.

Clark, D. M. (1988). A cognitive model of panic attacks. In S. Rachman & J. D. Maser (Eds.), *Panic: Psychological perspectives.* Hillsdale, NJ: Erlbaum.

Clark, D. M. (1993). Cognitive mediation of panic attacks induced by biological challenge tests. *Advances in Behaviour Research and Therapy, 15,* 75–84.

Cloitre, M., Heimberg, R. G., Liebowitz, M. R., & Gitow, A. (1992). Perceptions of control in panic disorder and social phobia. *Cognitive Therapy and Research, 16,* 569–577.

Cox, B. J., Endler, N. S., & Swinson, R. P. (1991). Clinical and nonclinical panic attacks: An empirical test of a panic–anxiety continuum. *Journal of Anxiety Disorders, 5,* 21–34.

Cox, B. J., Endler, N. S., Swinson, R. P., & Norton, G. R. (1992). Situations and specific coping strategies associated with clinical and nonclinical panic attacks. *Behaviour Research and Therapy, 30,* 67–69.

Craske, M. G. (1991). Phobic fear and panic attacks: The same emotional states triggered by different cues? *Clinical Psychology Review, 11,* 599–620.

Craske, M. G., Burton, T., & Barlow, D. H. (1989). *Simple phobics presenting for treatment: What are their fears?* Unpublished manuscript.

Cross-National Collaborative Panic Study, Second Phase Investigators. (1992). Drug treatment of panic disorder: Comparative efficacy of alprazolam, imipramine, and placebo. *British Journal of Psychiatry, 160,* 191–202.

Crowe, R. R., Noyes, R., Pauls, D. S., & Slymen, D. J. (1983). A family study of panic disorder. *Archives of General Psychiatry, 40,* 1065–1069.

de Loof, C., Zandbergen, J., Lousberg, H., Pols, H., & Griez, E. (1989). The role of life events in the onset of panic disorder. *Behaviour Research and Therapy, 27,* 461–463.

Dobson, K. S. (1985). The relationship between anxiety and depression. *Clinical Psychology Review, 5,* 307–324.

Dunner, D. L., Ishiki, D., Avery, D. H., Wilson, L. G., & Hyde, T. S. (1986). Effect of alprazolam and diazepam on anxiety and panic attacks: A controlled study. *Journal of Clinical Psychiatry, 47,* 458–460.

Eckman, P. (1992). Are there basic emotions? *Psychological Review, 99,* 550–553.

Ehlers, A., & Margraf, J. (1989). The psychophysiological model of panic attacks. In P. M. G. Emmelkamp, W. T. A. M. Everaerd, F. W. Kraaimaat, & M. J. M. van Son (Eds.) *Fresh perspectives on anxiety disorders.* Amsterdam: Swets & Zeitlinger.

Faravelli, C., & Pallanti, S. (1989). Recent life events and panic disorder. *American Journal of Psychiatry, 146,* 622–626.

Freedman, R. R., Ianni, P., Ettedgui, E., & Puthezhath, N. (1985). Ambulatory monitoring of panic disorder. *Archives of General Psychiatry, 42,* 244–250.

Goldstein, A. J., & Chambless, D. L. (1978). A reanalysis of agoraphobia. *Behavior Therapy, 9,* 47–59.

Gorman, J. M., Liebowitz, M. R., Fyer, A. J., & Stein, J. (1989). A neuroanatomical hypothesis for panic disorder. *American Journal of Psychiatry, 146,* 148–161.

Gotlib, I. H., & Cane, D. B. (1989). Self-report assessment of depression and anxiety. In P. C. Kendall & D. Watson (Eds.), *Anxiety and Depression: Distinctive and overlapping features* (pp. 131–169). New York: Academic.

Gray, J. A. (1982). *The neuropsychology of anxiety.* New York: Oxford University Press.

Gray, J. A. (1987). *The psychology of fear and stress.* New York: Cambridge University Press.

Gray, J. A. (1991). Fear, panic, and anxiety: What's in a name? *Psychological Inquiry, 2,* 77–78.

Harris, E. L., Noyes, R., Crowe, R. R., & Chaudhry, D. R. (1983). A family study of agoraphobia. *Archives of General Psychiatry, 40,* 1061–1064.

Hoehn-Saric, R., McLeod, D. R., & Zimmerli, W. D. (1988). Differential effects of alprazolam and imipramine in generalized anxiety disorder: Somatic versus psychic symptoms. *Journal of Clinical Psychiatry, 49,* 293–301.

Izard, C. E. (Ed.). (1977). *Human emotions.* New York: Plenum Press.

Izard, C. E. (1992). Basic emotions, relations among emotions, and emotion–cognition relations. *Psychological Review, 99,* 561–565.

Joyce, P. R., Bushnell, J. A., Oakley-Browne, M. A., Wells, J. E., & Hornblow, A. R. (1989). The epidemiology of panic symptomatology and agoraphobic avoidance. *Comprehensive Psychiatry, 30,* 303–312.

Judd, F. K., Burrows, G. D., & Hay, D. A. (1987). Panic disorder: Evidence for genetic vulnerability. *Australian and New Zealand Journal of Psychiatry, 21,* 197–208.

Kahn, R. J., McNair, D. M., Lipman, R. S., Covi, L., Rickels, K., Downing, R., Fisher, S., & Frankenthaler, L. M. (1986). Imipramine and chlordiazepoxide in depressive and anxiety disorders: II. Efficacy in anxious outpatients. *Archives of General Psychiatry, 43,* 79–85.

Kathol, R. G., Noyes, R., & Lopez, A. (1988). Similarities in hypothalamic–pituitary–adrenal axis activity between patients with panic disorder and those experiencing external stress. *Psychiatric Clinics of North America, 11,* 335–348.

Kendler, K. S., Neale, M. C., Kessler, R. C., Heath, A. C., & Eaves, L. J. (1992). Generalized anxiety disorder in women: A population-based twin study. *Archives of General Psychiatry, 49,* 267–272.

Klein, D. F. (1964). Delineation of two drug responsive anxiety syndromes. *Psychopharmacologia, 5,* 397–408.

Klein, D. F. (1981). Anxiety reconceptualized. In D. F. Klein & J. Rabkin (Eds.), *Anxiety: New research and changing concepts.* New York: Raven Press.

Klein, D. F. (1993). False suffocation alarms, spontaneous panics, and related conditions. *Archives of General Psychiatry, 50,* 306–317.

Klein, D. F., & Fink, M. (1962). Psychiatric reaction patterns to imipramine. *American Journal of Psychiatry, 119,* 432–438.

Klein, D. F., & Gorman, J. M. (1987). A model of panic and agoraphobic development. *Acta Psychiatrica Scandinavica, 76,* 87–95.

Lang, P. J. (1985). The cognitive psychophysiology of emotion: fear and anxiety. In A. H. Tuma & J. D. Maser (Eds.), *Anxiety and the anxiety disorders.* Hillsdale, NJ: Erlbaum.

Lang, P. J. (1988). Fear, anxiety, and panic: Context, cognition, and visceral arousal. In S. Rachman & J. D. Maser (Eds.), *Panic: Psychological perspectives.* Hillsdale, NJ: Erlbaum.

Levenson, H. (1973). Multidimensional locus of control in psychiatric patients. *Journal of Consulting and Clinical Psychology, 41,* 397–401.

Ley, R. (1987). Panic disorder: A hyperventilation interpretation. In L. Michelson & L. M. Ascher (Eds.), *Anxiety and stress disorders: Cognitive-behavioral assessment and treatment.* New York: Guilford Press.

Liebowitz, M. R., Gorman, J. M., Fyer, A. J., Levitt, M., Dillon, D., Levy, P., Appleby, I. L., Anderson, S., Palij, M., Davies, S. O., & Klein, D. F. (1985). Lactate provocation of panic attacks: II. Biochemical and physiological findings. *Archives of General Psychiatry, 42,* 709–719.

Lopatka, C. L. (1989). *The role of unexpected events in avoidance.* Unpublished manuscript.

Margraf, J., Ehlers, A., & Roth, W. T. (1986). Biological models of panic disorder and agoraphobia: A review. *Behaviour Research and Therapy, 24,* 553–567.

Margraf, J., Taylor, C. B., Ehlers, A., Roth, W. T., & Agras, W. S. (1987). Panic attacks in the natural environment. *Journal of Nervous and Mental Disease, 175,* 558–165.

Marks, I. M. (1987). *Fears, phobias, and rituals.* New York: Oxford University Press.

Maser, J. D., & Cuthbert, B. N. (1991). Emotions, their disorders, and precision in theory construction. *Psychological Inquiry, 2,* 58–71.

Mavissakalian, M. R., & Perel, J. M. (1989). Imipramine dose–response relationship in panic disorder with agoraphobia. *Archives of General Psychiatry, 46,* 127–131.

Mineka, S., Luten, A. G., & Pury, C. L. (1991). Is lack of control over emotions, or stressful life events, more important in disorders of emotion? *Psychological Inquiry, 2,* 83–86.

Nesse, R. M. (1987). An evolutionary perspective on panic disorder and agoraphobia. *Ethology and Sociobiology, 8,* 73S–83S.

Nesse, R. M., Curtis, G. C., Thyer, B. A., McCann, D. S., Huber-Smith, M. J., & Knopf, R. F. (1985). Endocrine and cardiovascular responses during phobic anxiety. *Psychosomatic Medicine, 47,* 320–332.

Norton, G. R., Cox, B. J., & Malan, J. (1992). Nonclincal panickers: A critical review. *Clinical Psychology Review, 12,* 121–131.

Norton, G. R., Dorward, J., & Cox, B. J. (1986). Factors associated with panic attacks in nonclinical subjects. *Behavior Therapy, 17,* 239–252.

Noyes, R., Crowe, R. R., Harris, E. L., Hamra, B. J., McChesney, C. M., & Chaudhry, D. R. (1986). Relationship between panic disorder and agoraphobia. *Archives of General Psychiatry, 43,* 227–232.

Noyes, R., Woodman, C., Garvey, M. J., Cook, B. L., Suelzer, M., Clancy, J., & Anderson, D. J. (1992). Generalized anxiety disorder vs. panic disorder: Distinguishing characteristics and patterns of comorbidity. *Journal of Nervous and Mental Disease, 180,* 369–379.

Nutt, D. J. (1989). Altered central alpha$_2$-adrenoceptor sensitivity in panic disorder. *Archives of General Psychiatry, 46,* 165–169.

Nutt, D., & Lawson, C. (1992). Panic attacks: A neurochemical overview of models and mechanisms. *British Journal of Psychiatry, 160,* 165–178.

Oatley, K., & Johnson-Laird, P. N. (1987). Towards a cognitive theory of emotions. *Cognition and Emotion, 1,* 29–50.

Ortony, A., & Turner, T. J. (1990). What's basic about basic emotions? *Psychological Review, 97,* 315–331.

Öst, L.-G. (1989). [Frequency of panic symptoms among injection phobics]. Unpublished raw data.

Pollack, M. H., & Rosenbaum, J. F. (1988). Benzodiazepines in panic-related disorders. *Journal of Anxiety Disorders, 2,* 95–107.

Pollard, A. C., Pollard, H. J., & Corn, K. J. (1989). Panic onset and major events in the lives of agoraphobics: A test of contiguity. *Journal of Abnormal Psychology, 98,* 318–321.

Rapee, R. M. (1993). Psychological factors in panic disorder. *Advances in Behaviour Research and Therapy, 15,* 85–102.

Rapee, R. M., Brown, T. A., Antony, M. M., & Barlow, D. H. (1992). Response to hyperventilation and inhalation of 5.5% carbon dioxide-enriched air across the DSM-III-R anxiety disorders. *Journal of Abnormal Psychology, 101,* 538–552.

Rapee, R. M., Litwin, E. M., & Barlow, D. H. (1990). Impact of life events on subjects with panic disorder and on comparison subjects. *American Journal of Psychiatry, 147,* 640–644.

Rapee, R. M., Sanderson, W. C., McCauley, P. A., & Di Nardo, P. A. (1992). Differences in reported symptom profile between panic disorder and other DSM-III-R anxiety disorders. *Behaviour Research and Therapy, 30,* 45–52.

Rescorla, R. A. (1988). Pavlovian conditioning: It's not what you think it is. *American Psychologist, 43,* 151–160.

Robins, L. N., Helzer, J. E., Weissman, M. M., Orvaschel, H., Gruenberg, E., Burke, J. D., & Regier, D. A. (1984). Lifetime prevalence of specific psychiatric disorders in three sites. *Archives of General Psychiatry, 41,* 949–958.

Roy-Byrne, P. B., Geraci, M., & Uhde, T. W. (1986). Life events and the onset of panic disorder. *American Journal of Psychiatry, 143,* 1424–1427.

Sanderson, W. C., Rapee, R. M., & Barlow, D. H. (1989). The influence of an illusion of control on panic attacks induced via inhalation of 5.5% carbon dioxide-enriched air. *Archives of General Psychiatry, 46,* 157–162.

Shear, M. K., Cooper, A. M., Klerman, G. L., Busch, F. N., & Shapiro, T. (1993). A psychodynamic model of panic disorder. *American Journal of Psychiatry, 150,* 859–866.

Taylor, C. B., Sheikh, J., Agras, W. S., Roth, W. T., Margraf, J., Ehlers, A., Maddock, R. J., & Gossard, D. (1986). Self-report of panic attacks: Agreement with heart rate changes. *American Journal of Psychiatry, 143,* 478–482.

Taylor, S., Koch, W. J., & McNally, R. J. (1992). How does anxiety sensitivity vary across the anxiety disorders? *Journal of Anxiety Disorders, 6,* 249–259.

Teasdale, J. D. (1993). Emotion and two kinds of meaning: Cognitive therapy and applied cognitive science. *Behaviour Research and Therapy, 31,* 339–354.

Telch, M. J., & Harrington, P. J. (1992, November). *Anxiety sensitivity and expectedness of arousal in mediating affective response to 35† carbon dioxide inhalation.* Paper presented at the meeting of the Association for Advancement of Behavior Therapy, Boston.

Telch, M. J., Lucas, J. A., & Nelson, P. (1989). Nonclinical panic in college students: An investigation of prevalence and symptomatology. *Journal of Abnormal Psychology, 98,* 300–306.

Torgersen, S. (1983). Genetic factors in anxiety disorders. *Archives of General Psychiatry, 40,* 1085–1089.

Van den Bergh, O., Vandendriessche, F., De Broeck, K., & Van de Woestijne, K. P. (1993). Predictability and perceived control during 5.5% CO_2-enriched air inhalation in high and low anxious subjects. *Journal of Anxiety Disorders, 7,* 61–73.

Watts, F. N. (1992). Applications of current cognitive theories of the emotions to the conceptualization of emotional disorders. *British Journal of Clinical Psychology, 31,* 153–167.

Weissman, M. M. (1990). Panic and generalized anxiety: Are they separate disorders? *Journal of Psychiatric Research, 24*(Suppl. 2), 157–162.

Wilkinson, G., Balestrieri, M., Ruggeri, M., & Bellantuono, C. (1991). Meta-analysis of double-blind placebo-controlled trials of antidepressants and benzodiazepines for patients with panic disorders. *Psychological Medicine, 21,* 991–998.

Wolpe, J., & Rowan, V. C. (1988). Panic disorder: A product of classical conditioning. *Behaviour Research and Therapy, 26,* 441–450.

Woods, S. W., Charney, D. S., Goodman, W. K., & Heninger, G. R. (1987). Carbon dioxide-induced anxiety: Behavioral, physiologic, and biochemical effects of 5% CO_2 in panic disorder patients and 5 and 7.5% CO_2 in healthy subjects. *Archives of General Psychiatry, 44,* 365–375.

Zajonc, R. B. (1980). Feeling and thinking: Preferences need no inferences. *American Psychologist, 35,* 151–175.

Zajonc, R. B. (1984). On the primacy of affect. *American Psychologist, 39,* 117–123.

Zinbarg, R. E., & Barlow, D. H. (1991). Mixed anxiety–depression: A new diagnostic category. In R. M. Rapee & D. H. Barlow (Eds.), *Chronic anxiety: Generalized anxiety disorder and mixed anxiety–depression.* New York: Guilford Press.

Zinbarg, R. E., & Barlow, D. H. (1992, November). *The construct validity of the DSM-III-R anxiety disorders: Empirical evidence.* Paper presented at the meeting of the Association for Advancement of Behavior Therapy, Boston.

4

Information-Processing
Views of Panic Disorder

Ronald M. Rapee

THE 1980s WITNESSED a tremendous surge of interest in research into the understanding and treatment of anxiety-related phenomena and the anxiety disorders; foremost among these were panic attacks and panic disorder, respectively. Over the past few years, a large number of models and theories have been presented to account for these conditions. A number of similarities among many of the theories are apparent, allowing them to be placed broadly into three general groups: biological/biochemical theories, emotion theory perspectives, and information-processing (cognitive) perspectives. Although each of these perspectives acknowledges and agrees upon certain basic features of panic attacks and panic disorder, there are a number of fundamental differences in the way each type of theory views these phenomena. In this chapter, I present the information-processing perspective and describe evidence in favor of this view, with particular emphasis on evidence that is difficult to explain from the alternative viewpoints.

THE INFORMATION-PROCESSING THEORY

Several authors have presented similar cognitive accounts of panic disorder (Clark, 1986; McNally, 1990; Margraf & Ehlers, 1989; Rapee, 1993). According to most cognitive views, individuals with panic disorder characteristically fear a particular set of physiological sensations. This characteristic is akin to, say, the fear reported by individuals with social phobia in response to social/evaluative situations, or by individuals with a specific phobia of small animals in response to a spider. In other words, when a socially phobic individual faces an audience, a fear reaction is generally triggered by this situation. In a similar way, when an individual with panic disorder perceives a certain physiological sensation (e.g., breathlessness), a fear reaction is typically triggered by this perceived cue.

The physiological sensations feared by individuals with panic disorder can be produced in a variety of ways, including exercise, surges of hormones such as adrenalin, hyperventilating, or (commonly) paying excessive attention to normal bodily changes. The idea of perception is important to the information-processing view. The simple existence of a particular sensation is not sufficient to trigger panic; rather, the sensation must be perceived by the individual. Thus, in some cases dramatic physiological change may not trigger panic in persons with panic disorder, because they may not notice the sensations (e.g., if their attention is taken up with a different task). On the other hand, individual with panic disorder often react to very subtle sensations that would not be noticed by most people. Importantly, the cognitive view sees these physiological sensations as simply triggers for the "panic" (fear reaction) experienced by the individuals *in response to* the sensations. Simply put, then, the cognitive view suggests that an unexpected (spontaneous) panic attack is no more than an anxiety/fear reaction to certain bodily symptoms. The confusing issue in panic disorder is that the feared stimuli (bodily symptoms) are also, in turn, part of the subsequent fear reaction. As a result, the panic attack *appears* to be spontaneous or unexpected, because the triggering stimulus is the same as the subsequent reaction; this makes it difficult for sufferers to identify the cause-and-effect sequence (Clark, 1986).

An important component of the cognitive view of panic disorder is the hypothesis that these individuals fear their own bodily sensations because they associate these sensations with immediately impending dramatic outcomes (e.g., heart attack, stroke, syncope, etc.). Thus it is predicted that individuals with panic disorder are particularly preoccupied and concerned with physical threats such as death, and that physical symptoms perceived by most people as innocuous are seen by these individuals as signals of impending physical catastrophe.

It is important to point out that modern cognitive views do not necessitate the conscious accessing of these associative processes (Rapee, 1993). Rather, it is likely that individuals engage in much of this attribution and association between perception of the stimulus and experience of the emotional reaction at an automatic, nonconscious level. Thus, it is not a necessary feature of the information-processing view that sufferers must be able to verbalize the causal chain of events. In fact, people often do not have conscious access to their motivations and influences (Wilson & Nisbett, 1978), although there are certainly situations in which they do.

Thus, in summary, according to the information-processing view, an unexpected panic attack occurs when an individual perceives a particular physiological sensation and associates this sensation with an immediately impending physical disaster. Individuals with panic disorder are likely to show a number of characteristics that increase the likelihood of their experiencing unexpected panic attacks. For example, they typically pay a lot of attention to monitoring their bodies; they are often highly aroused; and they are likely to be highly preoccupied with physical catastrophes. A diagrammatic representation of the information-processing model of panic disorder is presented in Figure 4.1.

CONTRAST WITH OTHER THEORIES

One of the major "battles" in the panic disorder literature has been between the proponents of cognitive or psychological theories and the proponents of biological or biochemical theories. There have been a number of biochemical theories of panic disorder, which, like the cognitive theories, have a few specific differences but a number of broad similarities

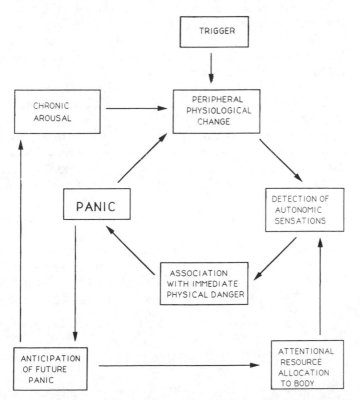

FIGURE 4.1. A model of the maintenance of panic disorder. From Rapee (1993, p. 98).

(Carr & Sheehan, 1984; Charney & Heninger, 1986; Gorman, Liebowitz, Fyer, & Stein, 1989; Klein, 1993; Pitts, 1969).

It must be stated at the outset that although it is common practice to assume that psychological and biological theories of psychopathology are in strict opposition to each other, this is not necessarily the case. If one takes a reductionist perspective, then all psychological phenomena are ultimately reducible to biochemical processes. This argument is paralleled in the areas of physics and chemistry. A water molecule can be described in terms of its chemical properties (the binding of hydrogen and oxygen) or its physical properties (the electronic balance between atomic particles). One would not say that either of these descriptions is "wrong" or that they oppose each other in any way—simply that they are different levels of explanation. Similarly, the biochemical and psychological perspectives on psychopathology can be seen as simply different levels of explanation. There are times when either perspective may have greater heuristic value in a particular situation. Thus, the view taken here is that biochemical and cognitive theories of panic disorder are not necessarily in fundamental disagreement. That is, to point to the importance of noradrenalin in producing panic attacks is not necessarily incompatible with the importance of expectancies of a heart attack in producing a panic attack. However, a number of aspects of each point of view, which are specific features of the theories themselves and not inevitable consequences of a "biochemical" or "psychological" view, are in disagreement. It is to these features that much of the rest of this chapter is devoted.

The other major dispute with the information-processing view of panic disorder has come from Barlow (1988), who has proposed a view of panic disorder from an emotion theory perspective. The emotion theory perspective is more fundamentally similar to the cognitive view than are the current biological perspectives. Nevertheless, there remain some basic differences that are in some respects central to theories of all the anxiety disorders. Thus, discussion of the differences between the cognitive and emotion theory views of panic disorder may be important in order to generate essential research.

In the remainder of this chapter, I discuss a number of issues for which different predictions are made by the information-processing view and the other perspectives. As much as possible, research evidence bearing on each issue is evaluated; alternatively, research questions requiring investigation are highlighted.

PANIC VERSUS GENERALIZED ANXIETY

Probably the most basic issue on which most proponents of the information-processing view disagree with both the emotion theory and biological perspectives is the distinction between "panic" and "generalized anxiety." This distinction is basically analogous to the distinction made by a number of authors between "fear" and "anxiety."

According to the biological view, chronic or generalized anxiety is a process that is biologically different from the intense, sudden surge of a panic attack (Klein, 1967, 1993). This point of view has recently been incorporated into the DSM-IV (American Psychiatric Association, 1994). Causally, generalized anxiety has typically been connected with the benzodiazepine/GABA receptor complex (Cowley & Roy-Byrne, 1991) while panic has been attributed to activity in the noradrenergic or in some cases serotonergic neurotransmitter systems (Charney & Heninger, 1986; Evans, 1989).

At a more psychological level of analysis, the emotion theory perspective has postulated a difference between anxiety and fear/panic. According to Barlow (1988), panic (or fear) is a "primitive alarm in response to present danger" (p. 70) and consists purely of high negative affect and arousal. On the other hand, anxiety is viewed as a "diffuse cognitive-affective structure" (p. 71) in response to future danger that involves both affective components (high negative affect) as well as cognitive components (such as a sense of uncontrollability and maladaptive shifts in attention). While both anxiety and panic are components of all the anxiety disorders, anxiety is more typically a component of generalized anxiety disorder, and panic is more typically a component of phobic disorders and panic disorder (Barlow, 1988).

In contrast to these points of view, the information processing perspective does not necessarily postulate a qualitative distinction between fear and anxiety. Continuity between fear and anxiety is not actually a necessary component of the cognitive view, and some authors do postulate a distinction (Öhman, 1993). However, a qualitative difference between fear and anxiety is certainly not an essential component of such theories. It is important to point out that postulating a lack of difference between two supposedly distinct emotional states is not to say that the overall conditions of panic disorder and generalized anxiety disorder do not have their differences. Indeed, there appear to be marked differences between panic disorder and generalized anxiety disorder as overall disorders. But this does not necessarily mean that fear and anxiety are fundamentally distinct states.

Evidence on whether fear/panic attacks and chronic/generalized anxiety are qualitatively distinct is very difficult to gather. One of the main difficulties is that few authors appear to have seen this as an important issue. However, its importance is found first in distinguishing the emotion theory and information-processing views, and also in a number of differential predictions affecting most of the anxiety disorders. The emotion theory perspective acknowledges that certain associations, attitudes, and beliefs can increase the likelihood of a panic attack or even trigger one, but the panic attack itself is seen as a unique emotional phenomenon that does not involve cognitive components. On the other hand, the cognitive view sees attitudes and beliefs as an integral component of the overall panic attack/anxious reaction. Thus, if the association with physical threat can be broken, then, according to the cognitive view, panic attacks should no longer occur. On the other hand, emotion theory predicts that breaking the association between physical sensations and threat may reduce the likelihood of panic attacks but will not necessarily stop them. Unfortunately, such hypotheses are extremely difficult to test. Certainly, there is evidence that cognitive therapy alone can attenuate panic attacks (Margraf, Barlow, Clark, & Telch, 1993), but treatment outcome cannot logically be used to support etiological theories.

Evidence on the distinction between "fear" and "anxiety" is minimal, and many authors have simply assumed that these terms refer to two distinct emotional states without considering this an empirical question (Beck & Emery, with Greenberg, 1985; Charney & Redmond, 1983; Uhde et al., 1984). The most widely cited evidence is the biochemical dissection work, in which it has been hypothesized that chronic anxiety responds to alleviation by benzodiazepines but not tricyclics, whereas panic attacks respond to alleviation by tricyclics and not benzodiazepines (Klein, 1967). The biochemical perspective's assumption of a distinction between panic attacks and chronic anxiety is still fundamentally based on this evidence, even though most researchers would now question its validity. A number of studies have shown that panic attacks do respond to benzodiazepines (Ballenger et al., 1988; Charney & Woods, 1989; Noyes et al., 1984); conversely, some work has attested to the anxiety-relieving properties of the tricyclics (Schweitzer & Rickels, 1991). In addition, some laboratory evidence has demonstrated that panic attacks can be produced by infusions of flumazenil, a benzodiazepine receptor antagonist (Nutt, Glue, Lawson, & Wilson, 1990).

Thus, what evidence remains for a distinction between anxiety and panic? Barlow (1988) points to two forms of somatic/physiological evidence. In several studies, individuals with panic disorder have been found to report a set of somatic symptoms differing from that reported by individuals with generalized anxiety disorder (Anderson, Noyes, & Crowe, 1984; Rapee, 1985). Typically, panic patients report more symptoms related to cardiovascular or respiratory changes (e.g., breathlessness, dizziness, chest pain, etc.). However, as mentioned above, a distinction between panic disorder and generalized anxiety disorder as overall conditions is very different from a distinction between panic and anxiety as qualitatively independent emotional constructs. It is very likely that individuals with panic disorder have a different attentional focus, a different interpretive bias, or even different physiological triggers from those of individuals with generalized anxiety disorder, but this does not provide evidence for a distinction between fear and anxiety within these individuals. For example, there is also evidence that the somatic symptoms experienced by subjects with panic disorder and social phobia are different (Amies, Gelder, & Shaw, 1983; Reich, Noyes, & Yates, 1988); yet most authors would agree that both of these disorders are based on fear responses.

More convincing is the evidence Barlow provides of a possible physiological difference between panic and chronic anxiety. In an ambulatory monitoring study by Freedman, Ianni, Ettedgui, and Puthezhath (1985), a comparison was made between episodes of "panic" and periods of "background anxiety," which were matched in terms of their subjective intensity. The panic episodes were associated with sudden increases in heart rate, whereas the anxiety episodes tended to involve fairly consistent heart rates. Of course, the difficulty for data such as these lies in determining the temporal sequence of the physiological and subjective parameters. According to emotion theory, the abrupt increases in heart rate represent a qualitatively unique episode of "panic" and thus accompany or even follow the subjective experience. On the other hand, the cognitive view would see these episodes as possibly random experiences, which, importantly, are *triggers* for a fear/anxiety reaction (labeled a "panic attack"). In support of this latter view, a number of researchers have found that sudden increases in heart rate can occur frequently and not be labeled "panic attacks" (Kenardy, Evans, & Oei, 1989; Shear et al., 1992; Taylor et al., 1986). Presumably, whether a heart rate surge triggers anxiety depends on whether the individual perceives the change. Nevertheless, final answers to this issue will depend on far more fine-grained temporal sequencing in ambulatory monitoring studies—a technique that has become considerably more feasible with the development of portable computer monitoring systems (Kenardy & Adams, 1993).

In summary, there appears to be no conclusive evidence demonstrating a qualitative difference between chronic anxiety and panic (fear). In the absence of such evidence, one should presumably revert to the more parsimonious position of a single emotional entity. Thus, "panic attacks" and "chronic anxiety" should be seen as different labels for the same basic emotion, differing possibly along such parameters as temporal features and intensity.

HIGHER CENTRAL NERVOUS SYSTEM INVOLVEMENT

Most biological theories of panic attacks posit the importance of a single major neurotransmitter system and/or the involvement of a single brain area, usually in lower-order areas such as the brainstem (Charney & Heninger, 1986; Gorman et al., 1989; Klein, 1993). For example, one attempt to produce a comprehensive neuroanatomical model of panic disorder hypothesized that an acute panic attack is "generated by a neural discharge in the brainstem" (Gorman et al., 1989, p. 150). Higher central nervous system (CNS) involvement was proposed to be necessary only for anticipatory anxiety (limbic system) and phobic avoidance (prefrontal cortex).

From a different perspective, Barlow (1988) proposes that higher CNS involvement is important in the probability of panic, but that the actual panic attack is a pure emotion, devoid of cognition.

The primary evidence cited for the importance of a single neurotransmitter system in panic disorder is the ability to produce panic attacks in the laboratory through the stimulation of these systems. Biochemical induction of panic attacks in panic disorder subjects has been demonstrated across a large number of studies in a variety of laboratories (van den Hout, 1988; Rapee, 1995). The majority of studies have utilized indirect stimulation of specific neurotransmitter systems through the use of such procedures as inhalations of carbon dioxide (CO_2), infusions of sodium lactate, and voluntary hyperventilation. However, a few studies have provided more direct evidence for the involvement of specific neurotransmitter systems through the infusion of such chemicals as yohimbine (an alpha$_2$ adrenergic receptor antagonist) and flumazenil (a benzodiazepine receptor antagonist) (Charney, Heninger, & Breier, 1984; Nutt et al., 1990).

It is clear that a variety of so-called "biological challenge procedures" can produce panic attacks in the laboratory. However, the mechanism by which this occurs is vital to the theoretical perspective supported. According to the biological view, challenge procedures produce panic attacks because they directly stimulate the neurotransmitter system responsible for panic attacks. In contrast, the information-processing view hypothesizes that such methods simply produce those somatic sensations that are feared by individuals with panic disorder. The panic attack (anxiety) is then experienced in response to those sensations and is mediated by associations with impending physical disaster (Clark, 1993; van den Hout, 1988; Rapee, 1995). Thus, information-processing theories would view the biological challenge as equivalent to a behavioral test in which individuals are simply exposed to the stimuli they fear (in this case, somatic sensations).

Support for this latter position has come from a number of studies demonstrating that manipulating expectancies, beliefs, or attitudes (through the use of instructions) can alter the response to biological challenge procedures in individuals with panic disorder (Clark, 1993;

Rapee, 1995). For example, Margraf, Ehlers, and Roth (1989) asked two groups of severe agoraphobics to hyperventilate. One group was told that the task was a "fast-paced breathing task," while another group was told that the task was a "panic attack test." The subjects who were expecting a panic attack responded more to the hyperventilation than the subjects who were not expecting panic, on both subjective and physiological measures. In another study looking at the effects of a different psychological variable, two groups of subjects with panic disorder inhaled 5.5% CO_2 in air and were told that they would be able to control the amount of gas they received if, and only if, a light in front of them was illuminated. One group had the light illuminated upon gas delivery, whereas the other did not. The "illusion of control" subjects were significantly less likely to have a panic attack, even though both groups demonstrated equivalent increases in CO_2 levels (Sanderson, Rapee, & Barlow, 1989).

Similarly there are also some data indicating that the propensity for individuals with panic disorder to experience a panic attack in response to biological challenge is markedly attenuated by behavioral treatment (Shear et al. 1991). During behavioral treatment, subjects are taught to control their panic attacks and to alter their beliefs so that physical sensations are no longer associated with impending catastrophe. Any brainstem-level biochemical abnormality is presumably not addressed. The fact that panic patients who undergo such a treatment program are less likely to panic in response to biological challenge provides further support for the involvement of higher CNS centers in acute panic attacks.

Finally, some work with nonclinical populations suggests that panic attacks can be produced by biological challenge procedures in subjects who presumably do not have the biochemical predisposition but who are psychologically predisposed. The Anxiety Sensitivity Index (ASI; Reiss, Peterson, Gursky, & McNally, 1986) is a questionnaire measure of the tendency to associate somatic sensations with danger (see McNally, Chapter 8 this volume). According to the information-processing view, high scorers on this measure should be more likely than low scorers to panic in response to biological challenge procedures. However, if all subjects are nonclinical, they should presumably all have equivalent biochemical apparatus. A number of studies have demonstrated that nonclinical subjects who score high on the ASI respond with greater distress to a brief period of hyperventilation than subjects who score low on the ASI (Donnell & McNally, 1989; Holloway & McNally, 1987; Rapee & Medoro, 1994).

Thus, consistent with the information-processing view, and in contrast to the biochemical and (to some extent) emotion theory views, it appears that higher-order CNS factors do play a central role in the experience of panic attacks in response to biological challenge.

ONSET OF PANIC DISORDER

Although it is not an essential component of any theory, the onset of panic disorder is differentially predicted by each. The biological view sees panic disorder as a disease process in the brainstem. Thus, there should be no predisposing factors or predictive signs, except possibly for milder panic attack symptoms. In a similar fashion, emotion theory predicts that the initial "false alarm" is more likely to occur in a background of stress, but that there are typically no learned associations to initiate the spiral (Barlow, 1988). In contrast to these perspectives, the information-processing view would predict that the first panic attack must still be based on an expected threatening physical outcome. Although this may at times be based on rapid traumatic learning (e.g., observing a loved one having a heart attack), it is more likely that subtle learning will occur over a long period of time, and therefore that evidence of an association between physical cues and threatening outcomes will be apparent before the initial experience of panic attacks.

Research evidence bearing on this issue is scarce, largely because of the difficulty of conducting accurate retrospective or (preferably) prospective studies. However, two studies have generated some data on the question of premorbid characteristics.

In a retrospective interview study, individuals with panic disorder were found to report significantly more hypochondriacal concerns and other anxious features before the onset of their first panic attack than were nonclinical comparison subjects (Fava, Grandi, & Canestrari, 1988). These results indicate that subjects who eventually experienced repeated unexpected panic attacks showed high levels of concern with and presumably attention to their bodily sensations before ever experiencing an attack. Thus, attention to physical symptoms could not have been purely a result of experience with panic attacks and may have reflected a general predisposing characteristic of somatic concern.

A more recent study compared subjects with panic disorder, subjects with infrequent panic attacks, subjects with other anxiety disorders, and nonclinical controls on a retrospective questionnaire assessing their childhood experiences with somatic threat-related information (Ehlers, 1993). The results showed that both the panic disorder subjects and the infrequent panickers reported more observation of illness and sick-role behavior in their early childhood than did the other groups.

These data suggest that individuals with panic disorder report high levels of physical concerns *before* onset of their first panic attack—a feature that is not predicted by either the emotion theory or the biological perspective. Of course, long-term prospective studies are needed, to answer this question properly, in which individuals with high levels of somatic concerns but without panic attacks are followed up to see whether they are the ones who develop panic disorder. One study along these lines has already been conducted: Nonclinical subjects scoring high on the ASI (described above) at time 1 were more likely to experience an initial panic attack and to meet criteria for panic disorder 3 years later (time 2) than were subjects who scored low on the ASI (Maller & Reiss, 1992). Again, this study suggests that personality features reflecting a concern with somatic sensations preceded the later experience of panic attacks, a result which is not predicted by either the biological or emotion theory perspectives.

SPONTANEITY OF PANIC ATTACKS

An issue very similar to the one discussed above is the notion of the onset of individual panic attacks. According to the information-processing view, panic attacks (anxious reactions) *must* be preceded by the perception of one or more somatic sensations. As described earlier, because the triggers for fear (somatic sensations) are also often part of the fear reaction (e.g., palpitations), individuals often may not notice the distinction of the initial cue, and this may produce an illusion of "spontaneity." In contrast, the biological view posits the existence of truly "spontaneous"[1] panic attacks, which presumably are the results of random misfirings in the disordered neurotransmitter system. In an intermediate fashion, the emotion theory perspective acknowledges that most later panic attacks are "learned alarms" precipitated by the perception of certain somatic sensations, but that at least some panic attacks are likely to be "false alarms" occurring in an uncued fashion.

At least two studies have asked individuals with panic disorder to report retrospectively on the sequence of events in their panic attacks (Ley, 1985; Wolpe & Rowan, 1988). In both cases, most subjects reported the experience of physical symptoms that *preceded* the experience of affect. However, both studies used small numbers of subjects and retrospective, nonblind interview procedures. It is unlikely that such a complex question could ever be answered by means of such procedures.

Empirical validation of these hypotheses is extremely difficult to demonstrate. As mentioned earlier, detailed ambulatory studies using portable computer sampling may provide some evidence, but the speed of the processes involved in panic attacks is so rapid that definitive answers to this question may never be obtained.

GENETIC FACTORS

Given that the biological perspective sees panic disorder as a distinct disease process, it is generally assumed that the predisposition to the biochemical disorder is genetically mediated. Indeed, a number of authors have proposed a specific genetic component in panic disorder (Pauls, Bucher, Crowe, & Noyes, 1980; Surman, Sheehan, Fuller, & Gallo, 1983). A similar prediction is made by Barlow (1988) regarding the experience of "false alarms." In contrast, the information-processing perspective postulates that panic attacks are nothing more than anxiety reactions to somatic sensations and that they parallel similar anxiety reactions in other disorders. Thus, a specific gene for panic disorder is highly improbable. Rather, any potential genetic component must be a general mediator of a much broader construct, such as arousal, anxiety, or emotionality.

A number of family studies have demonstrated a strong familial basis for panic disorder (Crowe, Noyes, Pauls, & Slymen, 1983). Furthermore, some of these studies have demonstrated that the familial penetrance is a specific one, such that individuals with panic disorder are more likely to have family members with panic disorder but not other anxiety disorders (Noyes, Clarkson, Crowe, Yates, & McChesney, 1987). Although such data may be consistent with a genetic basis for panic disorder, these studies have all been *family* studies; as such, they have not controlled for the effects of environmental variables, including modeling and other forms of learning. There is abundant evidence that anxiety can be modeled (Bandura & Rosenthal, 1966; Cook & Mineka, 1989). Thus family concordance for anxiety disorders, even specific concordance, is hardly surprising and is certainly not inconsistent with an information-processing view.

Stronger (but not conclusive) evidence for a genetic involvement can be garnered through twin studies. Unfortunately, few twin studies have specifically examined panic disorder. The most widely cited twin study (Torgersen, 1983), has been interpreted by a number of authors as indicative of a genetic basis for panic disorder. However, the results of this study clearly showed that "no [monozygotic] twin pairs [were found] in which both twins had the same anxiety disorder" (Torgersen, 1983, p. 1086). Some post hoc evidence was cited suggesting a higher concordance for monozygotic twins over dizygotic twins for disorders involving panic attacks as opposed to generalized anxiety. However, the use of DSM-III criteria, with their concomitant hierarchical structure, means that there was most likely a major difference in severity between these disorders.

In a similar large-scale study of 446 twin pairs, using a structured clinical interview and experienced interviewers to arrive at diagnoses (Andrews, Stewart, Allen, & Henderson, 1990), evidence was found for a genetic contribution to the broad construct of neuroticism. However, there was no evidence for a unique genetic contribution to any specific anxiety disorder. Further evidence for a genetic contribution to a general neurotic syndrome is presented in Chapter 1 of this volume.

Thus, although well-controlled studies are rare, the evidence to date is not supportive of a specific genetic basis for panic disorder. Rather, the evidence appears to indicate a genetic component in a general tendency to be emotionally reactive. Whether this general emotional reactivity is manifested as panic disorder presumably depends on a number of environmental factors, including the specific learning history of the individual.

CONCLUSION

To date, there are still a number of gaps in our knowledge about panic disorder. Theories and models of all types have their limitations. In this chapter, I have attempted to marshal evidence I believe is more consistent with those theories that can broadly be grouped under the generic heading of information-processing or cognitive theories, in contrast to predictions from biochemical or emotion theory perspectives. The key issues, as I see them, are the lack of clear evidence for a distinction between fear (panic) and anxiety; the mediating influences of higher-order functions in the response to biological challenge procedures, and thus in the experience of panic attacks; the importance of premorbid characteristics and learning; and the lack of evidence for a specific genetic component. Nevertheless, none of these issues has been conclusively settled to date, and more systematic research is required in each case. In addition, there are certain areas in which detailed research would greatly benefit the development of more comprehensive theories. In particular, more information is desperately needed on the long-term development of panic disorder and on the temporal anatomy of individual panic attacks. Advances in technology and theory should greatly aid research in these areas.

NOTE

1. "Spontaneous" in this context presumably refers to its apparent characteristics, since nothing is truly spontaneous (i.e., without cause).

REFERENCES

American Psychiatric Association. (1994). *Diagnostic and statistical manual of mental disorders* (4th ed.). Washington, DC: Author.

Amies, P. L., Gelder, M. G., & Shaw, P. M. (1983). Social phobia: A comparative clinical study. *British Journal of Psychiatry, 142,* 174–179.

Anderson, D. J., Noyes, R., Jr., & Crowe, R. R. (1984). A comparison of panic disorder and generalized anxiety disorder. *American Journal of Psychiatry, 141,* 572–575.

Andrews, G., Stewart, G. W., Allen, R., & Henderson, A. S. (1990). The genetics of six neurotic disorders: A twin study. *Journal of Affective Disorders, 19,* 23–29.

Ballenger, J. C., Burrows, G. D., DuPont, R. L., Jr., Lesser, I. M., Noyes, R., Jr., Pecknold, J. C., Rifkin, A., & Swinson, R. P. (1988). Alprazolam in panic disorder and agoraphobia: Results from a multicenter trial. I. Efficacy in short-term treatment. *Archives of General Psychiatry, 45,* 413–422.

Bandura, A., & Rosenthal, T. (1966). Vicarious classical conditioning as a function of arousal level. *Journal of Personality and Social Psychology, 3,* 54–62.

Barlow, D. H. (1988). *Anxiety and its disorders: The nature and treatment of anxiety and panic.* New York: Guilford Press.

Beck, A. T., & Emery, G., with Greenberg, R. L. (1985). *Anxiety disorders and phobias: A cognitive perspective.* New York: Basic Books.

Carr, D. B., & Sheehan, D. V. (1984). Panic anxiety: A new biological model. *Journal of Clinical Psychiatry, 45,* 323–330.

Charney, D. S., & Heninger, G. R. (1986). Abnormal regulation of noradrenergic function in panic disorders. *Archives of General Psychiatry, 43,* 1042–1054.

Charney, D. S., Heninger, G. R., & Breier, A. (1984). Noradrenergic function in panic anxiety: Effects of yohimbine in healthy subjects and patients with agoraphobia and panic disorder. *Archives of General Psychiatry, 41,* 751–763.

Charney, D. S., & Redmond, D. E., Jr. (1983). Neurobiological mechanisms in human anxiety: Evidence supporting central noradrenergic hyperactivity. *Neuropharmacology, 22,* 1531–1536.

Charney, D. S., & Woods, S. W. (1989). Benzodiazepine treatment of panic disorder: A comparison of alprazolam and lorazepam. *Journal of Clinical Psychiatry, 50,* 418–423.

Clark, D. M. (1986). A cognitive approach to panic. *Behaviour Research and Therapy, 24,* 461–470.

Clark, D. M. (1993). Cognitive mediation of panic attacks induced by biological challenge tests. *Advances in Behaviour Research and Therapy, 15,* 75–84.

Cook, M., & Mineka, S. (1989). Observational conditioning of fear to fear-relevant versus fear-irrelevant stimuli in rhesus monkeys. *Journal of Abnormal Psychology, 98,* 448–459.

Cowley, D. S., & Roy-Byrne, P. P. (1991). The biology of generalized anxiety disorder and chronic anxiety. In R. M. Rapee & D. H. Barlow (Eds.), *Chronic anxiety: Generalized anxiety disorder and mixed anxiety-depression.* New York: Guilford Press.

Crowe, R. R., Noyes, R., Pauls, D. L., & Slymen, D. (1983). A family study of panic disorder. *Archives of General Psychiatry, 40,* 1065–1069.

Donnell, C. D., & McNally, R. J. (1989). Anxiety sensitivity and history of panic as predictors of response to hyperventilation. *Behaviour Research and Therapy, 27,* 325–332.

Ehlers, A. (1993). Somatic symptoms and panic attacks: A retrospective study of learning experiences. *Behaviour Research and Therapy, 31,* 269–278.

Evans, L. (1989). Some biological aspects of panic disorder. *International Journal of Clinical Pharmacology Research, 9,* 139–145.

Fava, G. A., Grandi, S., & Canestrari, R. (1988). Prodromal symptoms in panic disorder with agoraphobia. *American Journal of Psychiatry, 145,* 1564–1567.

Freedman, R. R., Ianni, P., Ettedgui, E., & Puthezhath, N. (1985). Ambulatory monitoring of panic disorder. *Archives of General Psychiatry, 42,* 244–248.

Gorman, J. M., Liebowitz, M. R., Fyer, A. J., & Stein, J. (1989). A neuroanatomical hypothesis for panic disorder. *American Journal of Psychiatry, 146,* 148–161.

Holloway, W., & McNally, R. J. (1987). Effects of anxiety sensitivity on the response to hyperventilation. *Journal of Abnormal Psychology, 96,* 330–334.

Kenardy, J., & Adams, C. (1993). Computers in cognitive-behaviour therapy. *Australian Psychologist, 28,* 189–194.

Kenardy, J., Evans, L., & Oei, T. P. S. (1989). Cognitions and heart rate in panic disorders during everyday activity. *Journal of Anxiety Disorders, 3,* 33–43.

Klein, D. F. (1967). Importance of psychiatric diagnosis in prediction of clinical drug effects. *Archives of General Psychiatry, 16,* 118–126.

Klein, D. F. (1993). False suffocation alarms, spontaneous panics, and related conditions: An integrative hypothesis. *Archives of General Psychiatry, 50,* 306–317.

Ley, R. (1985). Agoraphobia, the panic attack and the hyperventilation syndrome. *Behaviour Research and Therapy, 23,* 79–81.

Maller, R. G., & Reiss, S. (1992). Anxiety sensitivity in 1984 and panic attacks in 1987. *Journal of Anxiety Disorders, 6,* 241–247.

Margraf, J., Barlow, D. H., Clark, D. M., & Telch, M. J. (1993). Psychological treatment of panic: Work in progress on outcome, active ingredients, and follow-up. *Behaviour Research and Therapy, 31,* 1–8.

Margraf, J., & Ehlers, A. (1989). Etiological models of panic: Psychophysiological and cognitive aspects. In R. Baker (Ed.), *Panic disorder: Theory, research and therapy.* New York: Wiley.

Margraf, J., Ehlers, A., & Roth, W. T. (1989). Expectancy effects and hyperventilation as laboratory stressors. In H. Weiner, I. Florin, R. Murrison, & D. Hellhammer (Eds.), *Frontiers of stress research.* Toronto: Huber.

McNally, R. J. (1990). Psychological approaches to panic disorder: A review. *Psychological Bulletin, 108,* 403–419.

Noyes, R., Jr., Anderson, D. J., Clancy, J., Crowe, R. R., Slymen, D. J., Ghoneim, M. M., & Hinrichs, J. V. (1984). Diazepam and propranolol in panic disorder and agoraphobia. *Archives of General Psychiatry, 41,* 287–292.

Noyes, R., Jr., Clarkson, C., Crowe, R. R., Yates, W. R., & McChesney, C.

M. (1987). A family study of generalized anxiety disorder. *American Journal of Psychiatry, 144,* 1019–1024.

Nutt, D. J., Glue, P., Lawson, C., & Wilson, S. (1990). Flumazenil provocation of panic attacks: Evidence for altered benzodiazepine receptor sensitivity in panic disorder. *Archives of General Psychiatry, 47,* 917–925.

Öhman, A. (1993). Fear and anxiety as emotional phenomena: Clinical phenomenology, evolutionary perspectives, and information processing mechanisms. In M. Lewis & J. M. Haviland (Eds.), *Handbook of emotions.* New York: Guilford Press.

Pauls, D. L., Bucher, K. D., Crowe, R. R., & Noyes, R., Jr. (1980). A genetic study of panic disorder pedigrees. *American Journal of Human Genetics, 32,* 639–644.

Pitts, F. N., Jr. (1969). The biochemistry of anxiety. *Scientific American, 220,* 69–75.

Rapee, R. M. (1985). Distinctions between panic disorder and generalised anxiety disorder: Clinical presentation. *Australian and New Zealand Journal of Psychiatry, 19,* 227–232.

Rapee, R. M. (1993). Psychological factors in panic disorder. *Advances in Behaviour Research and Therapy, 15,* 85–102.

Rapee, R. M. (1995). Psychological factors influencing the affective response to biological challenge procedures in panic disorder. *Journal of Anxiety Disorders, 9,* 59–74.

Rapee, R. M., & Medoro, L. (1994). Fear of physical sensations and trait anxiety as mediators of the response to hyperventilation in nonclinical subjects. *Journal of Abnormal Psychology, 103,* 693–699.

Reich, J., Noyes, R., & Yates, W. (1988). Anxiety symptoms distinguishing social phobia from panic and generalized anxiety disorders. *Journal of Nervous and Mental Disease, 176,* 510–513.

Reiss, S., Peterson, R. A., Gursky, D. M., & McNally, R. J. (1986). Anxiety sensitivity, anxiety frequency and the prediction of fearfulness. *Behaviour Research and Therapy, 24,* 1–8.

Sanderson, W. C., Rapee, R. M., & Barlow, D. H. (1989). The influence of perceived control on panic attacks induced via inhalation of 5.5% CO_2-enriched air. *Archives of General Psychiatry, 46,* 157–162.

Schweitzer, E., & Rickels, K. (1991). Pharmacotherapy of generalized anxiety disorder. In R. M. Rapee & D. H. Barlow (Eds.), *Chronic anxiety: Generalized anxiety disorder and mixed anxiety–depression.* New York: Guilford Press.

Shear, M. K., Fyer, A. J., Ball, G., Josephson, S., Fitzpatrick, M., Gitlin, B., Frances, A., Gorman, J., Liebowitz, M., & Klein, D. F. (1991). Vulnerability to sodium lactate in panic disorder patients given cognitive-behavioral therapy. *American Journal of Psychiatry, 148,* 795–797.

Shear, M. K., Polan, J. J., Harshfield, G., Pickering, T., Mann, J. J., Frances, A., & James, G. (1992). Ambulatory monitoring of blood pressure and heart rate in panic patients. *Journal of Anxiety Disorders, 6,* 213–221.

Surman, O. S., Sheehan, D. V., Fuller, T. C., & Gallo, J. (1983). Panic disorder in genotypic HLA identical sibling pairs. *American Journal of Psychiatry, 140,* 237–238.

Taylor, C. B., Sheikh, J., Agras, W. S., Roth, W. T., Margraf, J., Ehlers, A., Maddock, R. J., & Gossard, D. (1986). Ambulatory heart rate changes in patients with panic attacks. *American Journal of Psychiatry, 143,* 478–482.
Torgersen, S. (1983). Genetic factors in anxiety disorders. *Archives of General Psychiatry, 40,* 1085–1089.
Uhde, T. W., Boulenger, J. P., Post, R. M., Siever, L. J., Vittone, B. J., Jimerson, D. C., & Roy-Byrne, P. P. (1984). Fear and anxiety: Relationship to noradrenergic function. *Psychopathology, 17,* 8–23.
van den Hout, M. A. (1988). The explanation of experimental panic. In J. Rachman & J. D. Maser (Eds.), *Panic: Psychological perspectives.* Hillsdale, NJ: Erlbaum.
Wilson, T. D., & Nisbett, R. E. (1978). The accuracy of verbal reports about the effects of stimuli on evaluations and behavior. *Social Psychology, 41,* 118–131.
Wolpe, J., & Rowan, V. C. (1988). Panic disorder: A product of classical conditioning. *Behaviour Research and Therapy, 26,* 441–450.

Information-Processing and Emotion Theory Views of Panic Disorder: Overlapping and Distinct Features

Martin M. Antony
David H. Barlow

IN HIS CHAPTER on information-processing views of panic disorder (PD), Rapee has discussed the benefits of viewing PD from this perspective and compared the relative merits of his view to those of models based on a biological view and on emotion theory. Overall, we agree with many of the points made by Rapee in Chapter 4. The emotion theory view of panic shares many features with an information-processing perspective. In fact, as outlined in our chapter, the emotion theorists (e.g., Peter Lang) who inspired Barlow's (1988) model of PD clearly view emotion from an information-processing perspective based on current theories of memory. However, despite the overlap between our perspective and that of Rapee, we would argue that unidimensional models such as those based exclusively on cognitive theory are incomplete, and that any attempt to reduce the richness of emotional experience to a series of attributions and appraisals will have the same consequences as biological reductionism. Furthermore, we disagree with Rapee's arguments regarding several specific issues.

Rapee acknowledges that psychological phenomena can be viewed from a variety of perspectives that employ different levels of explanation (e.g., cognitive, biological, biochemical, etc.). Furthermore, he argues that one perspective may have advantages over others for explaining specific aspects of a given disorder. Despite this assertion, Rapee and other cognitive theorists have paid relatively little attention to the role of the biological factors in PD. As argued in our chapter, a comprehensive model of PD should be able to account for findings from a broad range of perspectives, including biological, cognitive, and learning perspectives. Emotion-based theories meet this goal (Barlow, 1988).

According to Rapee, one difference between theories based on information-processing theory and emotion theory is the hypothesized role of cognition. Rapee states that "if the association with physical threat can be broken, then, according to the cognitive view, panic attacks should no longer occur" (p. 82). Furthermore, he argues that emotion theory predicts that breaking this association may decrease the likelihood of panicking, but will not necessarily prevent panic attacks. Essentially, we agree with this analysis. To be more precise, Barlow's (1988) model predicts that effective cognitive-behavioral treatment for PD should decrease the frequency of learned alarms (the majority of panic attacks in PD), in addition to reducing anticipatory anxiety and agoraphobic avoidance. However, according to Barlow's model, a patient who is treated for PD may still be expected to have occasional episodes of panic (false alarms) following periods of extreme stress. Because treatment studies have tended to measure patients' "panic-free status" during relatively brief assessment periods (usually only 1 to 4 weeks), it is possible that a high percentage of patients who are considered to be "panic-free" at follow-up will still experience occasional autonomic rushes between follow-up assessments, especially if they experience stressful life events. More recent evidence examining the follow-up period subsequent to successful cognitive-behavioral treatment of PD in a longitudinal rather than a cross-sectional manner supports this assertion (Brown & Barlow, in press). Of course, after being treated successfully, patients should react to the occurrence of a false alarm differently than in the past. Presumably, they will no longer become anxious over having panic attacks, and the cycle of anxious apprehension and learned alarms will not recur.

Whereas Rapee argues that fear or panic and anxiety differ quantitatively only, we argue that there are important qualitative differences as well. As reviewed in our chapter and the chapter by Rapee, biological findings (e.g., from pharmacological treatment studies) have been mixed with respect to this issue, and we agree that evidence from this source is weak and post hoc. However, recent studies examining the phenomenological aspects of the two states (e.g., Zinbarg & Barlow, 1995) suggests that they do in fact represent different emotional phenomena. Rapee also ignores very strong findings from biological studies suggesting different neuroanatomical pathways for these emotional phenomena (e.g., Gray,

1991; Graeff, 1986). Also, an emotion theory view of PD suggests that panic, but not generalized anxiety, should be associated with a strong behavioral disposition (e.g., and urge to escape). Phenomenologically, this seems a clear clinical distinction (Barlow, Brown, & Craske, 1994), but it has not been well studied. Finally, it seems curious, at least, that the terms "anxiety" and "panic," which have been utilized differentially since the time of Cicero (Eysenck, 1991) by all major theorists in this area, including Freud, should have no differential meaning or referents in current usage.

In several places, Rapee argues that Barlow (1988) views panic as a "pure emotion" that is "devoid of cognition." The meaning of the term "cognition," as Rapee uses it, is ambiguous. Clearly, cognitions accompany fear. Most clinical patients report cognition of terror, urges to escape, and the like; also, much information is processed as part of the fear/panic response cycle (including cues, etc.). Although the emotion theory view of PD suggests that fear can occur without conscious appraisal, we would not argue that emotional states are devoid of cognition or information processing. Nonconscious processing of information is an essential component of Barlow's model. Furthermore, we would agree with the position that conscious appraisal may precede emotional reactions; however, we would argue that the experience of emotion need not always be preceded by conscious appraisal (Zajonc, 1980, 1984), and that the information processed as part of an affective or emotional reaction is probably qualitatively different (Teasdale, 1993).

According to Rapee, evidence that nonclinical subjects who report heightened anxiety sensitivity panic in response to biological challenges is contrary to what might be predicted by biological and emotion theory formulations of PD. Specifically, Rapee argues that according to biological and emotion theorists, nonclinical subjects should not have a biochemical predisposition to experience panic attacks and therefore should not panic. It should be noted that Barlow's (1988) model would argue that nonclinical panickers, like patients with PD, do in fact have a biological predisposition to experience panic attacks (i.e., false alarms). What distinguishes individuals with nonclinical and clinical levels of panic is a psychological vulnerability to developing anxious apprehension and the other features associated with PD.

Rapee argues against a specific genetic basis for PD; he suggests that at most, genetic factors may contribute to a general tendency to be emotionally reactive, which in turn may predispose individuals to develop any of a broad range of disorders. However, recent family and genetic studies have cast some doubt on that hypothesis. Goldstein et al. (1994) found that relatives of probands with PD were more likely to meet criteria for PD specifically that other disorders, with the possible exception of social phobia. This finding suggests that the familial nature of PD is disorder-specific. Skre, Torgersen, Lygren, and Kringlen (1993) found a similar pattern in a twin study showing that PD tends to be more prevalent in twins of PD patients, whereas generalized anxiety disorder (GAD) tends to be more prevalent in twins of GAD patients. Furthermore, the fact that the concordance ration for monozygotic versus dizygotic twins was greater than 2:1 for both PD and GAD supports the hypothesis that genetic factors at least partially mediate the familial nature of these disorders.

Finally, in an even more convincing study, Kendler, Neale, Kessler, Heath, and Eaves (1992) examined the contributions of genetic and environmental factors to the development of agoraphobia and other phobic disorders. Furthermore, the authors broke these influences down into those that contributed to the development of all phobic disorders (common factors) and those that contributed to the development of specific disorders. For patients with agoraphobia, environmental influences accounted for 64% of the variance in factors common across phobic disorders, whereas genetic influences accounted for 7% of the variance in common factors. With respect to disorder-specific influences, genetics accounted for 29% of the variance, whereas environment accounted for 0% of the variance. So, contrary to Rapee's hypothesis, genetic contributions were more relevant for the disorder-specific features of agoraphobia (e.g., perhaps the tendency to experience false alarms following periods of stress), whereas environmental influences were more important for the variables that contribute to the development of all phobic disorders. Nevertheless, we would agree with Rapee's conclusion from Andrews, Stewart, Allen, and Henderson (1990) that the primary genetic contribution to anxiety disorders is to a more general vulnerability to "neuroticism," and that the genetic contribution to specific disorders such as PD is of a considerably smaller magnitude (see also Barlow, 1988).

To summarize, we believe that the information-processing models of PD are sufficient to explain several aspects of the disorder. However, they lack the scope to serve as comprehensive models of PD. Specifically, they do not account sufficiently for findings from biological research (e.g., genetics studies, studies of the neurobiology of emotions). Furthermore, we disagree with Rapee's belief that the terms "panic" (or "fear") and "anxiety" refer to the same emotional state; this seems to disregard a range of evidence from different sources. Ascertaining and considering fundamental differences between fear or panic and anxiety, as well as their functional relationships, will be a very important step in any theoretical development pertaining to the anxiety disorders generally and to PD more specifically. Finally, we agree with Rapee's assertion that many of the features that distinguish between the information-processing and emotion theory views of PD have not been adequately researched.

REFERENCES

Andrews, G., Stewart, G. W., Allen, R., & Henderson, A. S. (1990). The genetics of six neurotic disorders: A twin study. *Journal of Affective Disorders,*
19, 23–29.

Barlow, D. H. (1988). *Anxiety and its disorders: The nature and treatment of*
anxiety and panic. New York: Guilford Press.

Barlow, D. H., Brown, T. A., & Craske, M. G. (1994). Definitions of panic attacks and panic disorder in DSM-IV: Implications for research. *Journal*
of Abnormal Psychology, 103, 553–564.

Brown, T. A., & Barlow, D. H. (in press). *Long-term outcome in cognitive-*
behavioral treatment of panic disorder: Clinical predictors and alternative
strategies for assessment. Journal of Consulting and Clinical Psychology.

Eysenck, H. J. (1991). Neuroticism, anxiety, and depression. *Psychological In-*
quiry, 2, 75–76.

Goldstein, R., Weissman, M. M., Adams, P. B., Horwath, E., Lish, J. D., Charney, D., Woods, S. W., Sobin, C., & Wickramaratne, P. J. (1994). Psychiatric disorders in relatives of probands with panic disorder and/or major
depression. *Archives of General Psychiatry, 51,* 383–394.

Graeff, F. G. (1986). The anti-aversive action of drugs. In N. A. Krasnegor, D.
B. Gray, & R. Thompson (Eds.), *Advances in behavioral pharmacology*
(Vol. 5). Hillsdale, NJ: Erlbaum.

Gray, J. A. (1991). Fear, panic, and anxiety: What's in a name? *Psychological*
Inquiry, 2, 77–78.

Kendler, K. S., Neale, M. C., Kessler, R. C., Heath, A. C., & Eaves, L. J. (1992).
The genetic epidemiology of phobias in women: The interrelationship of
agoraphobia, social phobia, situational phobia, and simple phobia. *Archives*
of General Psychiatry, 39, 273–281.

Skre, I., Torgersen, S., Lygren, S., & Kringlen, E. (1993). A twin study of DSM-
III-R anxiety disorders. *Acta Psychiatrica Scandinavica, 88,* 85–92.

Teasdale, J. D. (1993). Emotion and two kinds of meaning: Cognitive therapy
and applied cognitive science. *Behaviour Research and Therapy, 31,*
339–359.

Zajonc, R. B. (1984). On the primacy of affect. *American Psychologist, 39,*
117–123.

Zinbarg, R. E., & Barlow, D. H. (1995). *The structure of anxiety and the DSM-*
III-R anxiety disorders: A hierarchical model. Manuscript submitted for
publication.

Panic Disorder and Psychological Dimensions

RONALD M. RAPEE

ANTONY AND BARLOW, in Chapter 3 of this volume, have provided a clear and cogent account of the emotion theory of panic disorder as earlier detailed by Barlow (1988). As I have suggested in Chapter 4, there are strong similarities between this and the information-processing view of panic disorder. In fact, the two perspectives make similar predictions in terms of the importance of interoceptive cues, the accompanying thought processes, the importance of external triggers, and the appropriate treatment techniques. The two views, however, differ in terms of the causal roles afforded to some of these factors and in terms of the basic nature of the phenomenon.

The central tenet of emotion theory, as set forth by Antony and Barlow in Chapter 3, is that fear is a basic emotion that is fundamentally different from anxiety. A true panic attack is actually the experience of pure fear, which is qualitatively different from the anxious apprehension that may precede or follow this fear. In other words, panic attacks and anticipatory anxiety are discontinuous and will posess a number of unique features. In contrast, as I have outlined in Chapter 4, the information-processing view sees panic attacks as a type of anxiety—namely, that which is experienced in response to somatic cues. In fact, I would go so far as to say that the term "panic attack" has been a hindrance by confusing research through its implication of a qualitatively unique phenomenon (see Rapee, 1993).

Early in their chapter, Antony and Barlow provide clear descriptions of the phenomena of fear and anxiety. According to these authors, both are future-oriented feelings that occur in response to uncontrollable threat or danger. The key descriptive difference appears to be based on the temporal distance of the threat. Fear is said to occur in response to very proximal danger,[1] whereas anxiety presumably occurs in response to a threat that is some time away. Given this description, it is hard to see how one can justify a qualitative difference. Time exists on a continuum, and it is not clear why a time of, say, 5 minutes and one of 15 minutes should result in two qualitatively different states. There is certainly considerable precedent for predicting that the *intensity* of the experienced emotion will increase as the temporal proximity to the perceived threat decreases, but why the quality of the emotion should suddenly change at a particular point is not so clear. Nevertheless, the clarity of each theory's position allows for the formulation of clear hypotheses. For example, in a situation where an individual is waiting for the occurrence of a major threat and is given clear temporal cues, emotion theory would predict that at a particular point in time, there should be a sudden surge in the measured variables (heart rate, subjective report, etc.). In contrast, information-processing theory would predict that these measures of anxiety should show a simple inverse relationship with the temporal proximity of the threat and with the perception and interpretation of that threat.

Antony and Barlow make an excellent point by stating that anger and excitement share physical symptoms but that few would consider them to be qualitatively identical. In taking this point a little further, we could ask this: How, indeed, can we decide that anger and excitement are different emotions? There are two parameters that distinguish these emotions most obviously. First, anger and excitement are elicited by different triggers; second, anger and excitement are experienced by individuals as subjectively different. When we apply these parameters to fear and anxiety, it again appears that they are not qualitatively distinct. Fear and anxiety are both elicited by threat cues. In addition, anxiety-disordered clients typically have great difficulty determining where anxiety "ends" and fear "begins," and these terms are often used interchangeably by the lay public—something that cannot be said about excitement and anger.

Antony and Barlow point to a number of sources of evidence that they claim support their view of a qualitative distinction between fear and anxiety. However, none of these pieces of evidence provide conclusive support for a qualitative view. Differences between individuals with panic disorder and generalized anxiety disorder in drug response (for which, by the way, there is no empirical support; see Chapter 4), symptomatology, or onset cannot be used to investigate differences in emotions, because both disorders can involve experience with both emotions. Thus, any observed differences may be attributable to differences between the composite disorders, rather than to differences between the actual emotions. No one is arguing that there are no differences between the anxiety disorders. Genetic studies also fail to demonstrate differences, even between disorders. As I note in Chapter 4, the widely cited study by Torgersen (1983) failed to identify any "[monozygotic] twin pairs in which both twins had the same anxiety disorder" (p. 1086). This study only found a difference in genetic inheritance between the DSM-III category of generalized anxiety disorder (which was a "wastebasket" category) and all other anxiety disorders. More recent carefully conducted studies have failed to find evidence for the specific inheritance of any anxiety disorders; rather, they find evidence in favor of a genetic involvement in general neurosis (see Andrews, Chapter 1, this volume).

Probably one of the main differences between the information-processing model and most other models of panic disorder is the emphasis on what might be described as a continuum developmental approach. The information-processing account holds that the phenomena underlying panic attacks are simply extensions of normal functioning that lie at one end of a continuum and that develop across the individual's lifespan. Thus, it is predicted that vulnerability to experience panic attacks is to be found in attitudes and beliefs that grow from the developmental history of the individual. This is in contrast to theories that see the vulnerability to panic attacks as lying in a latent biological apparatus. A study by Maller and Reiss (1992), in which individuals who scored high on a measure of fear of somatic sensations were significantly more likely to experience panic attacks in the following 3 years than individuals who scored low on that measure, seems more consistent with the former perspective.

The emotion theory of panic attacks described by Antony and Barlow makes a number of testable predictions and is well supported by evidence. Indeed, it shares many similarities with the information-processing view, and the similarities between these views are more numerous than the differences. The main difference appears to lie in the need to specify two qualitatively distinct emotions, as opposed to the more parsimonious option of describing panic attacks as anxiety-related phenomena. Recent evidence has begun to identify individuals' tendencies to conceptualize threatening outcomes along two dimensions, social threats and physical threats (Campbell & Rapee, 1993; Lovibond & Rapee, 1993), and to indicate differences between these threats. Conceptualizing so-called "panic attacks" simply as instances of a response to physical threat would allow for the parsimonious option of keeping this phenomenon within the lines of a general model of anxiety, without having to resort to the invocation of additional, complicating constructs.

NOTE

1. The authors actually state "immediate," but danger cannot be truly immediate unless the individual is currently in the process of being injured.

REFERENCES

Barlow, D. H. (1988). *Anxiety and its disorders: The nature and treatment of anxiety and panic.* New York: Guilford Press.

Campbell, M. A., & Rapee, R. M. (1993). The nature of feared outcome representations in children. *Journal of Abnormal Child Psychology, 22,* 99–111.

Lovibond, P. F.m & Rapee, R. M. (1993). The representation of feared outcomes. *Behaviour Research and Therapy, 31,* 595–608.

Maller, R. G.m & Reiss, S. (1992). Anxiety sensitivity in 1984 and panic attacks in 1987. *Journal of Anxiety Disorders, 6,* 241–247.

Rapee, R. M. (1993). Psychological factors in panic disorder. *Advances in Behaviour Research and Therapy, 15,* 85–102.

Torgersen, S. (1983). Genetic factors in anxiety disorders. *Archives of General Psychiatry, 40,* 1085–1089.

5

Cognitive-Behavioral Approaches to the Understanding of Obsessional Problems

PAUL M. SALKOVSKIS

OBSESSIVE–COMPULSIVE DISORDER (OCD) as seen in the clinic is a particularly severe and disabling problem. Recent epidemiological studies also suggest that OCD may also be much more common in the general population than was previously believed (e.g., Robins et al., 1984). Community rates in the range of 1.9–3.2% have recently been reported. Fortunately, the last 25 years have seen the development and wide application of demonstrably effective psychological treatment in the form of behavior therapy. Although the same period has also seen a wide range of other psychological explanations for OCD, none of these have resulted in effective treatment development, and there have been surprisingly few useful experimental studies (e.g., Beech & Liddel, 1974; Reed, 1985).

In this chapter, the relative merits of two different approaches to cognitive reconceptualization of OCD are considered: general deficit models and the specific cognitive-behavioral hypothesis. The cognitive-behavioral theory is then described in greater detail, and research and clinical implications are outlined.

BACKGROUND TO
THE COGNITIVE-BEHAVIORAL APPROACH

The Development of Behavior Therapy
for Obsessional Patients

Mowrer (1947, 1960) described a two-factor model (i.e., encompassing both classical and operant conditioning) in order to account for fear and avoidance behavior in problems such as phobias and obsessions. He suggested that in such anxiety problems, fear of specific stimuli is acquired through classical conditioning and maintained by operant conditioning processes, because the organism learns to reduce aversive stimuli initially by escaping and later by avoiding the fear-associated conditioned stimuli. Solomon and Wynne (1954) made the further important observation in animal experiments that if stimuli had become classically conditioned by previous association with strongly aversive stimuli, then avoidance responses to the conditioned stimuli were extremely resistant to extinction. That is, they demonstrated that avoidance responses continued unabated long after any pairing of conditioned stimuli with aversive consequences had ceased. The avoidance behavior observed under these circumstances tended to become stereotyped in a fashion analogous to the behavior of obsessional patients. Only when the avoidance behavior was blocked did high levels of anxiety reappear; these animals would persistently attempt to continue the avoidance/escape behavior for a considerable time after the behavior was blocked, although these efforts eventually ceased (see also Wolpe, 1958).

Rachman and associates (see Rachman & Hodgson, 1980, for a detailed review) conducted a series of key experimental studies with obsessional patients to examine the applicability of this model. As predicted by their adaptation of the two-process theory, they found (1) that elicitation of the obsession was associated with increased anxiety and discomfort; (2) that if the patients were then allowed to ritualize then anxiety and discomfort almost immediately decreased; and (3) that if the ritualizing was delayed, anxiety and discomfort decreased ("spontaneously decayed") over a somewhat longer period (up to 1 hour). This work was the experimental foundation for the treatment that came to be known as "exposure with response prevention" (ERP), following the earlier work of Meyer (1966).

Behavioral treatment of OCD is therefore based on the hypothesis that obsessional thoughts have become associated, through conditioning, with anxiety that has subsequently failed to extinguish. Sufferers have developed escape and avoidance behaviors (e.g., obsessional checking and washing) that have the effect of preventing extinction of the anxiety (Rachman & Hodgson, 1980). This view leads simply and elegantly to the behavioral treatment known as exposure and ERP, in which the person is (1) exposed to stimuli that provoke the obsessional response and (2) helped to prevent avoidance and escape (compulsive) responses (Steketee & Foa, 1985; Salkovskis & Kirk, 1989; Foa & Goldstein, 1978).

The Need to Include Cognitive Elements

The success of behavioral treatments of obsessional disorders has in large part been attributable to the combination of and interaction among empirically grounded theoretical work, well-conducted research studies, and the creative clinical application of theory and research. The reported effectiveness of behavioral treatment contrasted sharply with previous expectations of progressive worsening, with long-term hospitalization and leucotomy for the more severe cases, or with many years of psychodynamic treatment without real hope of "symptomatic" improvement.

Behavioral treatment was initially carried out in inpatient or other intensive treatment settings (Marks, Stern, Mawson, Cobb, & McDonald, 1980), and tended to be relatively expensive. However, more recent research suggests that the more generally adopted clinical practice of outpatient treatment emphasizing homework ("self-exposure") can be at least as effective (Marks, Lelliott, Basoglu, & Noshirvani, 1988). The practice of ERP treatment has been extended to its logical conclusion by Edna Foa's group (Riggs & Foa, 1993), with maximal levels of exposure combined with continuous (24-hour) response prevention in some studies. Such programs typically report "success rates" of 75% or better (Abel, 1993; Christensen, Hadzi-Pavlovic, Andrews, & Mattick, 1987), and there is evidence that those patients who do not respond to treatment can be predicted by the presence of depressed mood or very distorted beliefs (Foa, Steketee, Grayson, & Doppelt, 1983).

Success in the treatment of OCD usually that means the patients are "much improved" or "improved"; the proportion of patients who are fully relieved of their obsessional problems is considerably less. Treatment refusal and early dropouts are also common, reducing the figure obtaining the reported improvement to 50% or fewer of those suitable for inclusion and seeking treatment in clinical trials. Clearly, the proportion of patients who are completely rid of their problems is still smaller. The significant residual levels of social and occupational impairment at the end of treatment persist to longer-term follow-up, with little sign of further improvement (Kasvikis & Marks, 1988). Thus, despite extension of ERP to its fullest, there is considerable room for improvement both in the response rate for those offered treatment and in the extent to which patients are completely better at the end of treatment. Theoretically, exposure treatments, having given of their best, have little further to offer without a major rethinking of the problem of obsessions.

These limitations of behavioral treatment suggested the need for developing an alternative approach to the conceptualization and therapy of OCD while retaining the best features of behavioral treatment. Given that obsessional problems are, by definition, driven by unusual and distorted patterns of thinking, I have formulated a cognitive-behavioral hypothesis (Salkovskis, 1985, 1989b, 1989c) and used it to devise cognitive elaborations of existing behaviorally based therapy approaches (See also Rachman, 1976a, 1993.) Before I describe this cognitive-behavioral approach in detail, it is important to indicate why this approach was adopted rather than cognitive deficit or biological disease models, which have tended to be popular in other circles.

THE RELATIVE MERITS OF SPECIFIC VERSUS GENERAL THEORIES OF OBSESSIVE–COMPULSIVE DISORDER

OCD lends itself readily to cognitive and biological theorizing. Thoughts intrude uncontrollably; repetitive, stereotyped, and sometimes bizarre behavior is prominent and pervasive; patients report problems with memory and with decision making; and generalized disturbances of mood are frequently evident. It is therefore not surprising that several writers and researchers have proposed that there may be a general cognitive deficit in OCD, possibly related to structural/and or neurochemical disturbances.

Cognitive deficit theories of obsessional disorders have been based on one of two main views: (1) that obsessional patients are experiencing a general failure in cognitive control, or (2) that obsessional patients have poor general memory and decision-making abilities. These approaches both represent radical departures from behavior therapy, and no attempt has thus far been made to use these views to account for the effectiveness of ERP treatment. By contrast, the much more specific cognitive-behavioral hypothesis is related to the previously described behavioral theory, in that it proposes that the problem is a highly specific one related to normal functioning rather than a function of some general deficit. According to this cognitive-behavioral view, obsessional problems arise from a pattern of specific responses to key stimuli to which the sufferer has acquired emotional sensitivity. Other problems, such as reported memory and decision-making difficulties and "failures of inhibition," are regarded as secondary to the emotional arousal and particularly to the counterproductive coping strategies deployed by the sufferer. In other words, obsessional patients tend to try too hard to control their own cognitive functioning, and other cognitive functions suffer as a result of competition for processing resources. Some recent research provides support for this view. Maki, O'Neill and O'Neill (1994) found that (nonclinical) "checkers" performed similarly to "noncheckers" on tests of inhibitory control of cognition. However, checkers *perceived themselves* to be more susceptible to failures of cognitive control; this finding is consistent with the hypothesis that even in the absence of actual failures of control, these people will try to exert control over their perceived shortcomings in this area.

Biological models have developed over the same period as behavioral theories, and so far have invariably been predicated on general deficit concepts. Several different biological theories have been proposed, usually associating obsessional problems with lesions in a particular brain area (e.g., Insel, 1992) or postulating deficits in neurotransmitter systems (serotonin [5-HT] is the current favorite; Goodman, McDougle, & Price, 1992). Biological theories again postulate a generalized, neuronally based abnormality/deficit, and suffer from the usual problems of deficit theories. The strongest evidence for these theories comes from the response of obsessional patients to pharmacological treatment. Unfortunately, the theories themselves have been derived from observations of treatment response (e.g., the apparent effectiveness of clomipramine in treatment of OCD is the principal foundation for the 5-HT deficit theory). Such conclusions are based on a misunderstanding of scientific status of treatment results. Logically, only research that shows the *ineffectiveness* of treatment (such as serotonergic drugs) can specifically illuminate the mechanism of the treated disorder. Indeed, the failure of buspirone, a 5-HT_{1A} agonist, provides some embarrassment for the 5-HT theory. Recent biological research indicates an apparently intact 5-HT system in terms of the results of 5-HT neurochemical challenge tests (Barr, Goodman, Price, McDougle, & Charney, 1992). *A priori* predictions concerning mechanism can provide a little further information, but even this cannot be regarded as strong evidence. Structural theories posit abnormalities in structures such as the basal ganglia and orbito-frontal cortex. The basis for much of the recent biological theorizing lies in the observation that obsessive symptoms co-occur with Gilles de la Tourette's syndrome, a rare movement disorder believed to be neurologically based (Robertson, 1990). There have been several attempts to generalize genetic and neurophysiological findings from Tourette's syndrome to OCD. If, as is argued, a common neurological basis exists for the two disorders, it is difficult to explain why Tourette's symptoms are so uncommon among OCD patients.

Although the available evidence is most consistent with specific cognitive-behavioral theories, this is not to say that obsessional problems have no biological substrate. Fundamentally, all behavior—from the occurrence of a fleeting thought to the writing of a scientific article—has neurophysiological correlates. However, the implications of a complex and functional biological substrate are very different from the inference of a biological lesion or disease state. In the field of panic disorder, Gorman, Liebowitz, Fyer, and Stein (1989) have argued for a synthesis between biological and psychological work. It matters little, they contend, whether the problem is seen as a biological disease or as a cognitive-behavioral disease. The more important initial distinction is, of course, between the idea of disease and the more parsimonious concept of functional adaptation, which characterized psychological approaches to anxiety at least until the adoption of DSM-III. It is, of course, easy to see why disease approaches have had such appeal in attempts to understand particular psychological disorders such as panic and obsessive–compulsive problems. Superficially, the experience of such patients is hard to account for without the postulation of qualitatively distinct processes. The phenomenology of OCD *appears* to be so abnormal that it leads many to the otherwise unsupported conclusion that a qualitative abnormality must be involved.

Paradoxically, then, one of the main problems with general deficit theories is their inability to account for key aspects of the phenomenology of OCD. OCD sufferers do appear to have memory and decision-making problems. However, these are highly specific. Although a patient will check the door of his/her house many times, the same patient seldom has problems locking a broom cupboard door. The presence of a trusted other (e.g., a therapist or spouse) also removes the urge to check (Rachman, 1993). Likewise, with the fear of contamination there is a degree of specificity involved in the experience of an object as contaminating (e.g., by particular people or classes of people), which is difficult to account for as a general problem of deciding what is clean and what is contaminated. A similar situation holds for memory as well. The main evidence for memory problems has come from the work of Sher and colleagues (e.g., Sher, Frost, Kushner, Crews, & Alexander, 1989), who have correlated Maudsley Obsessional–Compulsive Inventory (MOCI) Checking scores with scores on the Wechsler Memory Scale (WMS), and report that both nonclinical and clinical "checkers" have lower WMS scores than subjects scoring low on the MOCI Checking scale. Curiously, obsessional patients do not have such memory impairment; nor, indeed, do such patients show any signs of problems with their memory *outside areas directly linked to their obsessional problems.* However, if a person is concerned about his or her memory, the person may check because of this concern. This means that at least two types of people will report checking: those who have a memory problem and make attempts to compensate for it, and those who are unduly concerned about their memory and attempt similar compensation. A possible explanation of Sher et al.'s (1989) findings is therefore that people who actually have general problems with poor memory tend to check more than those who do not. The evidence from clinical obsessional checkers indicates that they have no generalized memory deficit; the cognitive-behavioral hypothesis suggests that in these instances checking may arise from undue and highly focused concern about memory for particular things. Checking may also develop in other people who *know* that they tend to have a poor memory; these probably constitute Sher et al.'s "non-obsessional clinical checkers."

Finally, there is the matter of the effectiveness of therapy. For a general deficit theory to be truly viable as an explanation of OCD, it must first be able to account for the effectiveness of existing psychological treatment (i.e., ERP). Such an account leads directly to testable predictions concerning changes that should occur in the course of treatment. It seems most unlikely that a procedure that cuts down repetitions of checking and washing will enhance memory per se. Despite their evident simplicity and apparent face validity, general deficit theories do not currently add to the understanding of clinical obsessional problems. To be useful, generalized cognitive or biological theories must both account for the phenomenology of OCD and back this up with specific experimental evidence evaluating theoretically derived predictions. At this point, only the behavioral and cognitive-behavioral theories can provide comprehensive and testable accounts of the phenomenology of OCD.

THE COGNITIVE-BEHAVIORAL HYPOTHESIS

General Description

In common with the behavioral theory of OCD (Rachman, 1977), the cognitive-behavioral theory starts with the proposition that obsessional thinking has its origins in normal intrusive thoughts, rather than being qualitatively different. Intrusive thoughts occur in almost 90% of the general population, yet are indistinguishable in terms of content from clinical obsessions (Rachman & de Silva, 1978; Salkovskis & Harrison, 1984). According to the cognitive-behavioral theory, the difference between normal intrusive thoughts and clinical obsessions lies not in the occurrence or controllability of these thoughts, but in the way in which obsessional patients *interpret* intrusions as an indication that they may be responsible for harm or its prevention. The concept is comparable to the cognitive hypothesis of panic (Clark, 1986; Salkovskis, 1988), in which panic attacks are said to occur as a result of the misinterpretation of normal bodily sensations, particularly sensations of normal anxiety. Most normal people experience such sensations, but only people who have an enduring tendency to interpret them in a catastrophic fashion will experience repeated panic attacks. By the same token, intrusive thoughts, impulses, images, and doubts are normal, but only people who have an enduring tendency to misinterpret their own mental activity as indicating personal "responsibility" will experience the pattern of discomfort and neutralizing that is characteristic of OCD.

For example, an obsessional young mother may believe that the occurrence of a thought such as "I will kill my baby" means that there is a risk that she will succumb to the action unless she does something to prevent it, such as avoiding being left alone with her child, seeking reassurance from people around her, trying to think positive thoughts to balance the negative ones, and so on. Thus, the *interpretation* of obsessional thoughts as indicating increased responsibility has a number of important effects in people suffering from OCD: (1) increased discomfort, anxiety, and depression; (2) greater accessibility of the original thought and other related ideas; and (3) behavioral "neutralizing" responses which constitute attempts to escape or avoid responsibility. These may include compulsive behavior, avoidance of situations related to the obsessional thought, seeking reassurance (thus diluting or sharing responsibility), and attempts to get rid of or exclude the thought from the mind. Each of these effects contributes not only to the prevention of extinction of anxiety, but also to a worsening spiral of intrusive thoughts that leads to maladaptive affective, cognitive, and behavioral reactions.

The cognitive-behavioral hypothesis therefore suggests that the problem in clinical obsessions is not poor mental control. Instead, it is hypothesized that obsessional patients tend to misinterpret aspects of their own mental functioning, including memory for actions, intrusive (obsessional) thoughts, and doubts, and that as a result they then try too hard to exert control. The discomfort experienced is a result of the patients' appraisal of the content and occurrence of intrusive thoughts. The increased frequency of intrusions in obsessional relative to nonobsessional individuals is in large part attributable to the behaviors (overt and covert) that are motivated by the appraisals made. These appraisals in obsessional patients center on distorted beliefs about responsibility. The distorted sense of responsibility that the sufferers attach to their activities (including intrusive thoughts and memories as well as overt behavior) leads them to attempt a pattern of mental effort characterized by both overcontrol and preoccupation.

"Responsibility" means here that the person believes that he or she may be, or come to be, the cause of harm (to self or others) unless he or she takes some preventative or restorative action. A group of researchers working on obsessions recently defined the "responsibility" appraisals of an obsessional individual as follows: "The belief that one has power which is pivotal to bring about or prevent subjectively crucial negative outcomes" (Salkovskis, Rachman, Ladouceur, & Freeston, 1992). It is this appraisal of the occurrence and content of intrusions as indicating personal responsibility that results in repeated "neutralizing" behavior. Neutralizing includes both overt behaviors (e.g., washing and checking) (Rachman, 1976a, 1993; Salkovskis, 1985, 1989c) and mental checking and restitution activity (e.g., "putting right" by saying prayers, thinking "good thoughts" in response to "bad thoughts," repeatedly running over details of events in memory) (Rachman, 1971; Salkovskis & Westbrook, 1989). The problem behaviors in obsessions therefore include not only obvious compulsive activities such as repeated checking and washing and their mental equivalents, but also attempts at thought suppression (which paradoxically may increase intrusions and preoccupation; see below). These responsibility-motivated neutralizing efforts reduce discomfort in the short term, but have the longer-term effect of increasing preoccupation and triggering further intrusions.

The Nature of Clinical Obsessions

It is hypothesized that clinical obsessions are intrusive cognitions, the occurrence *and* content of which patients interpret as indications that they may be responsible for harm to themselves or others unless they take action to prevent it. This interpretation results in attempts both to suppress and to neutralize the thought, image, or impulse. "Neutralizing" is defined as voluntarily initiated activity that is intended to have the effect of reducing the perceived responsibility and can be overt or covert (compulsive behavior or thought rituals). As a consequence of neutralizing activity, intrusive cognitions become more salient and frequent; they evoke more discomfort; and the probability of further neutralizing increases. By the same token, attempts to suppress a thought increase the likelihood of its recurrence.

The basis of obsessional problems is the occurrence of intrusive cognitions. Such intrusive cognitions mostly occur as an automatic process, probably linked to an individual's current concerns, and constitute a universal human phenomenon. Intrusive cognitions acquire emotional significance as a result of the way in which they are appraised. It therefore follows that intrusions are initially emotionally neutral, but can take on positive, negative, or no emotional significance, depending on the person's prior experience and the context in which intrusions occur (Edwards & Dickerson, 1987b; England & Dickerson, 1988).

Part of the appraisal of an intrusion will concern the implications of an intrusion and the need for further action. If the intrusion is appraised as having no implications, further processing is unlikely. At least two aspects of the intrusion are subject to appraisal: the occurrence and content. If appraisal suggests a specific reaction (including attempts to suppress or avoid the thought), controlled processing will follow (Anderson, 1985). Behavioral reactions (overt or covert) to intrusive cognitions result in such cognitions becoming salient and therefore acquiring priority of processing. Thus, when an intrusive cognition or its content has some direct implications for the reactions of the individual experiencing it, processing priority will increase, and further appraisal and elaboration will become more likely. This results in the strategic deployment of attention toward the control of mental activity. These attempts include trying to be sure of the accuracy of one's memory, to take account of all factors in one's decisions, to prevent the occurrence of unacceptable material, and to ensure that an outcome has been achieved when the difference between achieving it and not achieving it is imperceptible (e.g., as in deciding that one's hands are properly clean after washing to remove contamination).

Under most circumstances, personally relevant ideas will therefore tend to persist and be the subject of further thought and action; irrelevant ideas can be considered, but no further thought or action will ensue. However, sometimes unpleasant or upsetting cognitions cannot be resolved and become more persistent, as in depression, anxiety, and worry (Figure 5.1a). In instances where the occurrence of a particular type of thought is appraised as an indication that the individuals have become responsible for harm to themselves or others, then the occurrence and content of the thought become both a source of discomfort and an imperative signal for action intended to neutralize the thought and the potentially harmful consequences of its occurrence (Figure 5.1b). This specific acquisition of meaning in terms of "responsibility" distinguishes obsessional cognitions from anxious and depressed cognitions.

Appraisal of responsibility and consequent neutralizing can arise from a sensitivity to responsibility arising from a failure to control thoughts, and from an increase in the level of perceived personal responsibility. The majority of nonclinical subjects do not regard the occurrence of intrusive thoughts as being of special significance. Once neutralizing responses to intrusive thoughts are established, however, they are maintained by the association with the perception of reduced responsibility and discomfort, while the recurrence of the intrusive cognitions becomes more likely as a result of the other processes described above. Thus, obsessional problems will occur in individuals who are distressed by the occurrence of intrusions and who also believe that the occurrence of such cognitions indicates personal responsibility for distressing harm unless corrective action is taken.

The appraisal of intrusive thoughts as having implications for responsibility for harm to self or others is therefore seen as important, because

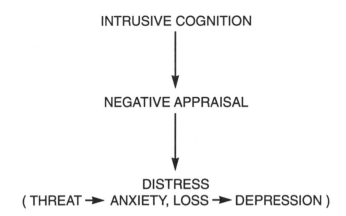

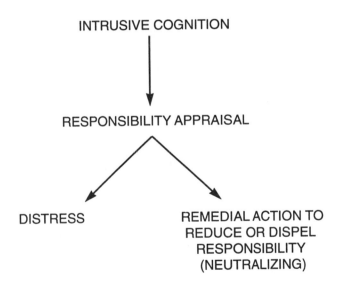

FIGURE 5.1. Appraisal of Intrusive Cognitions (5.1a–above; 5.1b–below)

appraisal links the intrusive thought with both distress *and* the occurrence of neutralizing behavior. If the appraisal solely concerns harm or danger without an element of responsibility, then the effect is more likely to be anxiety or depression; this may become part of a mood–appraisal spiral (Teasdale, 1983), but should not result in clinical obsessions without the additional component of the responsibility–neutralizing link. Hearing someone else making blasphemous statements or talking about harming one's children may not be upsetting in itself. This is not to say that if one perceives what is said as personally significant (e.g., "Perhaps this person wants to harm my children"), some emotional response (anxiety or anger) would not be expected. However, without the specific appraisal of *responsibility,* an obsessional episode should not result.

An obsessional pattern is seen as particularly likely in vulnerable individuals when intrusions are regarded as self-initiated (e.g., resulting in appraisals such as "These thoughts might mean I want to harm the children; I must guard against losing control"). The useful comparison here is between the effects of asking an obsessional checker to lock the door and to watch someone else locking the same door. This responsibility effect is clearly demonstrated by the experiments conducted by Roper and Rachman (1975) and Roper, Rachman, and Hodgson (1973). In these important experiments, situations that usually provoked checking rituals in obsessional patients (e.g., locking the door) produced little or no discomfort or checking when the therapist was present, in sharp contrast to the effects of having to deal with such situations alone (see Rachman, 1993, for a detailed description of responsibility–checking links).

Thus, the core of the cognitive-behavioral formulation is to be found in the occurrence of neutralizing behavior elicited by the appraisal of responsibility. That is, "if the automatic thoughts arising from the intrusion do not include the possibility of being in some way responsible . . . then neutralising is very unlikely to take place, and the result is likely to be heightened anxiety and depression rather than an obsessional problem" (Salkovskis, 1985, p. 579). Part of this appraisal arises from the occurrence of the intrusion itself linked with beliefs about thoughts themselves—for example, "Not neutralising when an intrusion has occurred is similar or equivalent to seeking or wanting the harm involved in the intrusion to happen" or "Thinking something is as bad as doing it" (Salkovskis, 1985, p. 579). Under these circumstances, appraisal will then tend to be of the form "My thinking this thought means . . . ". In this way, an appraisal that is regarded as sensible is based on a thought that is itself regarded as senseless. It is, of course, quite common to be told by anxious patients that "I must be crazy because I have crazy thoughts, and I know that they are crazy thoughts."

The cognitive-behavioral hypothesis thus differs in major ways from theories of some general cognitive deficit. Rather than having a general failure of mental control, memory, or decision making, patients are hypothesized as being especially concerned about these areas. As a consequence, they try too hard to exert control over mental processes and activity in a variety of counterproductive and therefore anxiety-provoking ways. Efforts at overcontrol increase distress, because (1) direct and deliberate attention to mental activity can modify the contents of consciousness; (2) efforts to deliberately control a range of mental activities apparently and actually meet with failure and even opposite effects; (3) attempts to prevent harm and responsibility for harm increase the salience and accessibility of the patients' concerns with harm; and (4) neutralizing behavior directed at preventing harm also prevents disconfirmation (i.e., prevents the patients from discovering that the things they are afraid of will not occur), with the result that exaggerated beliefs about responsibility and harm do not decline.

THE "NORMALIZING" INFLUENCE OF BEHAVIORAL AND COGNITIVE-BEHAVIORAL THEORIES

The Normality of Obsessions

Implicit in the behavioral and cognitive-behavioral theories of obsessions is the proposition that obsessional thoughts are normal phenomena, which have come to acquire special significance in terms of the way in which they are appraised. This idea receives support from a series of experiments on "normal obsessions," in which it was found that unwanted and unacceptable intrusive thoughts occurred in up to 90% of nonclinical subjects (Rachman & de Silva, 1978; Salkovskis & Harrison, 1984; Parkinson & Rachman, 1980; Freeston, Ladouceur, Gagnon, & Thibodeau, 1991). This work implies that people suffering from obsessional disorders are not abnormal in terms of the occurrence of intrusions; instead, they are experiencing an exaggeration of normal anxiety in the way that people suffering from generalized anxiety disorder may be suffering from (excessive) worry, and even that people suffering from panic disorder may be showing a relatively extreme variant of the tendency to misinterpret bodily sensations catastrophically (Salkovskis, 1988). Thus, in obsessions as in other anxiety problems, difficulties arise not because of any disease-specific "lesion," but rather because of normal anxiety triggering off mechanisms that prevent the otherwise normal decay and disappearance of the anxiety. Clearly, treatment then centers first on identifying the source of the initial anxiety reaction and any factors contributing to the maintenance of such anxiety, and then on helping the sufferer deal with these maintaining factors. It follows that the treatment does not aim to abolish intrusive thoughts, because these are seen as normal in and of themselves, in much the same way as other anxiety treatments do not aim to prevent the experience of all anxiety. This "normalizing" approach to obsessions is, in my own experience, particularly empowering for the sufferer; it also has the advantage of probably being true.

The Normal Function of Intrusive Thoughts: The Good, the Bad, the Ugly, and the Irrelevant

Other types of anxiety are normalized within the cognitive-behavioral framework by considering the importance of threat evaluation in responding to potential danger. Given the normalizing emphasis of the cognitive-behavioral hypothesis of obsessions, it would seem important to clarify just what the normal function of intrusive thoughts might be. The present hypothesis has major implications for our understanding of the psychological function of intrusive thoughts.

An implication of the model proposed here is that the initial occurrence of intrusive thoughts is unrelated to unacceptability or discomfort, which results from the evaluation of the person experiencing the intrusive thought. It can be hypothesized that the occurrence of intrusions reflects thoughts about people's areas of current concern or interest, and represents an important aspect of their active problem-solving capacity. Ideas occur constantly, and many are of considerable value. The comparison with problem-solving approaches is instructive, particularly as it has been suggested that this type of problem solving is a fundamental psychological process (Anderson, 1985). The best results of "brainstorming," in which people attempt to generate potential solutions to their current situation, are obtained when no attempt is made to censor the flow of ideas, because to do so would inhibit ideas and lead to premature rejection of potentially useful solutions. In order to evaluate an idea as useful or useless, further processing and cognitive rehearsal have to be carried out. This analysis of problem solving as a psychological process can clarify the value of generating ideas, regardless of their later evaluation. Furthermore, ideas that are "unacceptable" under normal circumstances can, under changed or extreme conditions, become useful and acceptable. Only when a particular set of beliefs suggests that such unfettered consideration of the full range of ideas can be harmful does the occurrence of such ideas become problematic.

This account also explains the intrusiveness of obsessional thoughts. For ideas to be useful, they have to be noticed and evaluated; hence the compelling nature of this class of thoughts. The tendency for disturbed mood to increase the occurrence of intrusions (Reynolds & Salkovskis,

1992) then serves an important and positive psychological function. Ideas are needed most urgently when there are indications that psychological or physical equilibrium is threatened. A problem-solving system that is responsive to emotional arousal would be particularly adaptive.

If it is assumed that the concept of an "idea generator" explains the occurrence of intrusive thoughts, then it can also account for the association between neutralizing behavior and the persistence of intrusions. It is clear that at most times people experience sequences of thoughts — some useful and relevant, others not. The vast majority of these thoughts do not persist; those that do tend to be particularly *salient*. Salience is evaluated early, and if the intrusive thought is not salient, then it is not processed further. On the other hand, intrusions with potentially important implications for what people are doing or are going to do will be subjected to further processing, regardless of their initial acceptability. Further processing and elaboration result in the content of the intrusive thought's being matched with and possibly incorporated into current concerns. If further processing suggests that there are consequences for voluntary action (including a possible requirement for future retrieval, further cognitive rehearsal, and processing), then the elaboration of the relevant concept will incorporate this and allocate processing priority to the concept. This applies equally to positively evaluated ideas (e.g., when a scientist solves a theoretical problem) and to negatively evaluated ones (e.g., when a person believes that he or she may have made a serious error). The overall effect is to facilitate future retrieval.

Figure 5.2 illustrates the simplest model to account for the factors hypothesized to determine the priority of processing of intrusive thoughts, whether positive or negative. Consistent with this view, Edwards and Dickerson (1987b) evaluated the occurrence and characteristics of positive and negative intrusions in a nonclinical population, and found positive intrusions were somewhat more common. The primary characteristics of positive and negative intrusions were found to be very similar, as indexed by controllability, relation to external triggers, form, lifespan, and duration. The variables that differed were those that would be regarded as the result of secondary evaluations in the present analysis: subjects' rating of congruence with beliefs, general acceptability, and harmfulness. Also consistent with the present hypothesis, high scores on the Depression subscale of the Profile of Mood States were associated with decreased controllability in both negative and positive intrusions.

Thus, intrusive thoughts persist to the extent to which they have implications for intentional behavior on the part of the person experiencing them. If an intrusive thought has no implications for further deliberate thought and/or action (such as mental problem solving), it will not persist. On the other hand, if an intrusive thought *does* have implications

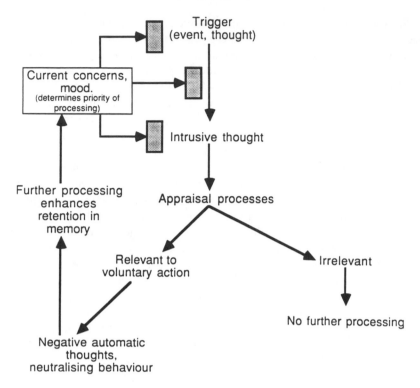

FIGURE 5.2. Factors involved in priority of processing of intrusions. Shaded box = Modulating influences.

for intentional behavior, then further processing will take place. A cognitive system that works in this way has several advantages; in particular, it allows the selection of important ideas from the welter of cognitive activity, and ensures that ideas most relevant to current concerns (positive or negative) will persist. In obsessions, these processes have gone awry because of attempts to overcontrol.

SPECIFIC ASPECTS OF
THE COGNITIVE-BEHAVIORAL HYPOTHESIS

Trying to Control Intrusive Thoughts

Experimental evidence on the paradoxical effects of overcontrol are nowhere more apparent than in attempts to suppress unwanted thoughts. By definition, people suffering from OCD try to suppress their obsessional thoughts. The idea that active attempts to suppress particular thoughts may result in more of the thoughts has long been an assumption in clinical practice. This concept is often used to help sufferers understand why obsessional thoughts occur so frequently, despite their attempts to suppress them. For example, as a behavioral experiment, obsessional patients are invited to try their hardest *not* to think of a giraffe; the subsequent occurrence of giraffe images is then used as the basis for educational discussion (Salkovskis & Kirk, 1989).

Recently, Wegner (1989; Wegner, Schneider, Carter, & White, 1987) has carried out a series of experiments on factors influencing mental control of emotionally neutral stimuli, with a praticular focus on thought suppression. The results of these studies suggested that efforts to suppress did not result in an initial enhancement, but that suppression was achieved in the short term. However, during the immediately subsequent period, an enhancement (described as a "rebound") *was* observed. By contrast, another group (Lavy and van den Hout, 1990) did find the expected paradoxical enhancement of emotionally neutral stimuli, and did not find a rebound. Subsequently, Clark, Ball, and Pape (1991) and Clark, Winton, and Thynn (1992) again failed to find an immediate enhancement effect, using vivid emotionally neutral stimuli (green rabbits) from a previously heard taped story. Clark and colleagues suggested that the studies that found enhancement had failed to control for the effects of the frequency with which the to-be-suppressed target was mentioned prior to the suppression task.

There are major methodological differences between such studies, and these present major problems of interpretation. For example, some studies used a thought-counting procedure, whereas others used "streaming," in which subjects are asked to verbalize their stream of consciousness (which is later coded, often with the "target" thought being represented as a percentage of total thoughts). Target stimuli have also varied in terms of how commonplace and relevant they are, ranging from green rabbits to kitchen utensils; most did not concern "intrusive" thoughts as usually defined, and did not focus on naturally occurring thoughts. A colleague and I (Salkovskis & Campbell, 1994) targeted personally relevant and naturally occurring negative intrusive thoughts, which subjects reported that they normally attempted to suppress to some extent. Thus, a characteristic of such intrusions was that subjects found them personally unacceptable and were self-motivated to remove or suppress such intrusions. In the study, 75 nonclinical subjects were allocated to one of five experimental conditions: thought suppression, mention control, and suppression under three different distraction conditions. This initial experimental period was followed by a standard "think anything" period. The design therefore allowed assessment of both suppression and rebound effects. Thought frequency was measured by means of a counter. This study showed that the subjects who wer asked simply to suppress experienced significantly more intrusive thoughts during both the first and the second experimental periods, compared to the mention control group. Distraction instructions significantly decreased frequency only when a specific engaging task was provided. Effects on evaluative components of the intrusive thoughts (discomfort and acceptability) were observed only in the condition that involved the specific distracting task.

Clearly, laboratory studies involving brief suppression periods (typically a few minutes) have limited applicability to obsessions, in which subjects describe struggling to exclude thoughts *most of the time.* In a study designed to investigate the longer-term impact of thought suppression in naturally occurring intrusive thoughts, we (Trinder & Salkovskis, 1994) asked subjects to record intrusions only, to suppress, or to "think through" over a period of 4 days. Again, suppression was found to enhance intrusion. This study is key in bridging the gap between the phenomenology of OCD and thought suppression experiments. A further important development is linking the effects of suppression to the perception of heightened responsibility, as described below.

Distorted Beliefs as the Foundation of Overcontrol

Appraisal

From a cognitive-behavioral perspective, both anxiety and avoidance/escape behaviors (including attempts to [over]control mental activity) are belief-driven (Salkovskis, 1991). That is, the perception of threat leads both to anxiety and to active attempts to achieve safety. In anxiety, appraisal is not confined to the perceived probability of danger, but can be represented as follows:

$$\text{Anxiety} \propto \frac{\substack{\text{Perceived likelihood} \\ \text{of anticipated danger}} \quad \times \quad \substack{\text{Perceived awfulness/cost} \\ \text{of anticipated danger}}}{\substack{\text{Perceived ability to} \\ \text{cope with danger}} \quad + \quad \substack{\text{Perceived external factors} \\ \text{that would assist ("rescue")}}}$$

The top line summarizes what is often referred to as "primary appraisal," the bottom line "secondary appraisal." In fact, the view presented here (derived from Beck & Emery with Greenberg, 1985) differs somewhat from that of Lazarus, in that the appraisal of coping and rescue is regarded as part of the initial appraisal of threat. Despite being virtually instantaneous, the appraisal of threat in a particular situation is clearly a complex process, based on a combination of past experience, present context, mood state, and so on. Although not truly mathematical, this "equation" neatly summarizes the idea that very low probabilities of danger may become very anxiety-provoking if associated with very high cost, and that efforts to control and cope with danger are part of the overall perception of threat. It seems likely that in OCD, patients may regard being "responsible" as being highly likely, and also perceive being responsible in any way as a particularly awful thing (see Salkovskis, 1989b for a clinical example).

Assumptions

The cognitive-behavioral theory proposes that people are predisposed to making particular appraisals because of assumptions that are learned over longer periods from childhood onward, or that may be formed as a result of unusual or extreme events and circumstances. Some assumptions characteristic of OCD patients are described in Salkovskis (1985, p. 579) and include the following:

> "Having a thought about an action is like performing the action."
> "Failing to prevent (or failing to try to prevent) harm to self or others is the same as having caused the harm in the first place."
> "Responsibility is not reduced by other factors such as something being improbable."
> "Not neutralising when an intrusion has occurred is similar or equivalent to seeking or wanting the harm involved in the intrusion to happen."
> "One should (and can) exercise control over one's thoughts."

If someone holds these attitudes very strongly, then the overt and covert behaviors characteristic of people suffering from obsessional problems tend to follow naturally.

"Thinking Errors"

The effects of these type of assumptions are often described in terms of "thinking errors" (Beck, 1976), which are characteristic distortions that influence whole classes of reactions. Thinking errors are not pathological in and of themselves; in fact, most people make judgments by employing a range of "heuristics," many of which can be fallacious (Nisbett & Ross, 1980).

The cognitive-behavioral hypothesis suggests that OCD patients show a number of characteristic thinking errors linked to their obsessional difficulties. Probably the most typical and important is the idea that "Any influence over outcome = responsibility for outcome." A particularly interesting possibility is the relationship between responsibility through action as opposed to inaction. As outlined above, I have suggested (Salkovskis, 1985, p. 579) that the belief that "Failing to prevent (or failing to try to prevent) harm to self or others is the same as having caused the harm in the first place" may be a key assumption in the generation of obsessional problems. Recently, Spranca, Minsk, and Baron (1991) demonstrated what they refer to as "omission bias" in nonclinical subjects. They showed that normal subjects judge responsibility for negative consequences to be diminished when an omission is involved, as opposed to when some specific action is involved in bringing about the negative consequence. This is true in normal subjects even when the element of intention (i.e., the extent to which the person wishes the "negative" outcome to occur) is controlled for. Thus, most people appear to regard themselves as more responsible for what they actively do than for what they fail to do. Clinical experience (and recent pilot work by our group) suggests that obsessional patients do not seem to show evidence of this type of omission bias. If this observation is experimentally validated, it opens up a range of new possiblities for the understanding of obsessional behavior.

The general belief that "Any influence over outcome = responsibility for outcome" could be expected to increase concern with omissions; consideration of the phenomenology of obsessional problems suggests several other more specific ways in which omissions may become relatively more important to a vulnerable individual. An important factor in judgments concerning responsibility is the perception of "agency," meaning that one has chosen to bring something about. Particular importance is usually given to "premeditation," in the sense of being able to foresee possible harmful outcomes. Thus:

> Responsible means 'to some extent culpable (either morally or in law according to the context) for *one's own* acts or omissions'. The ascription of responsibility in this sense on what we believe to have been the person's mental state at or before the time of the act or omission. 'Premeditation' usually makes an objectionable act seem more culpable. *If the actor foresaw a real possibility of his causing harm*—for example by his way of driving—his act or omission will be called 'reckless' and blamed accordingly. (*Oxford Companion to the Mind*, 1987, p. 681; emphasis added)

And:

> More often it is the actor's state of mind at the time of the act . . . that determines the degree to which he is regarded as blameworthy. If the act seems to have been quite accidental—if for instance he knocks over a child whom he did not see in his path—he is not blamed, unless we think that he should have been aware of this as a real possibility. (*Oxford Companion to the Mind*, 1987, p. 681)

One of the problems experienced by obsessional patients is that it is often in the nature of the condition that they frequently foresee a wide range of possible negative outcomes. That is, the intrusive thoughts often concern things that could go wrong unless dealt with (e.g., passing on contamination, having hurt someone accidentally, having left the door unlocked or the gas turned on). Sometimes obsessionals feel that it is not even permissible to try not to foresee problems/disasters, because this would mean that he or she had deliberately chosen this course, which again would increase responsibility. When aware of this, some patients regard it as a *duty* to try to foresee negative outcomes. However, if in any case a negative outcome *is* foreseen even as an intrusive thought, responsibility is established, because to do nothing the person would have to decide not to act to prevent the harmful outcome. That is, deciding *not* to act despite being aware of possible disastrous consequences becomes an active decision, making the person a causal agent in relation to those disastrous consequences. Thus, the occurrence of intrusive/obsessional thoughts transforms a situation where harm can only occur by omission into a situation where the person has "actively" chosen to allow the harm to take place. This may mean that the apparent absence of omission bias in obsessionals is mediated by the occurrence of obsessional thoughts.

Deciding not to do something results in a sense of "agency." Thus, a patient will not be concerned about sharp objects he or she has not seen, and will not be concerned if he or she did not consider the possibility of harm. However, if something is seen and it occurs to the person that he or she could or should take preventative action, the situation changes because *not* acting becomes an active decision. In this way, the actual occurrence of intrusive thoughts of harm and/or responsibility for it comes to play a key role in the perception of responsibility for the thoughts' contents. Suppression as described earlier will increase this effect further by increasing the thoughts in precisely the situations where the obsessional most wishes to exclude any intrusion. Thus, having locked the door, the person tries not to think that it could be open, experiences the thought again, and is therefore constrained to act or risk being responsible through having chosen not to check. The motivation to suppress will increase, but it is very difficult to suppress a thought that is directly connected to an action just completed; thus the action serves as a further cue for intrusion/suppression and so on, in the nightmarish way in which obsessionals find themselves being tortured.

Decision Making: Trying Too Hard

Many of the problematic areas for obsessional patients concern activities that are usually relatively automatic for other people, in that no particular conscious effort is devoted to them—for example, deciding when to stop washing, recalling what has been said during a conversation, or deciding whether a door is locked or the gas has been turned off. Again, obsessionals appear to be trying too hard in ways that interfere with the decision-making process itself. This problem may again be mediated by the occurrence of intrusions; to disregard intrusions concerning harm would be actively to disregard threat, as described above. Obsessionals tend to use two main solutions: (1) They repeat the action until they are sure that it "feels right," or (2) they conduct the activity in such a way as to ensure some objective token of "completeness." In both instances, the eventual outcome will tend to trump any intrusive doubts.

In the first instance, obsessionals use their affective state to confirm their decision to stop neutralizing activity. The basis for such judgments varies from person to person, but most commonly involves feeling "comfortable" to a particular level, having "the right attitude," or carrying out the neutralizing without experiencing the obsessional thought. In the first two of these instances, pre-existing mood disturbance (depression or anxiety) makes finishing particularly difficult, as the obsessional needs to achieve the sense of rightness regardless of general mood. Trying not to have the obsessional thought while ritualizing is a particularly difficult version of thought suppression, in that there is almost invariably a link between the obsession and the neutralizing activity. If someone washes because of a belief that he or she may be contaminated, terminating washing without thoughts of contamination presents special difficulties.

The set of strategies used to ensure completeness generally involves introducing some distinctive sequence that ensures that the neutralizing is recalled clearly enough "to be sure." Unfortunately, the frequency with which ordinary activities are carried out tends to result in difficulties in remembering any particular instance. The greater the repetition, the less distinctive any particular instance becomes. Patients adopt sequences to overcome this, but these become subject to the same doubts. A further complication is mental checking. Frequently, obsessionals describe going over things repeatedly in their minds. This can result in difficulties in remembering whether what is being recalled is actually having carried out the activity or an *image* of the activity. Shortcuts can be used to increase the distinctiveness, but almost by definition these rapidly lose their power. For example, a patient who tended to check came for an initial assessment with me. When asked how long it took to leave her car, she said that she would usually check for about 30 minutes. When asked about coming to this appointment, she said that she had only checked once for a few seconds by tugging the door handle in a rhythm that represented "ho-spi-tal," so that she was sure that she had done it. However, she also said that this strategy would only be effective on this visit, as she could not in future be sure whether she was recalling that day's appointment or a previous one.

TREATMENT IMPLICATIONS
OF THE COGNITIVE-BEHAVIORAL THEORY

Marks (1981) highlighted both the unstructured application of "cognitive" techniques and the limitations of the exposure-based approach when he argued that "calm, gentle, yet firm persuasion is helpful, but if the patient resists strongly, little can be done" (p. 97). Cognitive therapy can bring a systematic approach to the solution of this problem for the substantial proportion of patients for whom behavioral treatment can do little. Usually, where it is concluded that "little can be done," this in fact means that something *completely different* needs to be done. If, as seems likely, exposure is effective through bringing about belief change, cognitive strategies that combine and interact with behavioral techniques would seem optimal. Such an approach therefore not only would involve identifying and modifying the thoughts and beliefs that prevent the patient from engaging in or benefiting from exposure treatment, but also would take a general form indicated by the cognitive conceptualization (Salkovskis & Warwick, 1985, 1988; Salkovskis, 1989a). Modification of anxious or depressed mood concurrent with the obsessions can also be helpful (Salkovskis & Warwick, 1988).

The cognitive-behavioral theory predicts that successful treatment requires modification both of the beliefs involved in and leading to the misinterpretation of intrusive thoughts as indicating heightened responsibility, and of the associated behaviors involved in the maintenance of these beliefs. Prior to treatment, obsessional patients are distressed because they have a particularly threatening perception of their obsessional experience—for example, that their thoughts mean that they are child molesters, or that they are in constant danger of passing disease on to other people, and so on.[1] The essence of treatment is in helping the sufferers to construct and test a new, less threatening model of their experience. For instance, obsessional washers are helped to shift their view of their problem away from the idea that they might be contaminated (and therefore must ensure that they do not pass this on to someone else or come to harm themselves), and toward the idea that they have a specific problem to their *fears* of contamination. That is, patients are helped to understand their problem as one of thinking and deciding, rather than the "real-world" risks that they fear.

Most of the cognitive material is evoked and dealt with in the course of exposure, when the key beliefs are activated. The main elements of treatment are as follows:

1. Working with patients to develop a comprehensive cognitive-behavioral model of the maintenance of their obsessional problems. This involves the identification of key distorted beliefs and the collaborative

construction of a non threatening alternative account of their obsessional experience, to allow the patients to explicitly test beliefs about responsibility.

2. Detailed identification and self-monitoring of obsessional thoughts and patients' appraisal of these thoughtsm combined with exercises designed to help the patients to modify their responsibility beliefs on a minute-by-minute basis (e.g., by using a daily record of dysfunctional thoughts).

3. Discussion techniques for challenging appraisals and the basic assumptions upon which these are based. The aim is modification of the patients' negative beliefs about the extent of their own personal responsibility (e.g., by having the patients describe all contributing factors for a feared outcome and then depicting these factors' contributions in a pie chart).

4. Behavioral experiments that directly test appraisals, assumptions, and processes hypothesized to be involved in the patients' obsessional problems (e.g., demonstrating that attempts to suppress a thought lead to an increase in the frequency with which it occurs, or showing that beliefs such as "If I think, it I therefore want it to happen" are incorrect). All such behavioral experiments are idiosyncratically devised, in order to help patients test their previous (threatening) explanation of their experience against the new (nonthreatening) explanation worked out with their therapists.

5. Helping patients to identify and modify the underlying general assumptions (e.g., "Not trying to prevent harm is as bad as making it happen deliberately") that give rise to their misinterpretation of their own mental activity.

For example, some patients believe that if they imagine performing an act (such as stabbing their children), this increases the probability that they will carry out the action. Such patients are encouraged to test that belief by finding out directly whether thinking about things really can make them happen. The same patients may be later encouraged to try actively to bring about the feared consequence by adopting particular thinking patterns, in order to fully demonstrate the limits of their responsibility. This type of sequence is designed to help the patients reappraise their obsessional problem as being an understandable result of trying too hard to control their mental activity, rather than as one of being dangerously out of control and likely to act on their thoughts and therefore to cause harm. In cognitive therapy, the patients are thus helped to understand and test the way their beliefs and related efforts to prevent harm not only are unnecessary but also create the problems they experience. The aim is to allow them to see the problem as one of thinking, rather than one of actual danger of harm.

This style of therapy is particularly powerful in patients who are afraid of fully committing themselves to ERP, because the cognitive elements target the beliefs that produce distress as well as initiate and motivate compulsive behavior. Rather than simply asking patients to stop carrying out their compulsive behavior, cognitive therapy seeks to identify and challenge the misinterpretations that lead the patients to ritualize, so that stopping compulsive behavior is perceived by the patients as less dangerous and therefore irrelevant. The early development of cognitive therapy was in fact carried out with patients who were refusing or failing to respond to ERP (Salkovskis & Warwick, 1985). Direct modification of the misinterpretation of intrusive thoughts and related beliefs should also bring about a more complete and thorough change, as well as being more likely to engage the patients in treatment, with a consequent reduction in treatment refusal and dropout rates.

Apart from the specific development of cognitive-behavioral treatment for OCD in patients resistant to ERP (Salkovskis & Warwick, 1985), the cognitive-behavioral theory has also been applied to the development of an effective treatment for patients suffering from obsessional ruminations. Given the emphasis on the maintaining role of compulsive behavior in behavioral theory and treatment, patients who do not appear to ritualize are theoretically anomalous and impossible to treat with traditional methods. No behavioral treatment has been shown in controlled trials to be effective in the treatment of pure ruminators. Only 46% of patients treated in previous studies experienced 50% reduction in rumination frequency, and only 12% experienced a 50% reduction in distress (reviewed in detail in Salkovskis & Westbrook, 1989). The cognitive-behavioral theory indicates that *covert* compulsions are present, and that these need to be tackled in therapy. For example, a patient who pictures his or her child dead neutralizes this thought by thinking of the child alive, and mentally prays that this should not come about. Such covert compulsive behavior is rapid and difficult to identify and control, unlike handwashing or checking. These factors highlight the necessity of engaging the patient in the exercise of self-control over the identification and modification of ritualizing—a task for which cognitive therapy is particularly well suited.

The use of the cognitive conceptualization and of procedures such as those outlined above for OCD provides a framework for therapists to help such patients to detect, understand, and gain control over their mental compulsions. The covert nature of these rituals makes them difficult to stop without dealing with the patients' appraisal of the intrusions (and of the feared harm that could arise from *not* ritualizing). Cognitive-behavioral treatment both targets appraisal and uses an audiotape loop in order to maximize exposure and make response prevention easier for the patients. As an additional focus, an audiotape loop is used to provoke obsessional thoughts; subsequent within-session discussion identifies both the disturbing interpretations made by the patients and any impulses to control or neutralize these thoughts (Salkovskis, 1983; Salkovskis & Westbrook, 1989). Patients are taught to identify neutralizing (compulsive) behavior by attention to its effortful nature (in contrast to obsessional intrusions, which occur automatically). Cognitive techniques are used to modify the interpretations, and hence to reduce distress and facilitate the patients' attempts to cease to control mentally or neutralize obsessional thoughts. The use of the tape and cognitive procedures is then extended outside therapy sessions to specific focused homework exercises; in addition, patients are assisted in taking the exposure and belief change exercises into target (obsession-provoking) situations (by means of personal stereos with headphones). Early in treatment, homework involves daily tape-assisted exercises and thought answering at preset times. Subsequently, the same procedures are used in situations that are identified as usually provoking the obsessional thoughts. Later in treatment, patients will be helped to apply these techniques at times when the obsessional thoughts occur unexpectedly in the course of the day. The aim is to ensure complete emotional processing, in the sense that the obsessional patients come to see intrusive thoughts as a harmless (and potentially useful) aspect of normal psychological functioning. In a series of single-case experiments, we found that a combination of cognitive procedures and exposure aided by an audiotape loop were effective where more traditional habituation and thought-stopping techniques were not (Salkovskis & Westbrook, 1989).

SUMMARY AND CONCLUSION

Both phenomenology and current experimental studies are most consistent with the hypothesis that obsessional problems are the result of the specific appraisal of intrusive thoughts, rather than of a general neurological or cognitive deficit. Negative appraisals may give rise to deficits in some areas as a result of the strategies employed by obsessional patients (e.g., the effects on the Stroop test observed in anxious patients).

The principal aim of cognitive-behavioral treatment for obsessional problems therefore follows directly from the theory. Therapy aims to help patients conclude that obsessional thoughts, however distressing, are irrelevant to further action. Teaching the patients to control the occurrence of intrusive thoughts will be beneficial only if it alters the way in which their occurrence is interpreted, such as by convincing the patients that intrusive thoughts are at least partially under their own control and therefore of no special significance. Thus, the key to control of obsessional thoughts may be to learn that the exercise of such control is unnecessary.

Apart from the obvious therapy outcome trials, further experimental investigations are required into pathways to overresponsibility and the best ways to reduce responsibility in both the short and the long term. In addition, specific investigations are needed into ways in which the psychological formulation accounts for what appear to be general deficits, but which the cognitive-behavioral theory suggests are the results of the sufferers' trying too hard.

NOTE

1. This is similar to the treatment of panic patients who believe that their palpitations mean they are dying. Therapy is intended to help them to form and test a psychological model of their problem as arising from their misinterpretation.

REFERENCES

Abel, J. L. (1993). Exposure with response prevention and serotonergic antidepressants in the treatment of obsessive compulsive disorder: A review and implications for interdisciplinary treatment. *Behaviour Research and Therapy, 31,* 463–478.

Anderson, J. R. (1985), *Cognitive psychology and its implications.* New York: W. H. Freeman.

Barr, L. C., Goodman, W. K., Price, L. H., McDougle, C. J., & Charney, D. S. (1992). The serotonin hypothesis of obsessive–compulsive disorder: Implications of pharmacologic challenge studies. *Journal of Clinical Psychiatry, 53*(Suppl.), 17–28.

Beck, A. T. (1976). *Cognitive therapy and the emotional disorders.* New York: International Universities Press.

Beck, A. T., & Emery, G., with Greenberg, R. L. (1985). *Anxiety disorders and phobias: A cognitive perspective.* New York: Basic Books.

Beech, H. R., & Liddel, A. (1974). Decision making, mood states and ritualistic behaviour among obsessional patients. In H. R. Beech (Ed.), *Obsessional states.* London: Methuen.

Christensen, H., Hadzi-Pavlovic, D., Andrews, G., & Mattick, R. (1987). Behavior therapy and tricyclic medication in the treatment of obsessive–compulsive disorder: A quantitative review. *Journal of Consulting and Clinical Psychology, 55,* 701–711.

Clark, D. M. (1986). A cognitive approach to panic. *Behaviour Research and Therapy, 24,* 461–470.

Clark, D. M., Ball, S., & Pape, D. (1991). An experimental investigation of thought suppression. *Behaviour Research and Therapy, 29,* 253–257.

Clark, D. M., Winton, E., & Thynn, L. (1993). A further experimental investigation of thought suppression. *Behaviour Research and Therapy, 31,* 207–210.

Edwards, S., & Dickerson, M. (1987a). Intrusive unwanted thoughts: A two stage model of control. *British Journal of Medical Psychology, 60,* 317–328.

Edwards, S., & Dickerson, M. (1987b). On the similarity of positive and negative intrusions. *Behaviour Research and Therapy, 25,* 207–211.

England, S. L., & Dickerson, M. (1988). Intrusive thoughts: Unpleasantness not the major cause of uncontrollability. *Behaviour Research and Therapy, 26,* 279–277.

Foa, E. B., & Goldstein, A. (1978). Continuous exposure and strict response prevention in the treatment of obsessive–compulsive neurosis. *Behavior Therapy, 9,* 821–829.

Foa, E. B., Steketee, G., Grayson, J. B., & Doppelt, H. B. (1983). Treatment of Obsessive-compulsives: When do we fail? In Foa, E. B., & Emmelkamp, P. M. G. (Eds.), *Failures in Behavior Therapy.* New York: Wiley.

Freeston, M. H., Ladouceur, R., Gagnon, F., & Thibodeau, N. (1991). Cognitive intrusions in a non-clinical population: I. Response style, subjective experience and appraisal. *Behaviour Research and Therapy, 29,* 285–297.

Gregory, R. L. (Ed.). (1987). *Oxford Companion to the Mind* (p. 681). New York: Oxford University Press.

Goodman, W. K., McDougle, C. J., & Price, L. H., (1992). The role of serotonin and dopamine in the pathophysiology of obsessive–compulsive disorder. *International Clinical Psychopharmacology, 7*(Suppl. 1), 35–38.

Gorman, J. M., Liebowitz, M. R., Fyer, A. J., & Stein, J. (1989). A neuroanatomical hypothesis for panic disorder. *American Journal of Psychiatry, 146,* 148–161.

Insel, T. R. (1992). Neurobiology of obsessive-compulsive disorder: a review. *International Clinical Psychopharmacology, 7*(Suppl. 1), 31–34.

Kasvikis, Y., & Marks, I. M. (1988). Clomipramine, self-exposure, and therapist-accompanied exposure in obsessive–compulsive ritualizers: Two year follow-up. *Journal of Anxiety Disorders, 2,* 291–298.

Lavy, E., & van den Hout, M. (1990). Thought suppression induces intrusions. *Behavioural Psychotherapy, 18,* 251–258.

Maki, W. S., O'Neill, H. K., & O'Neill, G. W. (1994). Do nonclinical checkers exhibit deficits in cognitive control? *Behaviour Research and Therapy, 32,* 183–192.

Marks, I. M. (1981). *Cure and care of neurosis.* New York: Wiley.

Marks, I. M., Lelliott, P., Basoglu, M., & Noshirvani, H. (1988). Clomipramine, self-exposure and therapist aided exposure for obsessive-compulsive rituals. *British Journal of Psychiatry, 152,* 522–5334.

Marks, I. M., Stern, R. S., Mawson, D., Cobb, J., & McDonald, R. (1980). Clomipramine and exposure for obsessive rituals: I. *British Journal of Psychiatry, 136,* 1–25.

Meyer, V. (1966). Modification of expectations in cases with obsessional rituals. *Behaviour Research and Therapy, 4,* 273–280.

Mowrer, O. H. (1947). On the dual nature of learning—a reinterpretation of "conditioning" and "problem solving". *Harvard Educational Review, 17,* 102–148.

Mowrer, O. H. (1960). *Learning Theory and Behaviour,* New York: Wiley.

Nisbett, R. E., & Ross, L. (1980). *Human inference: Strategies and shortcomings of social judgement.* Englewood Cliffs, NJ: Prentice-Hall.

Parkinson, L., & Rachman, S. J. (1980). Are intrusive thoughts subject to habituation? *Behaviour Research and Therapy, 18,* 409–418.

Rachman, S. J. (1971). Obsessional ruminations. *Behaviour Research and Therapy, 9,* 229–235.

Rachman, S. J. (1976a). The modification of obsessions: A new formulation. *Behaviour Research and Therapy, 14,* 437–443.

Rachman, S. J. (1976b). The passing of the two stage theory of fear and avoidance. *Behaviour Research and Therapy, 14,* 125–131.

Rachman, S. J. (1978). Anatomy of obsessions. *Behavior Analysis and Modification, 2,* 253–278.

Rachman, S. J. (1993). Obsessions, responsibility and guilt. *Behaviour Research and Therapy, 31,* 149–154.

Rachman, S. J., & de Silva, P. (1978). Abnormal and normal obsessions. *Behaviour Research and Therapy, 16,* 233–238.

Rachman, S. J., & Hodgson, R. (1980). *Obsessions and compulsions.* Englewood Cliffs, NJ: Prentice-Hall.

Reed, G. F. (1985). *Obsessional experience and compulsive behaviour.* London: Academic Press.

Reynolds, M., & Salkovskis, P. M. (1992). Comparison of positive and negative intrusive thoughts and experimental investigation of the differential effects of mood. *Behaviour Research and Therapy, 30,* 273–281.

Riggs, D., & Foa, E. B. (1993). Obsessive-compulsive disorders. In D. H. Barlow (Ed.), *Clinical Handbook of Psycholgical Disorders.* New York: Guilford Press.

Robertson, M. (1990). Obsessional disorder and the Gilles de la Tourette Syndrome. In S. A. Montgomery, W. K. Goodman, & N. Goeting (Eds.), *Current approaches to obsessive-compulsive disorder.* London: Duphar.

Robins, L. N., Helzer, J, E., Weissman, M. M., Orvaschell, H., Gruenber, E., Burke, J. D., & Regier, D. A. (1984). Lifetime prevalence of specific psychiatric disorders in three sites. *Archives of General Psychiatry, 41,* 949–958.

Roper, G., & Rachman, S. J. (1975). Obsessional–compulsive checking: Replication and development. *Behaviour Research and Therapy, 13,* 25–32.

Roper, G., Rachman, S. J., & Hodgson, R. (1973). An experiment on obsessional checking. *Behaviour Research and Therapy, 11,* 271–277.

Salkovskis, P. M. (1983). Treatment of an obsessional patient using habituation to audiotaped ruminations. *British Journal of Clinical Psychology, 22,* 311–313.

Salkovskis, P. M. (1985). Obsessional–compulsive problems: A cognitive-behavioural analysis. *Behaviour Research and Therapy, 25,* 571–583.

Salkovskis, P. M. (1988). Intrusive thoughts and obsessional disorders. In D. Glasgow & N. Eisenberg (Eds.), *Current issues in clinical psychology* (Vol. 4). London: Gower.

Salkovskis, P. M. (1989a).Cognitive-behavioural factors and the persistence of intrusive thoughts in obsessional problems. *Behaviour Research and Therapy, 27,* 677–682.

Salkovskis, P. M. (1989b).. Obsessions and compulsions. In J. Scott, J. M. G. Williams, & A. T. Beck (Eds.), *Cognitive therapy: A clinical casebook.* London: Croom Helm.

Salkovskis, P. M. (1989c). Obsessions and intrusive thoughts: Clinical and non-clinical aspects. In P. Emmelkamp, W. Everaerd, F. Kraaymaat, & M. van Son (Eds.), *Annual series of European research in behaviour therapy: Vol. 4. Anxiety disorders.* Amsterdam: Swets.

Salkovskis, P. M. (1991). The importannce of behavior in the maintenance of anxiety and panic: A cognitive account. *Behavioural Psychotherapy, 19,* 6–19.

Salkovskis, P. M., & Campbell, P. (1994). Thought suppression in naturally occurring negative intrusive thoughts. *Behaviour Research and Therapy, 32,* 1–8.

Salkovskis, P. M., & Harrison, J. (1984). Abnormal and normal obsessions: A replication. *Behaviour Research and Therapy, 22,* 549–552.

Salkovskis, P. M., & Kirk, J. (1989). Obsessional disorders. In K. Hawton, P. M. Salkovskis, J. Kirk, & D. M. Clark (Eds.), *Cognitive-behavioural treatment for psychiatric disorders: A practical guide.* Oxford: Oxford University Press.

Salkovskis, P. M., Rachman, S. J., Ladouceur, R., & Freeston, M. (1992). *Proceedings of the Toronto Cafeteria.*

Salkovskis, P. M., & Warwick, H. M. C. (1985). Cognitive therapy of obsessive–compulsive disorder: Treating treatment failures. *Behavioural Psychotherapy, 13,* 243–255.

Salkovskis, P. M., & Warwick, H. M. C. (1988). Cognitive therapy of obsessive–compulsive disorder. In C.Perris, I. M. Blackburn, & H. Perris (Eds.), *The theory and practice of cognitive therapy.* Heidelberg: Springer-Verlag.

Salkovskis, P. M., & Westbrook, D. (1989). Behaviour therapy and obsessional ruminations: Can failure be turned into success? *Behaviour Research and Therapy, 27,* 149–160.

Solomon, R. L., & Wynne, L. C. (1960). Traumatic avoidance learning: The principles of anxiety conservation and partial irreversibility. *Psychological Review, 61,* 353–385.

Spranca, M., Minsk, E., & Baron, J. (1991). Omission and comission in judgment and choice. *Journal of Experimental Social Psychology, 27,* 76–105.

Sher, K. J., Frost, R. O., Kushner, M., Crews, T. M., & Alexander, J. E. (1989). Memory deficits in compulsive checkers: Replication and extension in a clinical sample. *Behaviour Research and Therapy, 27,* 65–69.

Steketee, G., & Foa, E. B. (1985). In D. H. Barlow (Ed.), *Clinical Handbook of psychological disorders: A step by step treatment manual* (1st ed.). New York: Guilford Press.

Teasdale, J. D. (1983). Negative thinking in depression: Cause, effect or reciprocal relationship? *Advances in Behaviour Research and Therapy, 5,* 3–25.

Trinder, H., & Salkovskis, P. M. (1994). Personally relevant intrusions outside the laboratory: Long term suppression increases intrusion. *Behaviour Research and Therapy, 32,* 833–842.

Wegner, D. M. (1989). *White bears and other unwanted thoughts: Suppression, obsession and the psychology of mental control.* New York: Viking.

Wegner, D. M., Schneider, D. J., Carter, S. R., & White, T. L. (1987). Paradoxical effects of thought supression. *Journal of Personality and Social Psychology, 53,* 5–13.

Wolpe, J. (1958). *Psychotherapy by reciprocal inhibition.* Stanford, CA: Stanford University Press.

6

Obsessive–Compulsive Disorder: A Neuropsychiatric Perspective

TERESA A. PIGOTT
KAREN R. MYERS
DAVID A. WILLIAMS

PATIENTS WITH OBSESSIVE–COMPULSIVE DISORDER (OCD) complain of recurrent, intrusive thoughts (obsessions) and/or repetitive, stereotyped behaviors (compulsions). The most common obsessions in patients with OCD include excessive concerns about contamination, somatic symptoms, symmetry, order, aggression, and sexual behaviors (Rasmussen & Eisen, 1988). Repetitive checking, washing, counting, confessing, hoarding, and arranging compulsions are the most common OCD behaviors (Rasmussen & Eisen, 1988). Most patients with OCD will have at least one of these OCD symptom constellations. Most, but not all, patients with OCD will have anxiety associated with their OCD symptoms.

OCD patients also have variable degrees of insight concerning the validity of their symptoms. For example, some OCD patients experience overwhelming and agonizing uncertainty connected to their symptoms. Such patients fear that their failure to "undo" aggressive OCD thoughts or behaviors will result in harm to other people. Other OCD patients do not experience significant anxiety, but instead complain of uncomfortable feelings of "incompleteness" or tension. Attempts to resist obsessive thoughts result in intensified tension and distress in these patients. Lastly, some OCD patients will consider their symptoms to be rational or realistic, despite evidence to the contrary. For example, some patients endorse intense contamination fears and multiple cleaning rituals, but do not appreciate that their OCD symptoms are inappropriate.

This variability in affective response and/or degree of insight in OCD patients has contributed toward the considerable controversy over whether OCD should remain classified as an "anxiety" disorder in psychiatric classification schemes (Rasmussen & Eisen, 1992; Baer, 1994a). In addition, recent epidemiological and treatment studies have suggested that OCD may be characterized by substantial heterogeneity in presentation and prognosis (Karno, Golding, Sorennson, & Burnam, 1988; Weissman et al., 1994).

The compulsive behaviors manifested by patients with OCD resemble some of the stereotyped behaviors exhibited by patients with Tourette's syndrome (TS), Sydenham's chorea, or partial complex seizures (Pauls & Leckman, 1986; Swedo, Rapaport, Cheslow, et al., 1989; Leckman, Walker, & Cohen, 1993). Data from neuroimaging and neuropsychological studies have also supported the presence of neurological dysfunction (particularly basal ganglia–frontal cortex abnormalities) in patients with OCD (Baxter, 1992; Behar et al., 1984; Goodman, McDougle, Price, et al., 1990).

Most antidepressant medications have direct but nonselective effects on central monoamines such as serotonin (5-HT), norepinephrine (NE), and dopamine (DA). However, antidepressant or anxiolytic efficacy does not correlate with specific effects on one monoamine in comparison to another (Richelson, 1988). That is, antidepressant agents that exhibit a greater effect on NE than on 5-HT or DA neurotransmission have antidepressant or anxiolytic effects similar to those of agents that exhibit higher 5-HT than NE or DA ratios. However, effective antiobsessive medications possess potent or selective effects on 5-HT in comparison to NE or DA neurotransmission (Insel, Mueller, Alterman, Linnoila, Murphy, 1985; Jenike, Baer, & Greist, 1990; Goodman, Price, Delgado, et al., 1990). Agents that possess selective NE or combined 5-HT and NE reuptake properties are not associated with consistent and significant antiobsessive benefit (Goodman, McDouble, & Price, 1992; Jenike, 1992). The relative importance of 5-HT versus NE or DA in antiobsessive efficacy has lead to the "5-HT hypothesis" of OCD. The 5-HT hypothesis implicates central 5-HT dysregulation as etiological in the development and pathophysiology of OCD.

Behavioral therapies (primarily exposure with response prevention and behavioral flooding procedures) are also successful in the treatment of patients with OCD (Baer, 1993). Of interest is the success of these two treatment modalities (behavioral and biological), despite their highly divergent theoretical underpinnings. The efficacy of specific psychopharmacological and behavioral treatments, coupled with the failure of traditional psychotherapy, has led to a shift in fundamental theories of etiology and in treatment strategies for patients with OCD.

With these issues in mind, we discuss the following areas in this chapter: (1) the association of OCD and neurological disorders; (2) neurobiological and neuropsychological studies in patients with OCD; (3) a proposed classification scheme for subtyping patients with OCD; and (4) OCD conceptualized as a neuropsychiatric disorder.

ASSOCIATION OF OBSESSIVE–COMPULSIVE DISORDER AND NEUROLOGICAL DISORDERS

Neurological disorders and/or lesions can be associated with the development of OCD symptoms. Over 60 years ago, survivors of postencephalitic Parkinson's syndrome were found to have a relatively high incidence of OCD symptoms (von Economo, 1931). Ritualistic behaviors and repetitive thoughts that are indistinguishable from primary OCD symptoms can occur after a brain infection such as herpes simplex encephalitis (Bhat, Satish, Chandra, Ravi, & Khanna, 1993). Certain toxic metabolic conditions such as amphetamine toxicity (Fischman, 1987) can also be associated with the development of OCD symptoms.

Even more common is the association between TS and OCD. TS is a chronic neurological disorder that is characterized by both multiple motor and phonic tics. It begins during childhood and is characterized anatomically by basal ganglion lesions. Recent systematic studies have reported that 30–50% of patients with TS are also afflicted with OCD (Pauls, Towbin, Leckman, Zahner, & Cohen, 1986; Frankel et al., 1986; Pitman, Green, Jenike, & Mesulam, 1987). There is also apparently a high rate of OCD and tics in the first-degree relatives of children with OCD (Leonard et al., 1992). These results suggest that in some cases, OCD and TS may be alternative manifestations of the same underlying illness or biological defect.

Patients with TS often describe premonitory feelings or urges that are relieved by performance of the tic, as well as a need to perform tics until they are felt to be "just right" (Leckman et al., 1993). This "just right" phenomenon is also described by many patients with OCD, suggesting that OCD patients with prominent "just right" compulsions or "incompleteness" may represent a distinct subtype of patients. This possibility is discussed in more detail later in this chapter (Rasmussen & Eisen, 1993; Baer, 1994).

The basal ganglion is a brain structure that has a major motor function. Focal damage to the basal ganglion has been associated with the development of abnormal choreiform movements and other neurological abnormalities (Kettle & Marks, 1986; Modell, Mountz, Curtis, & Greden, 1989). There is also evidence suggesting that basal ganglion dysfunction may be linked to the development and expression of OCD symptomatology (Rapaport & Wise, 1988; Stahl, 1988; Rapaport, 1991). The dissemination of streptococcal bacteria into the central nervous system can result in Sydenham's chorea. As many as one-third of children and adolescents diagnosed with Sydenham's chorea will also display prominent and typical OCD symptoms. Interestingly, one-half of patients with Sydenham's chorea have detectable antibodies to the caudate nuclei (part of the basal ganglion) and subthalamic neurons (Swedo, Rapaport, Cheslow, et al., 1989; Swedo et al., 1991). Discrete calcifications in the basal ganglion can occur as a complication of carbon monoxide poisoning (Kettle & Marks, 1986). Interestingly, survivors of carbon monoxide poisoning often exhibit prominent OCD behaviors, despite the absence of premorbid OCD or compulsive symptoms.

Neurosurgical data also support the importance of the basal ganglion in the pathophysiology of OCD. Stereotactic neurosurgical procedures such as capsulotomy, cingulotomy, limbic leucotomy, and subcaudate tractotomy are often effective in reducing symptoms in patients with intractable OCD symptoms (Jenike et al., 1991; Chiocca & Martuza, 1990; Sachdev, Hay, & Cumming, 1992). According to a recent review, 65% of OCD patients who underwent one of these neurosurgical procedures were rated as much improved or in remission from OCD symptoms. Only 12% of patients in the same report were unchanged or worse at follow-up (Mindus & Jenike, 1992). These results are particularly impressive, since such patients are required to be refractory to other treatment modalities for OCD before they can be considered for a neurosurgical intervention.

Effective neurosurgical procedures for the treatment of OCD involve lesions of the pathways between the basal ganglion, the limbic system, and the frontal lobes. For example, capsulotomy interrupts connections between the frontal cortex, thalamus, and basal ganglion and the anterior limb of the internal capsule (Modell et al., 1989). Cingulotomy is also highly effective for OCD and involves a lesion in the cingulum bundle. The efficacy of these operations in reducing OCD symptoms suggests that these overlapping brain areas are involved in the production of OCD symptoms. In fact, Martuza and colleagues (1990) have speculated that the functional neuroanatomy of OCD involves an OCD component (the anterior limb of the internal capsule) and an anxiety component that is mediated via the cingulum bundle (Mindus & Jenike, 1992).

Despite these observations concerning the importance of neurological processes and OCD symptoms, initial speculation about OCD's etiology emphasized psychoanalytic principles (Freud, 1915; Salzman, 1968). Unsuccessful repression of primary aggressive and libidinal drives was theorized to result in inappropriate reliance upon primitive defenses. Displacement and reaction formation were believed to emerge as common defenses to combat these "unacceptable" thoughts or impulses. For example, let us suppose that Mr. A. endorses substantial anxiety symptoms after the birth of his first child and a promotion at work. Mr. A. has a history of chronic difficulties with expressing anger in a direct manner. As the marital discord intensifies, Mr. A. begins to have irrational but intrusive concerns that he will stab his newborn son. He finds these obsessions to be intensely disturbing, but attempts to suppress them result in increased anxiety and doubt. Whenever thoughts of harming his son emerge, Mr. A. begins to perform counting rituals. He secretively counts and recounts the household knives in order to reassure himself that he has not acquired a "weapon." Mr. A. also begins to talk incessantly to his wife and family about his unwavering desire to have more children. The psychoanalytic formulation would suggest that Mr. A. has mixed feelings about becoming a father, but he is unable to acknowledge this ambivalence. Instead, Mr. A. decompensates and begins to rely on regressive coping strategies such as reaction formation (expressing a constant desire to have more children) and displacement (attempting to dislodge aggressive impulses by performing repetitive counting rituals). According to psychoanalytic theory, exploration of Mr. A.'s unconscious conflicts concerning aggression and control should eventually result in OCD symptom reduction. Unfortunately, most patients with OCD do not appear to experience significant reductions in symptomatology after either psychoanalytic or psychodynamic therapy.

In contrast, certain pharmacological or behavioral therapy techniques appear to be effective treatments for patients with OCD. The failure of traditional dynamic psychotherapy, coupled with the efficacy of some pharmacological or behavioral therapy interventions, has resulted in a fundamental shift in etiological theories of OCD. Instead of exploring the potential unconscious significance of OCD symptomatology, recent research investigations have focused on the potential importance of neurobiological processes in the production of OCD symptoms. As previously noted, prominent OCD symptoms can occur in many neurological conditions. In addition, stereotactic neurosurgical procedures can result in reduction of OCD symptoms. With these issues in mind, in the next section we review the available data concerning brain structure and function in patients with primary OCD.

NEUROLOGICAL AND NEUROBIOLOGICAL STUDIES

A number of methods may be utilized to evaluate the structural and functional integrity of the brain, including neurological examination, structural imaging studies, neuropsychological testing, and functional brain imaging studies. Most patients with OCD do not exhibit evidence of focal neurological dysfunction on physical examination, except for nonspecific and nonlocalizing "neurological soft signs" such as synkinesia (Behar et al., 1984) or poor fine motor coordination and predominantly "left-sided" abnormalities (Hollander et al.. 1990). Neither X-ray or magnetic resonance imaging examinations conducted in OCD patients have demonstrated evidence of structural brain abnormalities (Garber, Ananth, Chiu, Griswold, & Oldendorf, 1989; Kellner et al., 1991; Hoehn-Saric, 1993). However, a volumetric computed tomography brain scan analysis in a study of OCD patients revealed evidence of bilaterally decreased caudate nuclei volume in patients with OCD, compared to matched controls (Luxenberg et al. 1988).

When electrophysiological stimuli are administered, signs of hypervigilance and physiological arousal are common findings in patients with OCD compared to control subjects. For example, OCD patients exhibit enhanced reactions to novel stimuli on somatosensory (Shagrass, Roemer, Straumanis, & Josiassen, 1984) and auditory (Towey et al., 1990) evoked potentials. Brain evoked potentials demonstrate overarousal and overfocused attention in OCD. Moreover, electrophysiological studies are supportive of the growing body of evidence that suggests hyperactivation of cortical and/or subcortical regions (e.g., caudate nuclei) in OCD patients compared to controls (Towey et al., 1990, 1993).

Numerous but generally nonspecific abnormalities are present in most reports of neuropsychological testing conducted in patients with OCD (Flor-Henry, Yeudall, Koles, & Howarth, 1979). Evidence of prefrontal dysfunction in OCD patients is common in such testing. Specific findings have included visuospatial and visuoperceptual deficits (Insel, Donnelly, Lalakea, Alterman, & Murphy, 1983) or difficulty in shifting between perceptual sets in OCD patients (Rosen, Hollander, & Stannick, 1988). A verbal memory deficit may be present in nondepressed OCD patients, in comparison to psychiatrically healthy volunteers (Christensen, Kim, Dysken, & Hoover, 1992). Recent neuropsychological tests have also demonstrated evidence of a selective attentional deficit (Martinot et al., 1990; Stephanis, Rabavilas, & Papageorgiou, 1993).

Martin and colleagues (1993) developed a battery of neuropsychological tests that have demonstrated consistent defects in patients with basal ganglion disease such as Huntington's chorea. Although the basal ganglion has been implicated as important in the pathophysiology of OCD, there was no difference between OCD patients and controls who were administered this battery of tests (Martin et al., 1993). However, neurological abnormalities of these regions cannot necessarily be excluded by this study. Most neuropsychological test batteries are developed from studies conducted on patients with neurological dysfunction that is associated with structural or cortical brain damage such as dementia. Therefore, subtle or functional brain abnormalities in the basal ganglion may not be detectable by such investigations.

One study of regional cerebral blood flow conducted in patients with OCD demonstrated evidence of subcortical shunting (Zohar et al., 1989). Subsequent studies in OCD patients have suggested normal blood flow in the basal ganglia, although increased blood flow in the orbito-prefrontal cortex has been noted (Machlin et al., 1991; Rubin, Villanueva-Meyer, Ananth, Trajmar, & Mena, 1992; Hoehn-Saric, 1993). Positron emission tomography (PET) scans assess function by measuring metabolism in different areas of the brain. Patients with OCD appear to have fairly consistent abnormalities on PET scans in comparison to control subjects. Evidence of increased metabolism in the orbito-frontal region and/or basal ganglia of OCD patients relative to controls has been reported in several PET studies (Baxter et al., 1987, 1988; Baxter, 1992; Nordahl et al., 1989; Swedo, Schapiro, Grady, et al., 1989). Moreover, effective medication (Baxter et al., 1992; Benkelfat et al., 1990), as well as behavioral therapy (Baxter et al., 1992), is associated with normalization of these hypermetabolic brain regions in OCD patients. In addition, single photon emission computerized tomography (SPECT) studies have suggested elevated medial–frontal cerebral blood flow in patients with OCD (Machlin et al., 1991). This pattern appears to normalize after treatment with fluoxetine (Hoehn-Saric, Pearlson, Harris, Machlin, & Camargo, 1991). These results support the importance of the orbito-frontal region and/or basal ganglia areas in OCD.

There are numerous pathways between the areas of the frontal cortex and basal ganglion in the brain. Major neurotransmitters for these areas include 5-HT and DA. As noted earlier, 5-HT has been historically implicated in the pathophysiology of OCD. The "5-HT hypothesis" of OCD is based upon several areas of evidence, including peripheral markers of 5-HT function, pharmacological challenge tests, and (most convincingly) the relative preferential efficacy of 5-HT-reuptake-inhibiting antidepressants in comparison to non-5-HT-selective antidepressants in the treatment of OCD (Zohar & Insel, 1987; Benkelfat et al., 1989; Barr, Goodman, Price, McDougle, & Charney, 1992).

Peripheral measures of 5-HT, such as 5-HT content, reuptake, and [^{3}H]imipramine binding in blood platelets (Weizman et al., 1986), have been abnormal in some studies of OCD patients but not in others (Flament, Rapaport, Murphy, Lake, & Berg, 1987; Insel et al., 1985; Weizman et al., 1986). Cerebrospinal fluid (CSF) analyses in patients with OCD versus controls have yielded mixed results. Abnormal levels of the 5-HT metabolite 5-hydroxyindoleacetic acid (5-HIAA) were initially reported (Thoren, Asberg, Bertilsson, et al., 1980a; Insel et al., 1985), but more recent CSF studies have failed to demonstrate significant differences between OCD patients and controls (Altemus et al., 1992). Patients with OCD appear to have CSF levels of NE, DA, and their metabolites that are similar to those of controls (Thoren, Asberg, Bertilsson, et al., 1980; Insel et al., 1985; Altemus et al., 1992). Interestingly, reductions in OCD symptoms have been directly correlated with decreased levels of 5-HT in human platelets and 5-HIAA in CSF in some studies of OCD patients (Asberg, Thoren, & Bertilsson, 1982; Flament et al., 1987; Thoren, Asberg, Bertilsson, et al., 1980).

Panic disorder patients who receive acute does of pharmacological agents that alter noradrenergic function experience enhanced anxiogenic and hormonal responses, in comparison to control subjects. In contrast, noradrenergic agents such as lactate (Gorman et al., 1985), yohimbine (Rasmussen, Goodman, Woods, Heninger, & Charney, 1987) or clonidine (Hollander et al., 1988, 1991) do not elicit significantly different reactions in OCD patients and controls. Other agents that stimulate catecholaminergic function, such as CO_2 (Gorman et al., 1985), caffeine (Zohar et al., 1987), or amphetamine (Pigott, Grady, L'Heureux, et al., 1992), also fail to elicit significantly different responses in OCD patients and controls. However, pharmacological challenges utilizing agents that alter 5-HT function elicit significantly distinct behavioral and hormonal responses in patients with OCD and controls. The acute administration of serotonergic probes such as m-CPP (Zohar, Mueller, Insell, Zohar-Kadouch, & Murphy, 1987; Charney et al., 1988; Hollander et al., 1988, 1991, 1992; Pigott et al., 1993), fenfluramine (Hollander, DeCaria, Nitescu, et al., 1992), MK-212 (Bastani, Nash, & Meltzer, 1990), or tryptophan (Charney et al., 1988) demonstrates evidence of altered 5-HT function in OCD patients.

The 5-HT-reuptake-inhibiting antidepressants clomipramine, fluoxetine, fluvoxamine, paroxetine, and sertraline have all been shown to be effective in significantly reducing OCD symptoms in controlled medication trials (Goodman et al., 1992; Jenike, 1992; Greist, Jefferson, Koback, Katzelnick, & Serlin, 1995). In contrast, effective but non-5-HT-selective antidepressants, including nortriptyline (Thoren, Asberg, Crohnholm, Jornestedt, & Trachman, 1980), amitriptyline (Ananth, Pecknold, Van der Steen, & Englesmann, 1981), doxepin (Ananth, Solyom, & Solyom, 1975), desipramine (Zohar & Insel, 1987; Leonard, Swedo, Rapaport, Coffey, & Cheslow, 1988), and trazodone (Pigott, L'Heureux, Rubenstein, et al., 1992), lack significant antiobsessive properties in comparison to either placebo or clomipramine treatment. Unfortunately, improvement in OCD symptoms from baseline is generally partial even with effective treatment. For example, an approximately 40% mean reduction from baseline in OCD symptoms was noted during a multicenter clomipramine study (Clomipramine Collaborative Study Group, 1991). There is a considerable and similar delay in the onset of significant effects associated with effective OCD medications. Most studies have reported that at least 6 weeks of treatment are required in order to assess antiobsessive efficacy, regardless of the OCD medication used (Pigott et al., 1990). There are few comparative studies of effective OCD medications, but the available data suggest that clomipramine, fluoxetine, fluvoxamine, sertraline, and paroxetine appear to possess similar efficacy in reducing OCD symptoms (Rasmussen, Eisen, & Pato, 1993; Pigott, L'Heureux, & Murphy, 1993; Dominguez, 1992; Goodman, McDougle, & Barr, 1993: Greist et al., 1995).

Approximately 25% of patients with OCD will not respond to clomipramine or 5-HT-reuptake-inhibiting therapy. For these patients, various pharmacological treatments have been advocated, but few have proven to be significantly beneficial. Various medications have been implemented as potential adjuvant agents in conjunction with the 5-HT-reuptake-inhibiting antidepressants in an attempt to optimize and/or augment antiobsessive treatment in patients with OCD. The few controlled trials of adjuvant agents that have been conducted in patients with OCD have largely failed to demonstrate additional antiobsessive benefit (Grady et al., 1993; Pigott, Pato, L'Heureux, et al., 1991; Pigott, L'Heureux, Bernstein, et al., 1992; McDougle, Price, Goodman, Charney, & Heninger, 1991). It appears that long-term pharmacological treatment is necessary in most OCD patients to maintain benefit. The few systematic studies that have been conducted have consistently shown that relapse is rapid after discontinuation of medication in patients with OCD (Thoren, Asberg, Crohnholm, et al. 1980; Flament et al., 1987; Leonard, Swedo, et al., 1991; Pato et al., 1988; Pigott et al., 1990).

Although all of the effective antiobsessive medications are potent inhibitors of 5-HT reuptake, the magnitude of antiobsessive response does not correlate with the relative selectivity or potency of 5-HT reuptake inhibition (Jenike et al., 1990; Jenike, & Raush, 1994; Greist et al., 1995). Furthermore, a substantial subgroup of patients with OCD will not respond to 5-HT-reuptake-inhibiting antidepressants. This suggests that 5-HT reuptake inhibition is associated with antiobsessive efficacy but most likely is not the critical etiological factor. Instead, it is more likely that the "crucial" event that imparts significant antiobsessive properties occurs at a different site, perhaps in the G-protein complex or second-messenger cascade, and that the 5-HT reuptake site represents only a portion of the common pathway shared by effective antiobsessive agents.

In summary, evidence of neurological dysfunction is present in many studies of patients with OCD. The most compelling evidence emerges from functional neuroimaging studies such as PET scans. These studies support the importance of the prefrontal cortex and basal ganglion areas in the pathophysiology of OCD. In addition, data from pharmacological probe studies and controlled treatment trials suggest that altered 5-HT function exists in many patients with OCD. However, a substantial proportion of research studies conducted in OCD patients have yielded conflicting or inconsistent results; therefore, a comprehensive theory of the etiology of OCD remains elusive at this time. The following section proposes a scheme for the classification of OCD that may prove helpful in further addressing these critical issues.

PROPOSED SUBTYPES OF OBSESSIVE–COMPULSIVE DISORDER

Available data concerning shared phenomenology, comorbid conditions, and neurobiological characteristics may prove particularly helpful in identifying etiological factors in patients with OCD. In this section, we present a potential classification scheme for OCD patients that consists of three distinct OCD subtypes.

The phenomenology of OCD, including the most common content of obsessions and compulsions, has been reviewed earlier in this chapter. Comorbid psychiatric conditions are frequent and associated with further psychosocial impairment in many patients with OCD (Rasmussen & Eisen, 1988, 1992, 1993; Pigott et al., 1994; Weissman et al., 1994). The most common comorbid disorders that occur in patients with primary OCD are depression (Rasmussen & Tsuang, 1986) and additional anxiety diagnoses (Rasmussen & Eisen, 1988). Other comorbid conditions present in OCD patients include eating disorders (Rubenstein et al., 1992; Rasmussen & Eisen, 1988; Pigott, Altemus, et al., 1991; Kaye, Weltzin, Hsu, 1993), body dysmorphic disorder (Tanquary, Lynch, & Masand, 1992; Brady, Austin, & Lydiard, 1990; Hollander, Neville, Frenkel, Josephson, & Liebowitz, 1992), trichotillomania (Swedo, Leonard, Rapaport, et al., 1989), or delusional or schizophrenic disorders (Insel & Akiskal, 1986).

Extrapolating from these clinical characteristics, including symptom content and comorbid disorders, we propose the following OCD subtypes: (1) altered risk assessment disorder, (2) incompleteness/habit-spectrum disorder, and (3) psychotic-spectrum disorder. Inherent in this classification system is the assumption that distinct neurological and neurobiological processes may be involved in the production of the different OCD subtypes.

The first OCD subtype, altered risk assessment disorder, includes patients with OCD who exhibit prominent "pathological doubt," anxiety, and "undoing" behaviors. In pathological doubt, the ability to assess possible in contrast to probable consequences is severely impaired. This inability leads to paralyzing indecisiveness and extreme feelings of responsibility for actions. This pervasive doubt also results in escalating anxiety and ritualistic behaviors designed to "undo" or neutralize feared consequences. OCD patients with altered risk assessment often perform endless compulsive behaviors (checking locks, making sure that the stove is turned off, etc.) in an attempt to protect their families or other loved ones from harm. OCD patients with altered risk assessment recognize that their symptoms are excessive and irrational, but their inaccurate assessment of the consequences of their actions/impulses results in incapacitating anxiety. They cannot resist or suppress their OCD symptoms without experiencing this distress. Substantial rates of comorbid affective and anxiety disorders would be anticipated in this OCD subtype. In addition, OCD patients classified in this subtype may be particularly susceptible to developing eating disorders secondary to their altered risk assessment (they may assume that intake of even a small number of calories inevitably results in morbid obesity).

The second OCD subtype, incompleteness/habit-spectrum disorder, includes patients who have primary symptoms of incompleteness or perfectionism. Patients included in this OCD subtype describe their symptoms as coupled with feelings of rising tension (not necessarily anxiety), which is then "released" by performance of a ritual (e.g., finger tapping). These patients rarely have a sense of doom or impending catastrophe associated with their OCD symptoms. In fact, they often cannot articulate the rationale for their behaviors except to link them with a need to perform certain actions in "just the right way." Patients in this OCD subtype would be expected to have high rates of comorbid tics, TS, or trichotillomania. In fact, there is substantial empirical evidence already supporting the presence of this specific OCD subtype, based upon family studies (Pauls & Leckman, 1986; Leckman et al., 1993) and pharmacological treatment response (McDougle et al., in press; Goodman, McDougle, Price, et al., 1990; Jenike, Baer, Minichiello, Schwarz, & Carey, 1986).

The final OCD subtype, psychotic-spectrum disorder, includes any OCD patients who believe that most of their OCD symptoms are rational and reasonable. The content of the obsession and/or compulsions is less important than the patients' conviction regarding the reasonableness of the symptom(s). It might be expected that there would be a higher incidence of the following syndromes in this subtype: dysmorphophobia, psychogenic pain, and obsessional slowness. These patients are often classified as delusional or psychotic, and some evidence suggests that they represent a particularly treatment-resistant group (Insel & Akiskal, 1986). Patients who develop OCD symptoms after brain trauma, lesions, or infection often have symptoms that would be characterized as belonging to this subtype.

Dimensions of concomitant anxiety, conviction, and perfectionism differentiate the proposed OCD subtypes; the subtypes are independent of symptom content. For example, anxiety is the main trigger for the performance of compulsive behaviors in the first OCD subtype, whereas patients in the second OCD subtype experience a sense of tension or anxiety only when the performance of their compulsive behaviors is interrupted or blocked. Anxiety is generally absent in the third subtype of OCD patients, as they perceive their OCD symptoms as neither excessive nor worthy of resistance. Conviction, or belief in the rationality of OCD symptoms, also differs among the OCD subtypes. Patients in the first two OCD subtypes characterize their symptoms as irrational or excessive, whereas patients in the third subtype of OCD patients have a strong belief that their OCD symptoms are rational and reasonable. The presence of perfectionism is an integral part of the second OCD subtype, but may be absent in the other two OCD subtypes. Therefore, a patient manifesting a common OCD symptom such as repeated handwashing or cleaning rituals could be categorized in any of the three subtypes, depending upon certain characteristics.

For example, Mr. A. has repeated thoughts about contamination; he worries that he will accidentally contaminate his family, and that this will result in illness and possibly death. Mr. A. recognizes that his fears are excessive, but he only truly believes that his family is safe when he performs his cleaning and handwashing rituals. Consequently, Mr. A. becomes embroiled in an unending cycle of repetitive behaviors designed to prevent harm and maintain safety in his environment. Given these characteristics, Mr. A. would be categorized as having the first OCD subtype, altered risk assessment disorder.

Mr. B. also has excessive contamination concerns, along with cleaning and handwashing rituals. Mr. B. recognizes that these symptoms are irrational. However Mr. B. does not fear that if he fails to perform his rituals or attempts to resist his obsessions, "something terrible will happen." Instead, Mr. B. reports that he feels "uncomfortable" and "tense" if things are not "clean enough." He describes a sense of transitory relief when he is able to "complete" his rituals. Consequently, Mr. B.'s OCD symptoms result in a release of tension and a sense of completeness. Given these characteristics, Mr. B. would be categorized as having the second OCD subtype, incompleteness/habit-spectrum disorder.

Mr. C. exhibits excessive contamination concerns, as well as cleaning and handwashing rituals. However, Mr. C. does not consider his OCD symptoms excessive or irrational. He does not complain of anxiety and rarely attempts to resist his fears or rituals. Mr. C. denies that his rituals are associated with any attempts to avoid harm or to release "irresistible" urges. Given these characteristics, Mr. C. would be categorized as having the third OCD subtype, psychotic-spectrum disorder.

Although the proposed subtypes are speculative, they may be particularly helpful in selecting homogeneous samples of OCD patients for future research studies. In addition, the many discrepancies that exist in neurobiological research data on patients with OCD may in part have arisen from a failure to delineate valid subgroups of OCD patients. Most research studies in patients with OCD have included samples consisting of patients with diverse OCD symptomatology, frequent comorbid conditions, and differential levels of anxiety and insight associated with their OCD symptoms. Treatment-resistant patients with OCD also tend to be overrepresented in research samples, as they are most likely to be referred to tertiary treatment centers and are more likely to participate in investigational procedures because of the lack of effective treatment options.

Consequently, it is not surprising that consistent, replicable results have not yet emerged in most studies with OCD patients. Despite these limitations, the relatively impressive findings with neuroimaging techniques suggest the existence of neurobiological differences between patients with OCD and controls, and also indicate that these differences may be associated with therapeutic efficacy. In the next section, we return to the proposed OCD subtyping scheme when presenting the conceptualization of OCD as a neuropsychiatric illness.

A NEUROPSYCHIATRIC MODEL OF THE ETIOLOGY OF OBSESSIVE–COMPULSIVE DISORDER

In contrast to depression and other anxiety disorders, there are no current well-established animal models for OCD. Rapoport (1992) has proposed that canine acral lick dermatitis (ALD) may represent a useful model for OCD in terms of testing new pharmacological treatments for OCD. Canine ALD is a naturally occurring disorder characterized by excessive licking of paws or flanks that can lead to significant ulceration and infection. The disorder occurs almost exclusively in certain large dog breeds, and its repetitive, stereotypical characteristics suggest some degree of compulsivity that may be similar to compulsive behaviors manifested by patients with OCD. Interestingly, ALD apparently has a pharmacological response profile similar to that of OCD, in that 5-HT-uptake-blocking agents have been demonstrated to be effective, whereas non-5-HT-selective agents are ineffective (Rapaport, 1992). Unfortunately, this model is limited by several factors, including the fact that the etiology of ALD remains unknown. Further studies are needed to determine whether ALD may be associated with lesions and/or dysfunction of the frontal cortex–basal ganglia–thalamus circuitry. Such neurological dysfunction has been postulated as the source of phylogenetically mediated "grooming" behaviors that may become "uninhibited" in patients with OCD (Rapaport, 1991).

The basal ganglion and its connections with the thalamus and cerebral cortex have been implicated in most theories of OCD etiology. Evidence for the importance of this connection can be found in the fact that the basal ganglion has prominent control of motor behaviors, and in the previously described data suggesting that OCD patients exhibit basal ganglion dysfunction. However, recent research suggests that the basal ganglion is comprised of both a "motor" and a "memory" component. The motor system component is theorized to involve the connections between the cerebral cortex and basal ganglia, and is primarily mediated via dopaminergic pathways (Rolls & Williams, 1987; Modell et al., 1989). Disruption of these circuits is felt to be associated with movement disorders (Stahl, 1988). The memory component of the basal ganglia is theorized to involve connections to the cortex, thalamus, and amygdala. These pathways are probably serotonergic and may mediate emotional responses; disruptions of these pathways may thus be manifested as disturbed emotional responses (Stahl, 1988).

Stahl (1988) has theorized that the basal ganglion structure is responsible for receiving input, often conflictual, from the amygdala and hippocampus. After processing and prioritizing, this condensed information is transmitted via primary dopaminergic and serotonergic pathways to trigger the appropriate behavioral response to the environmental stimulus. Aberrant control of the basal ganglion's ability to select appropriate behavioral responses from its input, as well as an inability to suppress continuing sensory emotional input, may result in the production of OCD symptoms (Stahl, 1988). Rapoport and Wise (1988) have postulated a similar model, suggesting that basal ganglion dysfunction underlies the development of OCD. The development of obsessive thoughts and compulsive behaviors is thought to be secondary to abnormal processing of sensory input from the cerebral cortex to the basal ganglion.

Recent research in developmental neurobiology may also contribute valuable information to the theories concerning the pathophysiology of OCD. For example, although the human brain is relatively mature at birth from a gross morphological standpoint, substantial research studies reveal that it continues to undergo dramatic changes in microscopic anatomy (Cook & Leventhal, 1992). Indeed, the development of the nervous system appears to be highly dependent on a proper balance between genetically triggered events and the regulation of transcription by the microenvironment within the brain.

During normal brain development, it appears that the nervous system regulates itself by overproduction of neuronal processes and synapses, with subsequent retraction, rearrangement, and elimination of some neurons and synapses. For example, the number of neuronal synapses appears to peak at 18 months and to decline thereafter (Huttenlocher, 1982). Certain disorders (e.g., neurofibromatosis) involve failure to regulate

neuronal cell proliferation, with the subsequent formation of gross morphological brain lesions (Cook & Leventhal, 1992). It appears that human neurodevelopment involves a complex interaction among the genomic
substrate, neuroregulatory processes, and environmental factors. With
these complex interactions in mind, it is not difficult to conclude that even
minute perturbations in this "normal" neuronal development cascade (expression of genetic abnormalities, subtle neuronal dysregulation, and/or
the presence of environmental stressors) may lead to microscopic defects
in neuronal pathways, with subsequent neuropsychiatric manifestations.

At the same time that the anatomic nervous system is evolving, emotional development within the individual is occurring. This emotional development is apparently influenced by a variety of intrapersonal and
interpersonal factors. Although they have used different nomenclature and
stressed divergent influences, theorists of human development have long
emphasized the importance of resolving aggressive impulses and fears of
loss of control in order to achieve "normal" emotional development. Normal development encompasses the areas of impulse control and interpersonal confidence.

For example, Mahler (1975) has pointed out that toddlers enter the
stage of "rapprochement," which is characterized by "shadowing and dart-
ing" behaviors conceptualized to represent children's acting out their ambivalence about separating from their mothers. This stage occurs between
18 and 24 months, and failure to resolve this ambivalence results in a lack
of trust and self-esteem. In fact, Erikson (1963) called this vulnerable period in child development "autonomy versus shame and doubt." Even Freud
(1915) postulated that at approximately the same age, the developing child
must resolve conflicts concerning control and aggression. He postulated
that failure to navigate this stage successfully contributes to the formation of an obsessive–compulsive personality structure, in which qualities
such as orderliness, obstinacy, and parsimony predominate.

As previously summarized, it is unlikely that most patients with OCD
have demonstrable gross structural brain abnormalities. Yet patients with
OCD have demonstrated frequent evidence of subtle neurological dysfunction. These could easily result from relatively minor "glitches" in the regulation and modulation of the developing nervous system. It is interesting
to note that at the same time the issue of control is theorized to be the
focus of intrapsychic energies within the individual, the developing brain
contains the highest concentration of neuronal synapses and is undergoing dramatic shifts in neuronal organization.

Synthesizing developmental theories with developmental neurobiology, one could postulate that a complex interaction among genetic vulnerability, subtle neuronal dysregulation, and the intrapsychic focus on
control issues occurs during this critical developmental stage. That is, OCD

symptomatology may result from an interaction of the prominent focus on control, aggression, and doubt within the developing emotional substrate with subtle perturbations in neuronal pathways that involve critical information-processing and prioritization tasks.

OCD subtyping may be particularly helpful in identifying separate neurotransmitter dysregulation within the three proposed categories of patients with OCD. The first subtype, altered risk assessment disorder, may well result from dysregulated neuronal pathways that involve the memory component of the basal ganglion and its connections to the frontal cortex, thalamus, and amygdala. Since these pathways are primarily mediated via serotonergic subsystems, high levels of concomitant anxiety and comorbid affective disorder would be anticipated. OCD patients with altered risk asssessment would be predicted to exhibit evidence of 5-HT dysregulation via central or peripheral 5-HT indices and pharmacological challenge paradigms. PET and other functional neuroimaging studies obtained from this group of OCD patients would be expected to exhibit evidence of both basal ganglion and prefrontal cortex hypermetabolism, at least in the absence of active affective disorder.

OCD patients in this first subtype would be predicted to have good therapeutic responses, in terms of substantial OCD symptom reduction, to (1) 5-HT-reuptake-inhibiting medications, which would address the serotonergic dysregulation; and/or (2) behavioral therapy, which would help them to habituate to their anxiety and to overcome their distorted and overvalued ideations. Behavioral treatment such as exposure with response prevention would focus on uncoupling the feared consequence (e.g., contamination) from the undoing or neutralizing compulsion (e.g., handwashing).

The second OCD subtype, incompleteness/habit-spectrum disorder, is hypothesized to result from dysregulated neuronal pathways involving primarily the motoric component of the basal ganglion and its connections to the cerebral cortex. Since these pathways are primarily mediated via dopaminergic subsystems, one would predict relatively high rates of associated movement disorders (comorbid tic disorders, TS, etc.) and frequent neurological soft signs on physical examination. OCD patients in this subtype would be less likely to exhibit evidence of 5-HT dysregulation via central or peripheral 5-HT indices and pharmacological challenge paradigms, and in fact may instead demonstrate evidence of dopaminergic dysregulation. PET and other functional neuroimaging studies obtained from this group of OCD patients would be more likely to demonstrate basal ganglion than frontal cortex abnormalities.

OCD patient with incompleteness/habit-spectrum disorder would be less likely to respond to 5-HT-reuptake-inhibiting monotherapy than OCD patients in the first category. Instead, these patients would be more likely to respond to (1) a combination of 5-HT-reuptake inhibitor and a low-dose neuroleptic (the neuroleptic would provide DA-blocking effects, necessary for the postulated primary dopaminergic and motor components); (2) clomipramine, in contrast to other 5-HT reuptake inhibitors, since it also possesses some DA-blocking effects and thereby may even prove helpful as a monotherapy; and/or (3) behavioral therapy with a strong emphasis on response prevention, rather than the exposure component. These patients do not exhibit a feared consequence linked with a neutralizing behavior; rather, they exhibit a mounting urge without an identifiable feared consequence.

For the third subtype of OCD patients, those with psychotic-spectrum disorder, either structural or metabolic etiologies are hypothesized to be instrumental in the development of their OCD symptoms. These OCD patients may have more generalized neurological dysfunction, with disruption of both serotonergic and dopaminergic pathways connecting the basal ganglion, thalamus, and frontal lobes. One would predict relatively high rates of associated psychotic symptoms and superimposed hypochondriacal concerns. OCD patients with psychotic-spectrum disorder would be unlikely to exhibit evidence of specific neurotransmitter dysregulation, since the hypothesized neural dysfunction is though to be more diffuse than that in the first two subtypes. PET and other functional neuroimaging studies obtained from this group of OCD patients would be more likely to demonstrate nonspecific abnormalities or generalized frontal lobe dysfunction.

Psychotic-spectrum OCD patients would be likely to represent the most treatment-resistant group of OCD patients. In terms of pharmacotherapy, neuroleptics would probably result in some symptom reduction. However, since these patients by definition do not experience their OCD symptoms as excessive or irrational, one would anticipate that compliance with prescribed medication would be poor. Behavioral treatment would also be problematic, as these patients experience little anxiety and also have little internal motivation for changing behaviors that they view as reasonable or necessary. It is likely that effective treatment would require the presence of a strong, externally motivated factor (e.g., marital discord, impaired job performance, etc.).

Thus far, some research data support the utility of separating patients with OCD and a comorbid tic disorder or TS into a unified category (McDougle et al., 1993). Some data also suggest that OCD patients with psychotic features are more treatment-resistant than those without psychotic features (Insel & Akiskal, 1986). Although the remainder of the model presented lacks validation at this time, it represents an attempt to conceptualize OCD as a potentially heterogeneous disorder with several distinct subtypes. Certainly, separation of OCD into these subtypes may help to clarify etiological processes.

In summary, a wealth of available research data suggests that OCD is associated with neurological dysfunction. Our group is currently conducting neurobiological and treatment studies utilizing the proposed OCD subtyping scheme. We hope that these studies and future research will provide further data supporting the utility of this conceptualization of OCD as a neuropsychiatric disorder.

REFERENCES

Altemus, M. A., Pigott, T. A., Kalogeras, K., Demitrack, M. A., Dubbert, B., Murphy, D. L., & Gold, P. W. (1992). Elevations in AVP and CRH in obsessive–compulsive disorder: Pathophysiological implications. *Archives of General Psychiatry, 49*(1), 9–20.

Ananth, J., Pecknold, J., Van den Steen, N., & Englesmann, F. (1981). Double-bind study of clomipramine and amitriptyline in obsessive neurosis. *Progress in Neuropsychopharmacology, 5,* 257–261.

Ananth, J., Solyom, L., & Solyom, C. (1975). Doxepin in the treatment of obsessive–compulsive disorder. *Psychosomatics, 16,* 185–187.

Asberg, M., Thoren, P., & Bertilsson, L. (1982). Clomipramine treatment of obsessive–compulsive disorder: Biochemical and clinical aspects. *Psychopharmacology Bulletin, 18*(3), 13–21.

Baer, L. (1993). Behavior therapy for obsessive–compulsive disorder in the office-based practice. *Journal of Clinical Psychiatry, 54,* 10–15.

Baer, L. (1994). Factor analysis of symptom subtypes of obsessive-compulsive disorder and their relation to personality and tic disorders. *Journal of Clinical Psychiatry, 55,* 18–23.

Baer, L., Jenike, M., Black, D., Treece, C., Rosenfeld, R., & Greist, J. (1992). Effect of axis II diagnoses on treatment outcome with clomipramine in 54 patients with obsessive–compulsive disorder. *Archives of General Psychiatry,* 862–866.

Barr, L., Goodman, W., Price, L., McDougle, C., & Charney, D. (1992). The serotonin hypothesis of obsessive–compulsive disorder: Implications of pharmacologic challenge studies. *Journal of Clinical Psychiatry, 53*(4), 17–28.

Bastani, B., Nash, J., & Meltzer, H. (1990). Prolactin and cortisol responses to MK-212, a serotonin agonist, in obsessive–compulsive disorder. *Archives of General Psychiatry, 47,* 833–840.

Baxter, L. (1992). Neuroimaging studies of obsessive–compulsive disorder. *Psychiatric Clinics of North America, 15*(4), 871–884.

Baxter, L., Phelps, J., Mazziotta, J., Fuze, B., Schwarz, J., & Selm, C. (1987). Local cerebral glucose metabolic rates in obsessive–compulsive disorder: A comparison with rates in unipolar depression and in normal controls. *Archives of General Psychiatry, 44,* 211–218.

Baxter, L., Schwartz, J., Bergman, K., Szuba, M., Guze, B., Mazziotta, J., Alazraki, A., Selin, C., Ferny, H., Mumford, P., & Phelps, M. (1992). Caudate glucose metabolic rate changes with both drug and behavior therapy of obsessive–compulsive disorder. *Archives of General Psychiatry, 49,* 681–689.

Baxter, L., Schwartz, J., Mazziotta, J., Phelps, M., Pahl, J., Guze, B., & Fairbanks, L. (1988). Cerebral glucose metabolic rates in nondepressed patients with obsessive–compulsive disorder. *American Journal of Psychiatry, 145,* 1560–1563.

Behar, D., Rapaport, J., Berg, C., Denckla, M., Mann, L., Cox, C., Fedio, P., Zahn, T., & Wolfman, M. (1984). Computerized tomography and neuropsychological test measures in adolescents with obsessive–compulsive disorder. *American Journal of Psychiatry, 141,* 363–369.

Benkelfat, C., Murphy, D., Zohar, J., Hill, J., Grover, G., & Insel, T. (1989). Clomipramine in obsessive–compulsive disorder: Further evidence for a serotonergic mechanism of action. *Archivess of General Psychiatry, 46,* 23–28.

Benkelfat, C., Nordahl, T., Semple, W., King, C., Murphy, D., & Cohen, R. (1990). Local cerebral glucose metabolic activity in obsessive–compulsive disorder: Patients treated with clomipramine. *Archives of General Psychiatry, 47,* 840–848.

Bhat, M., Satish Chandra, P., Ravi, V., & Khanna, S. (1993). Obsessive–compulsive symptoms in herpes simplex encephalitis. *Proceedings of the 45th Annual Conference of the Indian Psychiatric Society,* Lucknow, India.

Black, D., Yates, W., Noyes, R., Phohl, B., & Kelley, M. (1989). DSM-III personality disorder in obsessive–compulsive study volunteers: A controlled study. *Journal of Personality Disorders, 3,* 58–62.

Brady, K., Austin, L., & Lydiard, R. (1990). Body dysmorphic disorder: The relationship to obsessive–compulsive disorder. *Journal of Nervous and Mental Disorders, 178*(8), 538–540.

Charney, D., Goodman, W., Price, L., Woods, S., Rasmussen, S., & Heninger, G. (1988). Serotonin function in obsessive–compulsive disorder: A comparison of the effects of tryptophan and *m*-CPP in patients and healthy subjects. *Archives of General Psychiatry, 45,* 177–185.

Chiocca, E., & Martuza, R. (1990). Neurosurgical therapy of obsessive–compulsive disorder. In *OCD: Theory and management.* Chicago: Year Book Medical Publishers.

Christensen, K., Kim, S., Dysken, M., & Hoover, K. (1992). Neuropsychological performance in obsessive–compulsive disorder. *Biological Psychiatry, 31,* 4–18.

Clomipramine Collaborative Study Group. (1991). Clomipramine in the treatment of patients with obsessive–compulsive disorder. *Archives of General Psychiatry, 48,* 730–738.

Cook, E., & Leventhal, B. (1992). Neuropsychiatric disorders of childhood and adolescence. In S. C. Yudovsky & R. E. Hales (Eds.), *Neuropsychiatry* (2nd ed.). Washington, DC: American Psychiatric Press.

Dominguez, R. (1992). Serotonergic antidepressants and their efficacy in obsessive–compulsive disorder. *Journal of Clinical Psychiatry, 53*(10), 56–59.

Erikson, E. (1963). *Childhood and Society.* New York: Norton.

Fischman, M. (1987). Cocaine and amphetamines. In H. Y. Meltzer (Ed.), *Psychopharmacology: The third generation of progress.* New York: Raven.

Flament, M., Rapaport, J., Murphy, D., Lake, C., & Berg, C. (1987). Biochemical changes during clomipramine treatment of childhood obsessive–compulsive disorder. *Archives of General Psychiatry, 44,* 219–225.

Flor-Henry, P., Yeudall, L., Koles, Z., & Howarth, B. (1979). Neuropsychological and power spectral EEG investigations of obsessive–compulsive disorder. *Biological Psychiatry, 14,* 119–130.

Frankel, M., Cummings, J., Robertson, M., Trimble, M., Hill, M., & Benson, D. (1986). Obsessions and compulsions in Gilles de la Tourette's syndrome. *Neurology, 36,* 378–382.

Freud, S. (1915). Instincts and their vicissitudes. In *Collected Papers of Sigmund Freud, Vol. IV.* London: Oxford Press, 195.

Garber, H., Ananth, J., Chiu, L., Griswold, V., & Oldendorf, W. (1989). Nuclear magnetic resonance of obsessive–compulisve disorder. *American Journal of Psychiatry, 146,* 1001.

Goodman, W., McDougle, C., Barr, L., & Price, L. (1993). Biological approaches to the treatment-refractory patient. In *1st International OCD Conference Abstracts.* Isle of Capri, Italy: Solvay Duphar.

Goodman, W., McDougle, C., & Price, L. (1992). Pharmacotherapy of obsessive–compulsive disorder. *Journal of Clinical Psychiatry, 53*(4), 29–37.

Goodman, W., McDougle, C., Price, L., Riddle, M., Pauls, D., & Leckman, J. (1990). Beyond the serotonin hypothesis: A role for dopamine in some forms of obsessive–compulsive disorder? *Journal of Clinical Psychiatry, 51*(8), 36–43.

Goodman, W., Price, L., Delgado, P., Palumbo, J., Krystal, J., Nagy, L., Rasmussen, S., Heninger, G., & Charney, D. (1990). Specificity of serotonin reuptake inhibitors in the treatment of obsessive–compulsive disorder. *Archives of General Psychiatry, 47,* 577–585.

Gorman, J., Liebowitz, M., Fyer, A., Dillon, D., Davies, S., Stein, J., & Klein, D. (1985). Lactate infusions in obsessive–compulsive disorder. *American Journal of Psychiatry, 142,* 864–866.

Grady, T. A., Pigott, T. A., L'Heureux, F., Hill, J. L., Bernstein, S. E., & Murphy, D. l. (1993). A double-blind study of adjuvant buspirone hydrochloride in fluoxetine-treated patients with obsessive–compulsive disorder. *American Journal of Psychiatry, 15,* 819.

Greist, J., Jefferson, J., Koback, K., Katzelnick, D., & Serlin, R. (1995). Efficacy and tolerability of serotonin transport inhibitors in obsessive–compulsive disorder: A meta-analysis. *Archives of General Psychiatry, 52,* 53–60.

Hoehn-Saric, R. (1993). Regional cerebral blood flow in obsessive–compulsive disorder patients before and during threatment with fluoxetine. In *1st International OCD Conference Abstracts.* Isle of Capri, Italy: Solvay Duphar.

Hoehn-Saric, R., Pearlson, G., Harris, G., Machlin, S., & Camargo, E. (1991). Effects of fluoxetine on regional cerebral blood flow in obsessive–compulsive disorder. *American Journal of Psychiatry, 148,* 1243–1245.

Hollander, E., DeCaria, C., Nitescu, A., Gorman, J., Klien, D., & Liebowitz, M. (1991). Noradrenergic function in obsessive–compulsive disorder: Behavioral and neuroendocrine responses to clonidine and comparison to healthy controls. *Psychiatry Research, 137,* 161–177.

Hollander, E., DeCaria, C., Nitescu, A., Gully, R., Suckow, R., Cooper, T., Gorman, J., Klein, D., & Liebowitz, M. (1992). Serotonergic function in obsessive–compulsive disorder: Behavioral and neuroendocrine responses to oral *m*-CPP and fenfluramine in patients and healthy volunteers. *Archives of General Psychiatry, 49,* 21–28.

Hollander, E., Fay, B., Cohen, R., Campeas, R., Gorman, J. M., & Liebowitz, M. R. (1988). Serotonergic and noradrenergic sensitivity in obsessive–compulsive disorder: Behavioral findings. *American Journal of Psychiatry, 145,* 1015–1018.

Hollander, E., Neville, D., Frenkel, M., Josephson, S., & Liebowitz, M. (1992). Body dysmorphic disorder: Diagnostic issues and related disorders. *Psychosomatics, 32*(2), 156–165.

Hollander, E., Schiffman, E., Cohen, B., River Stein, A., Rosen, W., Gorman, J., Fyer, A., Papp, L., & Liebowitz, M. (1990). Signs of central nervous system dysfunction in obsessive–compulsive disorder. *Archives of General Psychiatry, 48,* 278–279.

Huttenlocher, P. (1982). Synaptogenesis in the human visual cortex: Evidence for synapse elimination during normal development. *Neuroscience Letters, 33,* 699–705.

Insel, T., & Akiskal, H. (1986). Obsessive–compulsive disorder with psychotic features: A phenomenologic analysis. *American Journal of Psychiatry, 143,* 1527–1533.

Insel, T., Donnelly, E., Lalakea, M., Alterman, I., & Murphy, D. (1983). Neurological and neuropsychological studies of patients with obsessive–compulsive disorder. *Biological Psychiatry, 18,* 741–751.

Insel, T., Mueler, E., Gillin, J., Siever, L., & Murphy, D. (1983). Biological markers in obsessive–compulsive and affective disorders. *Journal of Psychiatric Research, 18,* 407–425.

Insel, T., Mueller, E., Alterman, I., Linnoila, M., & Murphy, D. (1985). Obsessive–compulsive disorder and serotonin: Is there a connection? *Biological Psychiatry, 20,* 1174–1188.

Jenike, M. (1992). Pharmacologic treatment of obsessive–compulsive disorder. *Psychiatric Clinics of North America, 15,* 895–919.

Jenike, M., Baer, L., Ballantine, H., Martuza, R., Tynes, S., Giriunas, I., Buttolph, M., & Cassem, N. (1991). Cingulotomy for refractory obsessive–compulsive disorder. *Archives of General Psychiatry, 48,* 548–555.

Jenike, M., Baer, L., Minichiello, W., Schwartz, C., & Carey, R. (1986). Concomitant obsessive–compulsive disorder and schizotypal personality disorder. *American Journal of Psychiatry, 143.,* 530–533.

Jenike, M., & Raush, S. (1994). Managing the patient with treatment-resistent obsessive–compulsive disorder: Current strategies. *Journal of Clinical Psychiatry, 55,* 11–17.

Jenike, M. A., Baer, L., & Greist, J. H. (1990). Clomipramine versus fluoxetine in obsessive–compulsive disorder: A retrospective comparison of side effects and efficacy. *Journal of Clinical Psychopharmacology, 10,* 122–124.

Jenike, M. A., Hyman, S., Baer, L., Holland, A., Minichiello, W. E., Buttolph, L., Summergard, P., Seymour, R., & Ricciardi, J. (1990). A controlled trial of fluvoxamine in obsessive–compulsive disorder: Implications for a serotonergic theory. *American Journal of Psychiatry, 147,* 1209–1214.

Karno, M., Golding, J., Sorenson, S., & Burnam, M. (1988). The epidemiology of obsessive–compulsive disorder in five U.S. communities. *Archives of General Psychiatry, 45,* 1094–1099.

Kaye, W., Weltzin, T., & Hsu, L. (1993). Relationship between anorexia nervosa and obsessive and compulsive behaviors. *American Journal of Psychiatry, 23*(7), 365–373.

Kellner, C., Jolley, R., Holgate, R., Lydiard, R., Austin, L., & Ballenger, J. (1991). Brain MRI in obsessive–compulsive disorder. *Psychiatry Research, 36,* 45–49.

Kettle, P., & Marks, I. (1986). Neurological factors in obsessive–compulsive disorder: Two case reports and a review of the literature. *British Journal of Psychiatry, 149,* 315–319.

Leckman, J., Walker, D., & Cohen, D. (1993). Premonitory urges in Tourette's Syndrome. *American Journal of Psychiatry, 150,* 98–102.

Leonard, H., Lenane, M., Swedo, S., Rettew, D., Gershon, E., & Rapaport, J. (1992). Tics and Tourette's syndrome: A two to seven year follow-up of 54 obsessive–compulsive disorder children. *American Journal of Psychiatry, 149,* 1244–1251.

Leonard, H., Swedo, S., Lenane, M., Rettew, D., Cheslow, D., Hamburger, S., & Rapaport. J. (1991). A double-blind desipramine substition during long-term clomipramine treatment in children and adolescents with obsessive–compulsive disorder. *Archives of General Psychiatry, 48,* 922–927.

Leonard, H., Swedo, S., Rapaport, J., Coffey, M., & Cheslow, D. (1988). Treatment of childhood obsessive–compulsive disorder with clomipramine and desmethylimipramine: A double-blind crossover comparison. *Psychopharmacology Bulletin, 24,* 43–45.

Luxenberg, J., Swedo, S., Flament, M., Friedland, R., Rapaport, J., & Rapaport, S. (1988). Neuroanatomical abnormalities in obsessive–compulsive disorder detected with quantitative x-ray computed tomography. *American Journal of Psychiatry, 145,* 1089–1093.

Machlin, S., Harris, G., Pearlson, G., Hoehn-Saric, R., Jeffrey, P., & Camargo, E. (1991). Elevated medial-frontal cerebral blood flow in obsessive–compulsive disorder patients: A SPECT study. *American Journal of Psychiatry, 148,* 1243–1245.

Mahler, M., Pine, F., & Bergman, A. (1975). *The psychological birth of the human infant.* New York: Basic Books.

Martin, A., Pigott, T. A., LaLonde, F. M., Dalton, I., Dubbert, B., & Murphy, D. L. (1993). Lack of evidence of Huntington's Disease-like cognitive dysfunction in obsessive–compulsive disorder. *Biological Psychiatry, 33,* 345–353.

Martinot, J., Allilaire, J., Majoyer, B., Hantouche, E., Huret, J., Legaut-Demare, F., Deslauriers, A., Hardy, P., Pappata, S., Baron, J., & Syrota, A. (1990). Obsessive–compulsive disorder: A clinical neuropsychological and position emission tomography study. *Acta Psychiatrica Scandinavica, 82,* 233–242.

Martuza, R., Chiocca, E., & Jenike, M. (1990). Stereotactic radiofrequency thermal cingulotomy for obsessive–compulsive disorder. *Journal of Neurology and Neuropsychiatry, 2,* 331–336.

Mavissaklian, M., Turner, S., Michelson, L., & Jacob, R. (1985). Tricyclic antidepressants in obsessive–compulsive disorder: Antiobsessional and antidepressant agents? *American Journal of Psychiatry, 142,* 572.

McDougle, C., Goodman, W., Leckman, J., Barr, L., Henninger, G., & Price, L. (1993). The efficacy of fluvoxamine in obsessive–compulsive disorder: Effects of comorbid tic disorder. *Journal of Clinical Psychopharmacology, 13,* 354–358.

McDougle, C., Price, L., Goodman, W., Charney, D., & Heninger, G. (1991). A controlled trial of lithium augmentation in fluvoxamine-refractory obsessive–compulsive disorder: Lack of efficacy. *Journal of Clinical Psychopharmacology, 11,* 175–184.

Mindus, P., & Jenike, M. (1992). Neurosurgical treatment of malignant obsessive–compulsive disorder. *Psychiatric Clinics of North America, 15*(4), 921–938.

Modell, J., Mountz, J., Curtis, G., & Greden, J. (1989). Neurophysiologic dysfuntion in basal ganglia/limbic striatal and thalamocortical circuits as a pathogenetic mechanisms of obsessive–compulsive disorder. *Journal of Neuropsychiatry, 1,* 27–36.

Nordahl, T., Benkelfat, G., Semple, W., Gross, M., King, A., & Cohen, R. (1989). Cerebral glucos metabolic rates in obsessive–compulsive disorder. *Neuropsychopharmacology, 2,* 23–28.

Pato, M., Zohar-Kadouch, R., Zohar, J., & Murphy, D. (1988). Return of symptoms after discontinuation of clomipramine in patients with obsessive–compulsive disorder. *American Journal of Psychiatry, 145,* 1521–1525.

Pato, M. T., Pigott, T. A., Hill, J. L., Grover, G. N., Bernsteing, S. E., & Murphy, D. L. (1991). Controlled comparison of buspirone and clomipramine in obsessive–compulsive disorder. *American Journal of Psychiatry, 148,* 127–129.

Pauls, D., & Leckman, J. (1986). The inheritance of Gilles de la Tourette's syndrome and associated behaviors: Evidence for autosomal dominant transmission. *New England Journal of Medicine, 315*(16), 993.

Pauls, D., Towbin, K., Leckman, J., Zahner, G., & Cohen, D. (1986). Gilles de la Tourette's syndrome and obsessive–compulsive disorder. Evidence supporting a genetic relationship. *Archives of General Psychiatry, 43,* 1180–1182.

Pigott, T., Grady, T., L'Heureux, F., Bernstein, S., Hill, J., & Murphy, D., (1992).

Amphetamine and amphetamine/metergoline challenges in patients with OCD. In *ACNP Annual Meeting Abstracts,* San Juan, Puerto Rico.

Pigott, T., L'Heureux, F., Dubbert, B., Bernstein, S., & Murphy, D. (1994). Obsessive–compulsive disorder: Comorbid conditions. *Journal of Clinical Psychiatry, 55*(10), 15–27.

Pigott, T. A., L'Heureux, F., & Murphy, D. (1993). Pharmacological approaches to treatment-resistant obsessive–compulsive disorder/patients. In *1st International OCD Conference Abstracts.* Isle of Capri, Italy: Solvay Duphar.

Pigott, T. A., Altemus, M. A., Rubenstein, C. S., Hill, J. L., Bihari, K., L'Heureux, F., Bernstein, S. E., & Murphy, D. L. (1991). Eating disorder symptoms in patients withobsessive–compulsive disorder. *American Journal of Psychiatry, 148*(11), 1552–1557.

Pigott, T. A., Hill, J. L., Grady, T. A., L'Heureux, F., Bernstein, S. E., Rubenstein, C. S., & Murphy, D. L. (1993). A comparison of the behavioral effects of oral vs. intravenous *m*-CPP administration in OCD patients and a study of the effects of metergoline prior to iv *m*-CPP. *Biological Psychiatry, 33*(1), 3–14.

Pigott, T. A., L'Heureux, F., Hill, J. L., Bihari, K., Bernstein, S. E., & Murphy, D. L. (1992). A double-blind study of adjuvant buspirone hydrochloride in clomipramine-treated OCD patients. *Journal of Clinical Psychopharmacology, 12,* 11–18.

Pigott, T. A., L'Heureux, F., Rubenstein, C. S., Bernstein, S. E., Hill, J. L., & Murphy, D. L. (1992). A double-blind, placebo controled study of trazodone in patients with obsessive compulsive disorder. *Journal of Clinical Psychopharmacology, 12*(3), 156–162.

Pigott, T. A., Pato, M. T., Bernstein, S. E., Grover, G. N., Hill, J. L., Tolliver, T. J., & Murphy, D. L. (1990). Controled comparisons of clomipramine and fluoxetine in the treatment of obsessive–compulsive disorder. *Archives of General Psychiatry, 47,* 1543–1550.

Pitott, T. A., Pato, M. T., L'Heureux, F., Hill, J. L., Grover, G. N., Bernstein, S. E., & Murphy, D. L. (1991). A controlled comparison of adjuvant lithium carbonate or thyroid hormone in clomipramine-treated OCD patients. *Journal of Clinical Psychopharmacology, 11*(4), 242–248.

Pitman, R., Green, R., Jenike, M,. & Mesulam, M. (1987). Clinical comparison of Tourette's disorder and obsessive–compulsive disorder. *American Journal of Psychiatry, 144,* 1166–1171.

Rapaport, J. (1991). The neurobiology of obsessive–compulsive disorder. *Neuropsychopharmacology, 5,* 1–10.

Rapaport, J., (1992). An animal model of obsessive–compulsive disorder. *Archives of General Psychiatry, 49,* 517–521.

Rapaport, J., & Wise, S. (1988). Obsessive–compulsive disorder: Evidence for basal ganglia dysfunction. *Psychopharmacology Bulletin, 3,* 380–384.

Rasmussen, S., & Eisen, J. (1988). Clinical and epidemiologic findings of significance to neuropharmacologic trials in obsessive–compulsive disorder. *Psychopharmacology Bulletin, 24,* 466–470.

Rasmussen, S., & Eisen, J. (1992). The epidemiology and clinical features of obsessive–compulsive disorder. *Psychiatric Clinics of North America, 15*(4), 743–758.

Rasmussen, S., & Eisen, J. (1993). Assessment of core features, conviction and psychosocial function in OCD. In *1st International OCD Conference Abstracts.* Isle of Capri, Italy: Solvay Duphar.

Rasmussen, S., Eisen, J., & Pato, M. (1993). Current issues in the pharacologic management of obsessive–compulsive disorder. *Journal of Clinical Psychiatry, 54,* 4–9.

Rasmussen, S., Goodman, W., Woods, S., Heninger, G., & Charney, D. (1987). Effects of yohimbine in obsessive–compulsive disorder. *Psychopharmacology, 93,* 308–313.

Rasmussen, S., & Tsuang, M. (1986). Clinical characteristics and family history in DSM-III obsessive–compulsive disorder. *American Journal of Psychiatry, 143,* 317–322.

Richelson, E. (1988). Synaptic pharmacology of antidepressants: An update. *McLean Hospital Journal, 43,* 6–16.

Rolls, E., & Williams, G. (1987). Sensory and movement-related neuronal activity in different regions of the primate striatum. In J. S. Schneider & T. I. Lidsky (Eds.), *Basel ganglia and behavior: Sensory aspects of motor functioning.* Toronto: Saunders.

Rosen, W., Hollander, E., & Stannick, V. (1988). Task performance variables in obsessive–compulsive disorder. *Journal of Clinical and Experimental Neuropsychology, 10,* 73.

Rubenstein, C., Pigott, T., L'Heureux, F., Hill, J., & Murphy, D. (1992). A preliminary investigation of the lifetime prevalence rate of anorexia and bulimia nervosa in patients with OCD. *Journal of Clinical Psychiatry, 53*(9), 309–314.

Rubin, R., Villanueva-Meyer, J., Ananth, J., Trajmar, P., & Mena, I. (1992). Regional xenon 133 cerebral blood flow and cerebral technetium 99m HMPAO uptake in unmedicated patients with obsessive–compulsive disorder and matched normal control subjects. *Archives of General Psychiatry, 49,* 695–702.

Sachdev, P., Hay, P., & Cummings, S. (1992). Psychosurgical treatment of obsessive–compulsive disorder. *Archives of General Psychiatry, 49,* 582–583.

Salzman, L. (1968). *Obsessional personality.* New York: Science House.

Shagrass, C., Roemer, R., Straumanis, J., & Josiassen, R. (1994). Distinctive somatosensory evoked potential features in obsessive–compulsive disorder. *Biological Psychiatry, 19,* 1507–1524.

Sher, K., Frost, R., Kushner, M., Crews, T., & Alexander, J. (1989). Memory deficits in compulsive checkers: Replication and extension in a clinical sample. *Behaviour Research and Therapy, 27,* 65–69.

Stahl, S. (1988). Basal ganglia neuropharmacology and obsessive–compulsive disorder: The obsessive–compulsive disorder hypothesis of basal ganglion dysfunction. *Psychopharmacology Bulletin, 24*(3), 370–374.

Stefanis, C., Rabavilas, A., Papageorgiou, C. (1993). Event related potentials and selective attention in obsessive–compulsive disorder. In *1st International OCD Conference Abstracts*. Isle of Capri, Italy: Solvay Duphar.

Swedo, S., Kilpatrick, K., Schapiro, M., Leonard, H. Cheslow, D., & Rapaport, J. (1991). Antineuronal antibodies in Sydenham's chorea and obsessive–compulsive disorder. *Pediatric Research, 29,* 364A.

Swedo, S., Leonard, H., Rapaport, J., Lenane, M., Goldberger, E., & Cheslow, D. (1989). A double-blind comparison of clomipramine and desipramine in the treatment of trichotillomania. *New England Journal of Medicine, 321,* 497–501.

Swedo, S., Rapaport, J., Cheslow, D., Leonard, H., Ayoub, E., Hosier, D., & Wald, E. (1989). High prevalence of obsessive–compulsive disorder symptoms in patients with Sydenham's chorea. *American Journal of Psychiatry, 146,* 246–249.

Swedo, S., Schapiro, M., Grady, C., Cheslow, D., Leonard, H., Kumar, A., Friedland, R., Rapaport, S., & Rapaport, J. (1989). Cerebral glucose metabolism in childhood-onset obsessive–compulsive disorder. *Archives of General Psychiatry, 46,* 518–523.

Tanquary, J., Lynch, M., & Masand, P. (1992). Obsessive–compulsive disorder in relation to body dysmorphic disorder. *American Journal of Psychiatry, 149(9),* 1283–1284.

Thoren, P., Asberg, M., Bertelsson, L., Mellstrom, B., Sjoqvist, F., & Traskman, L. (1980). Clomipramine treatment of obsessive–compulsive disorder, II: Biochemical aspects. *Archives of General Psychiatry, 37,* 1289–1294.

Thoren, P., Asberg, M., Crohnholm, B., Jornestedt, L., & Trachman, L. (1980). Clomipramine treatment of obsessive–compulsive disorder. I. A controled clinical trial. *Archives of General Psychiatry, 37,* 1281–1285.

Towey, J., Bruder, G., Hollander, E., Friedman, D., Erham, H., Liebowitz, M., & Sutton, S. (1990). Endogenous event-related potentials in obsessive–compulsive disorder. *Biological Psychiatry, 28,* 92–98.

Towey, J., Bruder, G., Tenke, C., Leite, P., Friedman, D., & Hollander, E. (1993). Brain evoked potential, clinical and neurological correlates of neurodysfunction in OCD. In *1st International OCD Conference Abstracts*. Isle of Capri, Italy: Solvay Duphar.

von Economo, C. (1931). *Encephalitis lethargica: Its sequelae and treatment.* London, England: Oxford University Press.

Weissman, M., Bland, R., Canino, G., Greenwald, S., Hwu, H., Lee, C., Newman, S., Oakley-Browne, M., Rubio-Stipec, M., Wickermaratne, P., Wittchen, H., & Yeh, E. (1994). The cross national epidemiology of obsessive–compulsive disorder. *Journal of Clinical Psychiatry, 55,* 5–10.

Weizman, A., Carmi, M., Hermesh, H., Shahar, A., Apter, A., Tyrano, S., & Rehavi, M. (1986). High affinity imipramine binding and serotonin uptake in platelets of eight adolescent and ten adult obsessive–compulsive disorder patients. *American Journal of Psychiatry, 143,* 335–339.

Zohar, J., & Insel, T. (1987). Obsessive–compulsive disorder: Psychobiological approaches to diagnosis, treatment, and pathophysicology. *Biological Psychiatry, 22,* 667–687.

Zohar, J., Insel, T., Berman, K., Foa, E., Hill, J., & Weinberger, D. (1989).
    Anxiety and cerebral blood flow during behavioral challenge: Dissociation
    of central from peripheral and subjective measures. *Archives of General
    Psychiatry, 46,* 505–510.
Zohar, J., Mueller, E. A., Insel, T. R., Zohar-Kadouch, R. C., & Murphy, D.
    L. (1987). Serotonergic responsivity in obsessive–compulsive disorder: Com-
    parison of patients and healthy controls. *Archives of General Psychiatry,
    44,* 946–951.

7

Obsessive–Compulsive Disorder: Anxiety Disorder or Schizotype?

THIS CHAPTER BEGINS by reviewing the clinical status of obsessive–compulsive disorder (OCD) and outlines both similarities and differences between OCD and the other anxiety disorders (OADs). Emphasis is placed on cognitive differences between these disorders, and it is suggested that such cognitive differences in patients with severe OCD and "overvalued ideas" may have some similarities to cognitive symptoms within the schizophrenic constellation of disorders. Any direct relationship between the two conditions is ruled out following a review of the available literature, but attention is drawn to the higher incidence of schizotypal personality disorder found in OCD patients. It is suggested via the dimensional theories of psychosis that OCD may be related to schizophrenia through the expression of increased numbers of subclinical schizotypal traits, particularly of a cognitive nature.

A description of empirical research begins with two psychometric studies that attempted to identify schizotypal traits in OCD and OAD subjects, using a range of 18 trait and symptom questionnaires. In both studies OCD subjects exhibited significantly greater schizotypal traits and symptoms, particularly those related to positive symptoms of schizotypy and cognitive disorganization.

In view of the psychometric findings, it was hypothesized that OCD subjects would perform schizotypically on cognitive experimental paradigms that have successfully discriminated high- and low-schizotype subjects and schizophrenics from other clinically diagnosed patients. One such paradigm is that of negative priming. Four negative priming experiments are described that consistently differentiated OCD from OAD subjects in a manner conforming to a hypothesis that OCD and schizotypy are related through a common exhibition of reduced preattentive cognitive inhibition.

These negative priming findings were further investigated within OCD and OAD samples by manipulating the speed of presentation of the stimuli. Although OCD subjects as a whole again behaved schizotypically within this experiment, the division into checkers and noncheckers revealed differential experimental effects in these two groups. The group of checkers exhibited a greater putative reduction of cognitive inhibition, which was less effectively compensated for as the processing of stimuli was mediated by more attended strategies of information processing.

A final experimental study is reported that attempted to analyze the putative effects of reduced cognitive inhibition for more attended strategies of suppression. OCD subjects, particularly checkers, exhibited significantly greater problems in conscious attempts to inhibit a neutral target stimulus. The chapter concludes with a discussion of the overall findings.

THE CLINICAL STATUS
OF OBSESSIVE–COMPULSIVE DISORDER

Obsessive–Compulsive Disorder and the Anxiety Disorders

Diagnostic classification is an attempt to arrange clinical phenomena into categories that share common attributes. Ideally, the members of each category express very similar symptoms and signs, etiology, pathophysiology, prognosis, and response to treatment (Marks, 1987). In this respect, the classification of OCD as an anxiety disorder has presented particular problems.

There are undoubted similiarities between OCD and the OADs. Most OCD and OAD patients experience discomfort in the presence of specific stimuli and make efforts to avoid these stimuli. This avoidance has the primary aim of reducing anxiety in both groups. OCD and OAD patients both commonly report such problems as generalized tension and anxiety, spontaneous panic, worry, and depressed mood. Both groups can be treated with exposure therapy.

However, there also appear to be important differences between OCD and OAD patients. There is an equal sex distribution of OCD sufferers; in the OADs, by contrast, females outnumber males two to one. The age of onset of OCD is significantly younger (Karno, Golding, Sorenson, &

Burnam, 1988). There also appear to be signficant differences in the bio-chemistry of the disorders. OCD symptoms, unlike OAD symptoms, are not made worse with the administration of anxiogenic compounds (Gorman et al., 1985; Rasmussen, et al., 1987). OCD patients are also refractory to anxiolytic medications, but usually have a selective responsivity to serotonergic medication. The response to placebo is high in anxiety states and low or absent in OCD (Montgomery, 1990).

Steketee, Grayson, and Foa (1987) compared the demographic, familial, and intrapersonal characteristics of OCD and OAD groups. OCD subjects demonstrated greater poverty and unemployment, more psychiatric symptoms (specifically depression and interpersonal discomfort), and increased feelings of inadequacy, hostility, and guilt. The authors concluded that OCD was also functionally more debilitating than OAD. Cameron, Thyer, Nesse, and Curtis (1986) compared the symptom severity and pattern of severity in a mixed group of 316 anxiety-disordered subjects, in order to test the validity of the disorders as discrete syndromes. Their results supported the grouping of these conditions within the general diagnostic category of anxiety disorders, "with the possible exception of OCD" (p. 1132).

At a purely functional level, for many clinicians the single most important and striking factor that differentiates OCD and OAD patients is the nature of the cognitive experience: the everyday intrusion into conscious thinking of intense, repetitive, personally abhorrent, absurd, and alien thoughts, leading to endless repetition of specific acts or to the rehearsal of bizarre and irrational mental and behavioral rituals. These repetitive thoughts are often evoked by stimuli that are more abstract than those seen in OAD patients (e.g., untidiness, contamination, danger), and the fear is one of vague consequences often unconnected to the eliciting stimuli (Marks, 1987).

The majority of OCD patients remain aware of the senselessness and futility of their obsessional thoughts and behaviors. However, for others the intensity and fixity of the irrational belief appears to have more in common with delusional states. These symptoms have tended to be categorized rather parsimoniously as "overvalued ideas" (Foa, 1979). Such features have led other authors to suggest the creation of separate diagnostic categories for these more apparently deluded OCD patients, including "obsessive compulsive disorder with psychotic features" (Insel & Akiskal, 1986), "schizoanancastic" disorder (Shakhlavov, 1988), "Schizo-obsessive" disorder (Jenike, Baer, Minichello, Schwartz, & Carey, 1986); "obsessive psychosis" (Weiss, Robinson, & Winnick, 1975; Robinson, Winnick, & Weiss, 1975), and "obsessive–compulsive psychosis" (Solyom, DiNicola, & Phil, 1985).

Obsessive–Compulsive Disorder and Schizophrenia

The suggestion that some patients with severe OCD express focal delusions leads logically to the proposition that a relationship might exist between OCD and the schizophrenias, since delusions are a Schneiderian first-rank symptom of schizophrenia (Schneider, 1959). This notion has periodically resurfaced in the clinical literature ever since Westphal (1878) suggested that the entire obsessive–compulsive syndrome is a variant or prodrome of schizophrenia.

Schizophrenia and OCD do have a number of features in common. They have similar age of onset (early 20s), and marriage and fertility rates in both groups are reduced. Historically, both have responded poorly to psychological and somatic treatments, though the recent developments of specific serotonergic drugs and the advances of cognitive-behavioral therapies for OCD have offered greater promise (Black & Noyes, 1990).

There is also evidence for an increased incidence of schizophrenia in patients originally diagnosed as exhibiting OCD, though there are obvious problems with diagnostic specificity in these studies. Of nine reports reviewed by Insel and Akiskal (1986), the mean incidence of schizophrenia in follow-up of OCD groups was 4.42%, compared to a lifetime risk of 1% for the development of schizophrenia in the general population.

The incidence of OCD symptoms in schizophrenia seems to be even more common, though it should be noted that there is also a generally raised incidence of other neurotic and personality disorder symptoms in schizophrenia. Rosen (1957) reviewed 848 schizophrenics and found that 3.5% exhibited marked OCD symptoms. Fenton and McGlashan (1986) reported that 13% of 163 chronic schizophrenic patients exhibited prominent OCD symptoms, and that the presence of OCD in schizophrenia is a powerful predictor of poor prognosis.

Experimental evidence for the existence of a relationship between OCD and the schizophrenias is very sparse. Flor-Henry, Yeudall, Koles, and Horwarth (1979) investigated neuropsychological and power-spectral electroencephalographic concomitants of OCD, and suggested similarities in psychophysiology between these groups. Ciesielski, Beech, and Gordon (1981) noted that the evoked potentials during cognitive processing of six out of eight OCD patients paralleled those reported in psychotic patients. This result was replicated by Beech, Ciesielski, and Gordon (1983).

Bannister and Fransella (1971) used repertory grid methods with OCD patients. Fransella (1974) reported that the results of OCD patients overlapped significantly with those of thought-disordered schizophrenic patients, but had little in common with neurotic patients. Related to this are the findings of abnormalities on the Wisconsin Card Scoring Test

(WCST) in OCD subjects. This test assesses a subject's ability to form, maintain, and shift cognitive sets, including the capacity to use feedback to modify inappropriate but previously rewarded responses. Harvey (1986) demonstrated greater total errors and marked preservative errors in a group of OCD patients on the WCST. A similar result was reported by Head, Bolton, and Hymas (1989). Other independent studies have reported comparable results for schizophrenic subjects (Fey, 1951; Malmo, 1974; Heaton, Baade, & Johnsen, 1978).

Despite these clinical demographic and experimental similarities, the majority of authors have expressed skepticism concerning a significant relationship between OCD and schizophrenia. Following a thorough review of the literature, Black (1974, p. 53) concluded, in the words of Rudin (1953) and Lewis (1957), that "there is no close affinity between OCD and schizophrenia." A similar conclusion was reached by Rachman and Hodgson (1980, p. 87), who quoted Ingram (1961): "It would be unwise to suggest obsessional illness and schizophrenia are closely linked."

Dimensional Models of Schizophrenia

If OCD is not diagnostically related to schizophrenia, it is nevertheless possible that there may be common ground at a functional level. This hypothesis becomes particularly plausible in the light of increasing evidence for dimensional theories of psychotic disorder, first postulated by Eysenck (1952). This work emphasizes that psychotic disorder is not a discrete entity, but that the predisposition to psychosis forms a continuum and series of continua.

There are essentially two views of this continuity hypothesis within schizophrenia research; these may be broadly described as a psychological and a psychiatric perspective. The former view has been most clearly associated with Claridge (1967, 1985, 1987). He proposes that the starting point for a schizophrenia continuum is normality or health; schizotypy is seen as a fully normal personality dimension. Crucial here is the idea that healthy diversity and disposition to illness are synonymous, forming an unbroken continuum of schizotypy. Illness is then construed as an aberration of otherwise normal functional processes; this aberration, it is proposed, begins in small and discontinuous steps, giving rise intially or when occurring in a mild degree to an appearance of continuity even at the illness level. This clinical dimension and the transition to it are reflected in the observed blurring of the boundaries between personality, personality disorder, and outright illness (Claridge, 1993).

In contrast, the quasi-dimensional psychiatric perspective (e.g., McGuffin & Thapar, 1992; Levinson & Mowry, 1991) concentrates on variations of clinical features within the illness domain, with schizotypal personality disorder (SPD) as its starting point leading to schizophrenia at the other end of the continuum.

Obsessive–Compulsive Disorder and Schizotypal Personality Disorder

All of the available literature thus far has focused on the search for clinical features of schizotypy, drawn from the diagnostic criteria for SPD, in OCD patients. As such, this evidence suggests the possibility of quasi-dimensional links between OCD and schizophrenia via SPD. A number of studies attest to the increased incidence of clinical schizotypal features in OCD patients. Insel and Akiskal (1986), Joffe, Swinson, and Regan (1988), and Solyom et al. (1985) all reported that 17% of their samples of OCD patients exhibited concomitant SPD. Jenike et al. (1986) suggested that 30% of their OCD patients expressed significant schizotypal features. Stanley, Turner, and Borden (1990) reported 28% of OCD patients with schizotypal features; of these, 8% met the full criteria for SPD. There is also evidence that the concomitance of OCD and high schizotypy predicts a less optimistic outcome for conventional therapies (Jenike et al. 1986).

QUESTIONNAIRE EVIDENCE LINKING OBSESSIVE–COMPULSIVE DISORDER AND SCHIZOTYPY

Our initial study (Enright & Beech, 1990) was based on the more fully dimensional viewpoint of a putative relationship between OCD and schizophrenia. This work aimed to assess the level of schizotypy in OCD measured by a battery of questionnaires designed to identify "psychosis proneness" in nonclinical subjects. The psychometric tool utilized in this research was the Composite Schizotypy Questionnaire (CSTQ; Bentall, Claridge, & Slade, 1989), which consists of 18 published scales as follows:

• The Eysenck Personality Questionnaire (EPQ): Extraversion (E), Neuroticism (N), Psychoticism (p), Lie (L) scales (Eysenck & Eysenck, 1975). Of major interest was the P scale. Although this is not a measure of schizotypy per se, it was hypothesized to offer a general indicator of psychosis proneness in normal subjects.
• Claridge's Schizotypy Questionnaire: STA and STB scales (Claridge & Broks, 1984). The STA scale is based on the characteristics of SPD and is designed to tap elements assumed to be genetically related to the spectrum of schizophrenic disorders. It samples unusual perceptual ex-

periences, magical thinking, paranoid ideation, and suspiciousness (Claridge & Hewitt, 1987). The STB characterizes borderline personality disorder and measures other elements of "borderline" syndromes that may be seen as stable psychopathological characteristics. Although not so directly related to schizophrenic symptomatology, the STB measures instability in a number of areas, including mood and self-image.

• The Chapman Group Scales: Social Anhedonia (SoAn), Physical Anhedonia (PhAn), Perceptual Aberration (PAb), Magical Ideation (MGI), and Hypomanic Personality (HoP) (Chapman, Chapman, & Raulin, 1976; Ekbald & Chapman, 1983, 1986). The first four of these scales were developed to measure different aspects of schizophrenia-like characteristics in the normal population.

• The Launay–Slade Hallucinatory Scale (LSHS; Launay & Slade, 1981). This scale was developed to measure hallucinatory experiences in the normal population.

• The Nielsen–Petersen Schizophrenism Scale (NPSS; Nielsen & Petersen, 1976). Items in this scale are based on characteristics of premorbid and early-stage schizophrenia (i.e., hypersensitivity and cognitive peculiarities).

• The Golden–Meehl Schizoidia Scale (GMSS; Golden & Meehl, 1979). This is a schizotypy scale based on items from the Minnesota Multiphasic Personality Inventory (Hathaway & McKinley, 1943); it produces a set of indicators, most of which discriminate between groups of schizoids and nonschizoids, but which are largely independent of one another within each group.

• The Foulds and Bedford Delusional Scales: Contrition (dC), Persecution (dP), Disintegration (dD), and Grandiosity (dG) (Foulds & Bedford, 1975). These scales were designed to measure the two highest levels of the authors' postulated hierarchy of mental illness. The whole system is comprised of four levels of increasing severity of symptomatology: depression; anxiety neurosis; integrated delusions (paranoia and melancholia, measured by the dC, dG, and dP scales); and disintegrated delusions (involved in schizophrenia and measured by the dD scale). In contrast to the other CSTQ scales, this instrument was designed to be used in clinical diagnosis rather than as a measure of psychotic characteristics in the general population.

We (Enright & Beech, 1990) compared OCD and a mixed group of OAD subjects, and found significantly greater incidence of schizotypal traits in OCD subjects on the majority of the CSTQ scales. We (Enright, Claridge, Beech, & Kemp-Wheeler, 1994) replicated this finding in a sample of 37 OCD and 62 OAD subjects drawn from each of the DSM-III-R (American Psychiatric Association, 1987) subcategories of anxiety disorder.

The results of this latter comparison are presented in Table 7.1. OCD subjects scored significantly higher than OAD subjects on 13 of the 18 schizotypy scales, notable exceptions being Eysenck's E, P, and L scales from the EPQ and Chapman's two anhedonia scales (SoAn and PhAn). Higher scores in the combination of these latter scales has often been linked to evidence of "negative" psychotic symptoms with psychometric schizotypy research (Raine & Allbutt, 1989; Kendler & Hewitt, 1992).

In contrast, OCD subjects were significantly different from OAD subjects on the CSTQ scales reflecting cognitive and perceptual aspects of schizotypy and those indicating a degree of cognitive disorganization. Jackson and Claridge (1991) reported mean STA and STB scores of 21.31 and 9.06, respectively, in a patient group who had been diagnosed as suffering from a schizophrenic illness but whose symptoms were currently in relative remission. In normal subjects, the mean STA and STB scores were 14.38 and 6.03, respectively. When these data are compared to those of our (Enright et al., 1994) main questionnaire study, there is an obvious alignment between OCD and schizophrenic patients and between OAD and normal subjects on these scales.

The OCD and OAD data were further analyzed with respect to the putative subfactors of schizotypy. In this regard, there is a growing body

TABLE 7.1. Scores on Individual Scales of the CSTQ for OCD and OAD Subjects

Scale	OCD		OAD		T
	Mean	(SD)	Mean	(SD)	
STA	22.18	(6.96)	15.48	(7.82)	4.30***
STB	10.03	(3.73)	6.45	(4.05)	4.37***
E	8.37	(5.28)	9.76	(4.85)	1.32
N	18.89	(3.50)	15.58	(5.36)	3.35***
P	3.59	(2.77)	2.92	(1.82)	1.46
L	7.97	(3.62)	7.90	(3.87)	0.09
SoAn	16.78	(5.74)	14.50	(6.94)	1.68
PhAn	18.37	(7.89)	15.64	(7.32)	1.75
HoP	14.21	(6.45)	11.70	(5.91)	2.01*
PAb	7.38	(6.22)	4.34	(4.48)	2.82**
MgI	7.51	(4.67)	4.11	(3.87)	3.90***
LSHS	4.78	(3.00)	3.03	(2.31)	3.26**
NPSS	10.19	(3.17)	7.02	(4.05)	4.07***
GMSS	4.43	(1.59)	3.20	(2.12)	3.02**
dC	1.97	(1.82)	0.79	(0.97)	4.21***
dP	1.16	(1.54)	0.50	(1.07)	2.53**
dD	1.00	(1.29)	0.34	(0.83)	3.11**
dG	1.30	(1.37)	0.56	(0.80)	3.36***

Note. For scale abbreviations, see text.
*$p < 0.05$. **$p < 0.01$. ***$p < 0.001$.

of evidence to suggest that the concept of schizotypy is multidimensional rather than unitary. Bentall et al. (1989) have attempted to analyze the subfactors of schizotypy using the CSTQ. Their principal-components analysis yielded a three-factor solution to the CSTQ when the Foulds and Bedford (1975) clinical scales were omitted. These factors were described by Bentall et al. as 'Positive Symptom' Schizotypy, Cognitive Disorganisation/Anxiety, and Introverted Anhedonia. When the Foulds and Bedford scales were included in the analysis, a four-factor solution was obtained, the first three factors remaining consistent and the fourth factor measuring an asocial component of schizotypy. A further factor analysis of the CSTQ has recently been undertaken by McCreery (1993), who found a four-factor solution similar to that of the original study, both including and omitting the Foulds and Bedford scales. These schizotypy factors are broadly similar to other psychometric studies using factor analysis to identify the principal components of schizotypy (Muntaner, Garcia-Sevilla, Fernandez, & Torrubia, 1988; Kendler & Hewitt, 1992).

We (Enright et al., 1994) applied the factor weightings for each of the individual scales of the CSTQ (taken from Bentall et al., 1989) to our OCD and OAD questionnaire data, to examine which of the subfactors of schizotypy would differentiate most clearly between the two groups. Results indicated that OCD subjects were significantly more schizotypal on all subfactors than were OAD subjects. The two groups were most distinct on the first two factors—those pertaining to postive psychotic symptomatology and cognitive disorganization. These data therefore further supported the proposition that OCD and the schizophrenia spectrum of disorders may be linked at a cognitive level.

THE NEGATIVE PRIMING PARADIGM

If OCD is related to schizophrenia on a schizotypal continuum, then logically it should be possible to demonstrate this association further, using laboratory tasks that have linked subjects high in schizotypal traits with those exhibiting schizophrenia. One such task is the negative priming (NP) paradigm.

NP extends the Stroop phenomenon (Stroop, 1935), which occurs when the analysis of sensory stimuli contains a conflict within this information. A typical example of this is the presentation of the color word "blue" written in the hue of red. The subject's response time to state the hue is typically longer than for congruous or unrelated word and hue.

The NP task presents a series of stimuli in which previously ignored information becomes the required response for the next trial—for instance, if the word "red" is presented written in a green hue. The subject is required to say "green" and ignore the nonrelevant word "red." If the next trial consists of a word written in a red hue, then the correct response is now "red." In normal subjects, this latter naming takes longer (i.e., is negatively primed) than a control condition when the prior distractor is unrelated to the subsequent target.

Cognitive psychologists have suggested that the NP effect can be attributed to a process of active inhibition of the ignored stimulus, which then delays the subsequent response when this stimulus becomes the target, since the subject must first overcome this inhibition (Lowe, 1979; Neill, 1977). This explanation provides an important theoretical overlap with explanations of schizophrenia. It has long been supposed that the schizophrenic nervous system shows deviant modulation of response to sensory and other information, probably because of the weakening of some inhibitory process (Claridge, 1967). Parallel formulations drawn from cognitive psychology refer to poor filtering of information, as articulated by Frith (1979) in his proposal that the positive symptoms of schizophrenia result from weakened preattentive inhibitory selection mechanisms, leading to a relative failure to "limit the contents of consciousness." (p. 225)

Consistent with this theoretical position is the idea that auditory hallucinations have their basis in real sounds that activate various logogens preconsciously (Morton, 1979). Initial processing may result in some incorrect interpretations, and conscious awareness of these provides the most pertinent information that an individual uses for attribution (Posner & Boies, 1971). Delusions arise because of the need to explain these irrelevant perceptions. Thought disorder is inferred from problems in speech and language, in which there is an inability to inhibit the alternative meanings of words not normally available to consciousness, leading to abnormal speech output.

Negative Priming with Schizophrenic and High-Schizotype Subjects

In normal and mixed neurotic subjects, Beech, Baylis, Smithson, and Claridge (1989) have demonstrated that the NP condition produces a slower reaction time (RT). However, in schizophrenic subjects this effect is abolished (Beech, Powell, McWilliam, & Claridge, 1989) and even reversed, with RT being facilitated in individuals who score high on schizotypy questionnaires (Beech & Claridge, 1987; Beech, Baylis, et al., 1989). This effect has been consistently replicated with different experimental stimuli, including color words (Beech, Baylis, et al., 1989; Beech, Powell, et al., 1989) and semantically related words (Beech, McManus, Baylis, Tipper, & Agar, 1991).

Beech (1987) theorizes that reduced NP in highly schizotypal and schizophrenic subjects reflects a common deficit of cognitive inhibition. Since the irrelevant stimuli on the previous trial are less effectively inhibited, they are more accessible as the correct response for the next trial. Less effective inhibitory processes in schizophrenic and high-schizotype subjects may therefore account for the faster relative reaction times on the priming task.

If a relationship exists between OCD and schizotypy, and therefore schizophrenia at some cognitive level, it would be logical to assume that this would become apparent with the NP experimental paradigm. If OCD can also be distinguished from the other categories of anxiety disorder with these methods, then it suggests that there may also be a fundamental difference in mechanisms of information processing between these groups, which might warrant reconsideration of their alignment in the current systems of diagnostic classification.

Negative Priming in Obsessive–Compulsive Disorder and Other Anxiety Disorders

The NP paradigm used in the following series of experiments consisted of four basic experimental conditions.

1. *Priming distractor:* The word or letter to be ignored became the target in the next trial.
2. *Control:* The ignored stimulus was unrelated to the target in the next trial.
3. *Repeated distractor:* The ignored stimulus was the same throughout the list and unrelated to the subsequent target.
4. *Neutral distractor:* The ignored stimulus was a series of crosses or a slash.

A derived measure of the amount of NP exhibited by a subject was calculated by subtracting the mean RT for the control condition from the mean RT of the priming distractor condition. Stimuli were presented as 12 trials under each of these four conditions; each trial consisted of 9 items. Condition 3 was used as a filler to reduce the chance of subjects' spotting the experimental manipulations in conditions 1 and 2.

The Pilot Study

We (Enright & Beech, 1990) first used the adapted Stroop NP technique with color words to demonstrate cognitive information-processing differences between OCD subjects and a heterogeneous group of OAD subjects. Most significant was the pattern of results. Whereas OAD subjects ex-

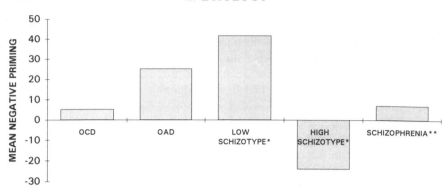

FIGURE 7.1. NP results from three studies: our pilot study (Enright & Beech, 1990 — OCD and OAD subjects); *Beech, Baylis, Smithson, and Claridge (1989 — subjects low and high in schizotypy); and **Beech, Powell, McWilliam, and Claridge (1989 — schizophrenic subjects).

hibited amounts of NP similar to those of normal subjects reported by Beech, Baylis, et al. (1989). OCD subjects' NP results were much closer to those exhibited by highly schizotypal and schizophrenic subjects (Beech, Baylis, et al., 1989; Beech, Powell, et al., 1989). NP data from these experiments are presented for comparison with our data in Figure 7.1.

In the light of these results, it seemed important to attempt to replicate and consolidate such findings, using other NP procedures previously utilized with highly schizotypal subjects. In addition, there is experimental evidence (Ciesielski et al, 1981; Beech et al., 1983) that OCD subjects can be increasingly differentiated from normal controls as the cognitive complexity of the experimental task increases. Our subsequent NP experimentation therefore sought to utilize tasks of increasing cognitive complexity. Lastly, in order to investigate the specificity of the reduced NP effect to OCD among the anxiety disorders, it was necessary to compare OCD subjects separately with groups of subjects drawn from each of the OAD subcategories. The following three experiments were therefore instigated. In each of the three experimental studies described below, the subject panel and apparatus used were the same. The order of presentation of the experiments was randomized for each subject, and a 15-minute rest period preceded each of the experiments.

A total of 37 OCD subjects (23 females and 14 males; mean age [$\bar{X}$] = 36.4 years), and 62 subjects with other anxiety disorders, participated in the study. The latter group contained subjects in the following DSM-III-R categories: 10 agoraphobia (8 female, 2 male; $\bar{X}$ = 40.3); 12 simple phobia (8, 4; $\bar{X}$ = 32.6); 11 panic disorder (3, 8; $\bar{X}$ = 35.7); 10 generalized anxiety disorder (7, 3; $\bar{X}$ = 39.6); 9 social phobia (2, 7; $\bar{X}$ = 31.2); and 10 posttraumatic stress disorder (5, 5; $\bar{X}$ = 45.8). All subjects met DSM-III-R criteria for their respective diagnoses.

The Negative Priming Paradigm Using Letters

Allport, Tipper, and Chmiel (1985) were the first to describe NP effects on a letters task with normal subjects. The experimental procedure involved reading consecutive single red letters aloud, while ignoring single green letters presented simultaneously and slightly overlapping.

Theoretically, it was assumed that the demands of information processing on this task are related principally to the physical analysis of the letter, which enables recognition. There is evidence that this level of analysis occurs at an early basic phase in the processing of sensory information, and it was therefore assumed that this task reflects a relatively simple cognitive demand (Lindsay & Norman, 1977).

We (Enright & Beech, 1993a) reported evidence of reduced NP in OCD subjects, using this letters task. OCD subjects clearly exhibited the least NP, as displayed in Figure 7.2. However, when amounts of NP in OCD and OAD subjects were compared, significant differences were limited to only three OAD subgroups: subjects with simple phobia, panic disorder, and social phobia.

The Adapted Stroop Negative Priming Task

The adapted Stroop NP task used in the pilot study was replicated with this much larger experimental sample. Since the processing of colors and color words is assumed to be cognitively more complex than the recognition of letters, this task represented a greater information-processing demand for the same subjects as in the previous experiment. We (Enright & Beech, 1993a) found that the OCD group exhibited the least amount of NP, as shown in Figure 7.3. This reduced NP was now significantly

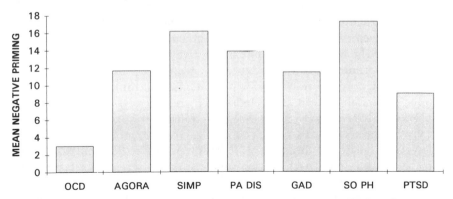

FIGURE 7.2. NP results for the OCD group and various OAD subgroups (AGORA, agoraphobia; SIMP, simple phobia; PA DIS, panic disorder; GAD, generalized anxiety disorder; SO PH, social phobia; PTSD, posttraumatic stress disorder) on the letters task.

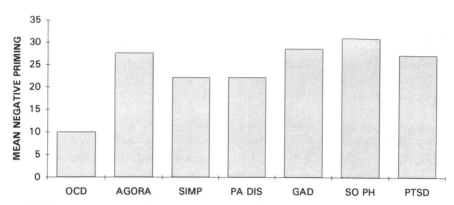

FIGURE 7.3. NP results for the OCD group and various OAD subgroups (see Figure 7.2 caption for abbreviations) on the adapted Stroop task.

different from that of four of the OAD subgroups: subjects with agoraphobia, generalized anxiety disorder, social phobia, and posttraumatic stress disorder.

Repetition and Semantic Negative Priming

The final task involved more complex semantic processing of target stimuli; it therefore represented a further extension of information-processing demand, compared with the previous two experiments. The experimental stimuli were 10 words, two drawn from each of the following five semantic categories: animals, furniture, tools, music, and the human body. The words were as follows: "dog," "cat," "table," "chair," "hammer," "spanner," "guitar," "trumpet," "hand," and "foot." Stimuli were presented as two words simultaneously and slightly overlapping, one red and one green. Subjects were instructed to ignore the green word in each pair and to categorize the red word into one of the five semantic categories. There were two priming conditions: Repetition negative priming (NP) occurred when the ignored distractor prime was identical to the subsequent probe (e.g., red "chair"/green "dog," followed by red "dog"); semantic negative priming (SNP) occurred when the ignored distractor prime was semantically related to the subsequent probe (e.g., red "chair"/green "dog," followed by red "cat"). Beech et al. (1991) reported reduced NP and SNP on this task in highly schizotypal subjects, compared to subjects low in schizotypal traits.

We (Enright & Beech, 1993b) found that OCD subjects exhibited results very similar to those of highly schizotypal subjects. Compared to the OAD subgroups, OCD demonstrated least NP and SNP, as shown in Figure 7.4. The amount of NP exhibited by OCD subjects differed

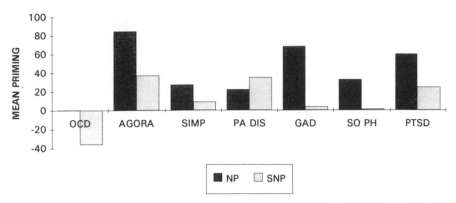

FIGURE 7.4. NP and SNP results for the OCD group and various OAD sub-groups (see Figure 7.2 caption for abbreviations) on the semantic processing task.

significantly from that of four OAD subgroups: subjects with agoraphobia, generalized anxiety disorder, social phobia, and posttraumatic stress disorder. The amount of SNP in OCD subjects differed significantly from that of all OAD subgroups.

The semantic facilitatory priming effect demonstrated that OCD subjects benefited from the ignored prime in naming the subsequent semantically related target. Beech et al. (1991) have suggested that this similar result in highly schizotypal subjects may reflect a difference in the relative strength of mechanisms of spreading facilitation (Collins & Loftus, 1975) and spreading inhibition (Roediger & Neely, 1982). The specific proposal is that high-schizotype subjects exhibit weaker inhibition to semantically related concepts activated in memory by the target stimuli. This suggests that certain stimuli previously associated with specific symptoms in OCD patients may more readily serve as a reminder of these obsessional thoughts or actions, because of a failure to inhibit such associations preattentively. This hypothesis is discussed in detail later in this chapter.

The Relationship among Negative Priming Results from the Three Experiments

Since the same group of subjects was used in all three NP experiments, derived priming measures were intercorrelated to examine whether each task was tapping a similar mechanism of cognitive inhibition. Our findings indicated that only the two measures from the semantic task were correlated significanly at the 5% level, both in the analysis of all subjects' results and in that of OCD subjects' results alone. Since the derived priming data from the semantic task were calculated by subtraction of the same control condition, care is warranted in the interpretation of this one significant finding. Statistical attempts to establish nonlinear relationships among the derived priming measures also proved nonsignificant in all but the data from the semantic task.

The lack of an interrelationship among derived NP results from the three experimental tasks suggests that each experimental task may reflect the employment of a different mechanism of cognitive inhibition, or differing levels of a number of processes of inhibition. OCD subjects exhibited a greater failure of inhibition on all tasks, suggesting deficits across the complete range of inhibition mechanisms tapped by these tasks.

Conclusions Regarding the Negative Priming Findings

The pilot study and the three experiments demonstrate the consistency of the differential NP effects between OCD and OAD subjects. Where comparative data were available, OCD subjects exhibited reduced NP (similar to that found in high-schizotype and schizophrenic subjects), whereas OAD subjects showed NP effects similar to those of low-schizotype subjects. The differentiation of OCD and OAD groups became greater as the cognitive task complexity increased. The theoretical explanation for these effects suggests that reduced NP reflects less effective cognitive inhibition of the nonrelevant stimulus.

Other authors have pointed to the importance of a putative abnormality in the balance between facilitatory and inhibitory cognitive processes in other psychological disorders (see Power, 1991, for a review). These include posttraumatic stress disorder (Horowitz, 1983), depresssion (Ingram, 1990), and anxiety (Williams, Watts, MacLeod, & Mathews, 1988). When empirical research has been conducted, these studies have tended to focus on cognitive processes involving emotionally charged experimental stimuli (either negative or threat-related words). It would seem likely from our failure to demonstrate a significant intercorrelation among different measures of priming that many different processes of inhibition may be in operation at different stages of pre- and postattentive processing. It would therefore be very premature to equate the suppression of disturbing thoughts in the anxiety literature with the putative processes of inhibition tapped by our NP tasks. The importance of our findings with OCD subjects (and of those previously reported for high-schizotype and schizophrenic subjects) is that evidence of reduced cognitive inhibition was demonstrated with emotionally neutral stimuli, suggesting a global deficit.

Finally, it should be noted that these data could not be explained with reference to any experimental group being consistently less accurate or faster within the experimental paradigm. There were no significant differences between OCD and OAD subjects in recorded error rates in any of the experimental tasks. This fact need not be surprising, since although one might expect greater cognitive confusion from reduced cognitive inhibition, the tasks were very focal and the uninhibited distractors served to facilitate rather than to disrupt performance in OCD subjects. The OCD and OAD groups did not differ significantly in their overal RTs to the stimuli across all experimental conditions. The OAD subgroups also did not differ significantly from one another in priming effects or errors in the letters or adapted Stroop task. On the semantic task, there was one signficant difference between OAD subgroups: The agoraphobia group differed significanly from the social phobia group regarding greater priming effects and greater numbers of errors.

NEGATIVE PRIMING AT DIFFERENT SPEEDS OF STIMULUS PRESENTATION

In order to understand the clinical implications of a theory of reduced cognitive inhibition in OCD, it may be important to try to identify at what stage in the processing of information the putative deficit occurs. Theorizing about the mechanism of NP has suggested that the process of cognitive inhibition operates at a preattentive level (Neill, 1977; Tipper, 1985). This propostion was investigated by Beech, Baylis, et al. (1989), who presented high- and low-schizotype subjects with NP stimuli at three different presentation speeds. They found that the reduced NP effect in high-schizotype subjects was confined to very short presentation speeds. Beech and his colleagues concluded that at the fastest presentation rates, the stimuli are acted upon by primarily automatic processes of selective attention (Posner & Snyder, 1975; Neely, 1977). Beech and colleagues have suggested that at longer presentation speeds, it becomes increasingly likely that conscious cognitive processing begins to assist the decision-making task, and these processes may have the capacity to overcome the earlier cognitive inhibition deficits.

Laplante, Everett, and Thomas (1992) demonstrated a similar effect of reduced cognitive inhibition tied to the faster rates of stimulus presentation in schizophrenic subjects, although the methodology of this study was rather different. They hypothesized that the rate of growth of inhibition in schizophrenics is abnormally slow and requires longer to reach levels that have a significant impact on NP tasks.

In order to investigate these effects in OCD we (Enright, Beech, & Claridge, in press) used a methodology similar to that of Beech, Baylis, et al. (1989) and compared 32 OCD subjects with 32 OAD subjects drawn from the generalized anxiety disorder, simple phobia, and social phobia subgroups. These latter OAD groups exhibited priming effects most similar to the OCD group, particularly on the most complex semantic NP task.

They were therefore selected to provide a stricter test of the cognitive inhibition deficit hypothesis in subsequent experimentation. The OCD group consisted of 16 "checkers," diagnosed by clinical interview and scoring 6 or above on the Maudsley Obsessional–Compulsive Inventory's Checking scale (MOCI-C), and 16 "noncheckers," OCD subjects scoring 2 or below on the MOCI-C. This selection of OCD subjects was designed to enable separate comparison of checkers and noncheckers, who have been reported to show cognitive differences in nonclinical and non-OCD experimental groups (Sher, Mann, & Frost, 1984; Sher, Frost, Kushner, Crews, & Alexander, 1989; Goodwin & Sher, 1992).

The NP experimental task utilized was the adapted Stroop paradigm. The task was performed three times. Stimuli were presented at 100, 250, and 350 milliseconds (ms). The order of presentation speeds was counterbalanced. The resulting amount of NP for the two groups at each of the three presentation speeds is presented in Figure 7.5. These data were consistent with the results of the previous work (Beech, Baylis, et al., 1989; Laplante et al., 1992). At a presentation speed of 100 ms, OCD subjects exhibited significantly reduced NP compared to OAD subjects. However, at 250 ms and 350 ms, there was no significant difference between experimental groups. In the Beech, Baylis, et al. (1989) study, highly schizotypal subjects differed from those low in schizotypal traits at 100 ms but not at 250 ms and 500 ms. It was concluded that the locus of the NP effect in OCD subjects is similar to that of highly schizotypal subjects, being tied to preattentive cognitive mechanisms and most significant at the fastest presentation rates. As the data were presented for longer, other more attended strategies of selective attention intervened, and both OCD and OAD groups exhibited similar priming effects.

These results became more intriguing when checkers were compared directly with noncheckers. Differential priming effects occurred: Noncheck-

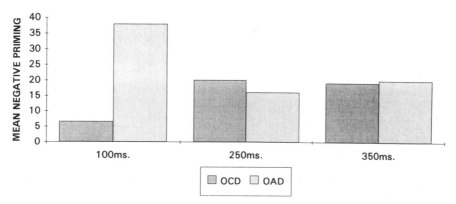

FIGURE 7.5. NP results at three presentation speeds for OCD and OAD subjects.

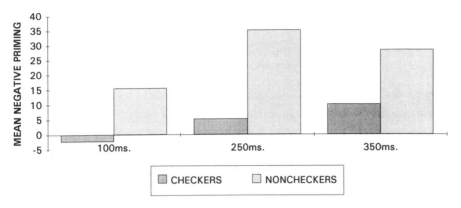

FIGURE 7.6. NP results at three presentation speeds for OCD checkers and non-checkers.

ers initially exhibited reduced NP at 100 ms, but the amount of NP approached levels similar to those of OAD subjects at 250 and 350 ms. The checkers, however, continued to exhibit significantly reduced levels of NP even at the slower presentation speeds. These data are presented in Figure 7.6.

In view of the way OCD subjects were assigned to checking and non-checking groups on the basis of MOCI-C scores, it was possible that the checking group would have also had generally higher MOCI total scores and that this fact (i.e., an increased general severity of OCD) may have accounted for the group differences. A second analysis of the OCD subjects' data was therefore undertaken—a split-half comparison of higher and lower MOCI total scores. No significant differences were found between the groups, suggesting that the different priming effects were specific to differential amounts of checking behavior.

These findings may have important implications for theories of the etiology of OCD. It would now seem that there may be a difference in degree of cognitive inhibition deficit apparent in checkers and noncheckers. The former group continued to exhibit a relative dysfunction of inhibition despite the slowing of presentation time, suggesting that the more attended processes of selective attention were unable to compensate as effectively for preattentive deficits. This may have occurred because the fundamental problem of inhibition failure is more severe, as measured by a greater reduction in NP at the fastest presentation speed in checkers relative to noncheckers. Another possibility is that the more conscious strategies of suppressing nonrelevant information in checking subjects are also less effective. The third hypothesis suggests that the rate of growth of inhibition in checkers is slower than that of other OCD subjects. The currently available data cannot clearly distinguish among these hypotheses, all of which may be correct.

COGNITIVE INTRUSIONS
AND CONSCIOUS SUPPRESSION PARADIGMS

Although intrusive thoughts in the general population are a universal phenomenon it is known that the frequency of occurence of such intrusions is significantly higher in OCD patients (Rachman & de Silva, 1978; Salkovskis & Harrison, 1984). This finding, incorporated with the current results, leads logically to speculation that reduced preattentive cognitive inhibition may be associated with the higher frequency of cognitive intrusions in OCD patients. The NP paradigm is concerned with the impact of external stimuli on the information-processing system; its relevance to clinical disorder may therefore be limited to those problems and symptoms that are generated by external stimuli.

Steketee, Grayson, and Foa (1985) suggested from a survey of OCD patients that 92% of obsessional washers' fears and 60% of checkers' fears were generated by external stimuli. This survey was based on clinical interviews aimed at identifying the strength of the association, high or low, between the OCD patients' fear responses and circumscribed external cues. The problems of a compulsive washer who is washing after having retrieved milk bottles from the front doorstep would therefore be recorded as "high" in external stimulation, whereas the problems of a person compelled to retrace a car journey for fear of having knocked down a cyclist, in the absence of dents in the car or loud bangs on the journey, would be recorded as "low" in external stimulation.

The distinctions above are concerned with the immediacy of the specific external stimuli in relation to the specific problem focus. However, this may not be an entirely accurate reflection of whether a problem or symptom is in fact internally or externally generated. An example of this difficulty lies in the first-rank symptoms of schizophrenic patients. These do not occur in the presence of what is reported (e.g., the sound of God's voice or the presence of the secret police); yet some authors have suggested that delusions (Frith, 1981), hallucinations (Morton, 1979), and thought disorder (Maher, 1972; Frith, 1981) may have their basis in external stimuli that are misinterpreted. Frith (1979) has suggested that this misinterpretation occurs as a result of a fundamental failure to control and limit the contents of consciousness, which is hypothesized to occur at least in part because of reduced cognitive inhibition in schizophrenic patients.

Second, since human memory is undeniably associative (Anderson & Bower, 1973), it may be that other external stimuli associated in the patient's mind with the specific problem can trigger obsessional behavior and thought just as readily as the presence of more obviously related triggers. Third, there is evidence (Wegner, Schneider, Knutson, & McMahon, 1991; Muris, Merckelbach, & de Jong, 1993) that when a person attempts to suppress an unwanted thought, environmental features or objects are often used as distractors. Subsequently, these distractors can paradoxically act as cues to the unwanted thought or image, and so can trigger further preoccupation. It is likely therefore that the driver wanting to distract himself or herself from the fear of having caused an accident will be using environmental distractors associated with being in a car. Thus a plethora of external cues may potentially trigger obsessive thoughts while driving, in the absence of stimuli directly associated with the actual feared event.

When unwanted thoughts achieve conscious representation, these must be ignored or suppressed. A number of studies have examined the effects of nonclinical subjects' conscious attempts to suppress unwanted thoughs and images. Of these studies, the best-known is the "white bear" paradigm originally reported by Wegner, Schneider, Carter, and White (1987) and subsequently methodologically revised by Merckelbach, Muris, van den Hout, and de Jong (1991). Subjects were asked to try not to think about a white bear (suppression) either before or after they had been primed to think about white bears (expression).

The findings within this and similar though suppression paradigms are mixed. For every reported result, other authors have both supported the finding and failed to replicate it. Essentially, controversy surrounds three purported experimental effects resulting from attempts to suppress target thoughts: (1) an "immediate enhancement effect," in which subjects were unable to suppress target thoughts completely when told to do so and in fact seemed to become preoccupied by them; (2) a "delayed rebound effect," in which subjects instructed to think specifically about the target though did so more frequently when they had previously suppressed the thought; and (3) an effect whereby subjects who had previously suppressed target thoughts had an accelerated tendency to report intrusions over a subsequent period of expression.

We (Enright, Beech, Kemp-Wheeler, & Claridge, 1995) compared the 32 OCD and 32 OAD subjects from the preceding experiment on the white bears suppression paradigm, utilizing the Merckelbach et al. (1991) methodology. None of the disputed experimental effects described above were found. This result was identical to that of Merckelbach et al. (1991). However, the OCD group exhibited significantly greater numbers of white bear intrusions in every experimental condition, compared to OAD subjects.

When the OCD group was subdivided into checkers and noncheckers, the former group exhibited greater numbers of intrusions, though this result just failed to reach significance at the 5% level. There was no difference in numbers of intrusions when OCD subjects were divided into groups of higher and lower total OCD symptoms. Numbers of total intrusions in all groups over the experimental periods of expression and suppression are shown in Table 7.2. (In view of the lack of significant effects of order — i.e., whether subjects first suppressed or expressed — these data have been collapsed across order for the purpose of clarity.)

The current working hypothesis for consistent findings of reduced NP in OCD subjects is that these occur as a consequence of reduced cognitive inhibition in OCD, which causes less effective inhibition of unwanted or irrelevent information at a preattentive level of information processing. This may occur as a consequence of a direct failure to inhibit the unwanted target stimulus preattentively, or as a consequence of a failure to inhibit intrusions associated with spreading semantic activation to the target from environmental stimuli. The hypothesis therefore may also begin to make sense of the greater significance of the semantic task of OCD subjects in the NP studies reported earlier.

If this hypothesis is correct, it implies that obsessional clients are constantly being influenced by unwanted and irrelevant stimuli in conscious thought. The specific unwanted thoughts they experience will be those that have become most associated with their current environmental stimuli. Presumably, in OCD patients many of these associations will have been made because specific environmental distractors have been used deliberately to focus the patients' minds away from the obsessive thoughts. Others will occur simply through having become associated with specific environments. This now may begin to explain the fact that some OCD patients (particularly checkers and washers) are more obsessional in environments that are well known to them, since many associations have been set up; it may also explain how OCD becomes focused, since all cues lead back to the same unwanted thoughts.

In order to minimize the distraction caused by these unwanted thoughts, the patients must then presumably resort to attended strategies of thought suppression, which will include further environmental focusing. These may have initial short-term benefits but quickly lead back to the target, because of the preattentive failure to inhibit intrusions with this semantic association. Conscious suppression has litle or no influence upon rates of intrusion, as demonstrated in the lack of difference in rates of intrusion when subjects in the white bears paradigm either suppressed or expressed. This then may lead to greater frustration and anxiety associated with the specific intrusion.

The cognitive inhibition failure in compulsive checkers extends into

TABLE 7.2. Mean Cognitive Intrusions for OCD and OAD Subjects, and for OCD Checkers and Noncheckers

Group	Suppression		Expression	
	Mean	(SD)	Mean	(SD)
OCD	21.1	(17.3)	21.7	(19.4)
OAD	10.2	(9.1)	9.2	(7.1)
Checkers	26.3	(21.4)	28.00	(24.3)
Noncheckers	15.7	(11.4)	13.9	(10.0)

more attended mechanisms of inhibition. Their greater failure to inhibit unwanted stimuli both preattentively and during more attended processing is clearly demonstrated in the greater numbers of white bear intrusions in OCD checkers within the white bear paradigm.

Wegner (1991) suggests a model, supported by experimental studies, to attempt to explain the mechanism of thought suppression. He posits two processes acting as components of a feedback system aimed at the control of thought. The cycle of suppression begins with a "controlled distractor search"—a conscious, attention-demanding search for thoughts unrelated to the unwanted thought. This active process involves a significant allocation of cognitive resources to the process of finding distractors and maintaining these in consciousness. Operating in parallel is a second process, "automatic target search"—a nonconscious process that searches for any sign of the unwanted thought, registers this failure in conscious thought, and thereby highlights the failure of suppression and the need for devoting further effort to controlled distractor search.

Wegner and Erber (1991) demonstrated that increasing cognitive load (by requiring subjects to perform simple cognitive tasks while also suppressing target thoughts) appeared to reduce the allocation of cognitive resources to the controlled distractor search and resulted in the automatic target search's encountering the unwanted thoughts more often. If we assume that clinically anxious subjects are generally under greater cognitive load as a consequence of high levels of anxiety, this may begin to account for the considerably greater numbers of unwanted intrusions in the clinical experimental groups than in the nonclinical groups of previous studies.

More important within Wegner's model, however, may be the potential impact of global putative cognitive inhibition deficits on cognitive load, as suggested by the NP results reported earlier. This then allows for either a direct relationship between levels of NP and intrusion rates, or (more likely) an indirect effect, since other factors will presumably constantly be influencing cognitive load. OCD subjects—in particular, checkers—

would therefore appear to be constantly under greater cognitive load, allowing the automatic target search greater freedom to access specific unwanted intrusive thoughts. This may begin to explain how the proposed global deficit of cognitive inhibition in OCD can be squared with the specificity of OCD symptoms. Under greater cognitive load, the sufferers inadvertently directs the increased efficiency of the automatic target search toward the specific obsessional focus that they are trying hardest to suppress, thereby increasing its frequency. Increased autonomic discomfort adds to cognitive load, and the cycle is further exacerbated.

AMALGAMATION OF CURRENT FINDINGS, AND INTERIM CONCLUSIONS

In summary, on psychometric measures of schizotypal traits (especially those related to positive symptoms and cognitive dysfuntional aspects of schizotypy), and on one schizotypy experimental paradigm, OCD subjects consistently exhibit results implying a link with high-schizotype and schizophrenic subjects. This is particularly true of OCD checkers.

The accumulated data in the current thesis point to the tentative suggestion that OCD patients (especially checkers) may experience greater numbers of unwanted thoughts because of a failure to inhibit intrusions associated with the spreading semantic activation from environmental stimuli (particularly those used as distractors) to unwanted thoughts. This hypothesis is particularly relevant to the OCD problems of checkers and washers, which are known to be more readily triggered by external cues. However, it would seem likely that the more covert OCD symptoms can also be triggered by external stimuli.

Clearly, the hypothesis that high-schizotype, schizophrenic, and OCD subjects all share a common global deficit of cognitive inhibition cannot yet account for the different presentations of these categories. High-schizotype subjects, though by definition at risk of developing psychopathology, are apparently able to compensate for a relative failure in the mechanism of inhibition with the expression of only mild symptoms. For the most part, OCD subjects retain integrated and rational thought processes outside of their obsessional focus. In these subjects, therefore, the failure of inhibition appears to become especially focused to produce OCD symptoms, while also exhibiting schizotypy to varying degrees. Finally, in schizophrenic subjects the breakdown of rational and integrated thought becomes complete; it is apparently associated with a failure to cope with uninhibited stimuli.

The future tasks for research in this area will be (1) to develop more subtle techniques for identifying different types and degrees of cognitive inhibition; and (2) to identify what factors mediate and modify the integration of excessive and unwanted sensory input, caused by a failure of cognitive inhibition, with previously stored information.

The evidence from the current research for a possible dimensional relationship between OCD and schizophrenia suggests that the model for theoretical development in OCD may be assisted with reference to parts of the schizophrenia literature (e.g., Hemsley, 1993), in which a gradual rapprochement between cognitive dysfunction theories and neuroanatomical models of sensory gating appears to be underway.

ACKNOWLEDGMENTS

My grateful thanks are due to Drs. Tony Beech and Gordon Claridge at the University of Oxford, for all of their help and advice with this research and in the preparation of this chapter.

REFERENCES

Allport, D. A., Tipper, S. P., & Chmiel, N. J. R. (1985). Perceptual integration and post-categorical filtering. In M. E. Posner & O. S. M. Marin (Eds.), *Attention and performance XI*. Hillsdale, NJ; Erlbaum.

American Psychiatric Association. (1987). *Diagnostic and statistical manual of mental disorders* (3rd ed., rev.). Washington, DC: Author.

Anderson, J. R., & Bower, G. H. (1973). *Human associative memory*. Washington, DC: V. H. Winston.

Bannister, D., & Fransella, F. (1971). A grid test of schizophrenic thought disorder. *British Journal of Social and Clinical Psychology, 5,* 95–102.

Beech, A. R. (1987). *Cognitive differences and schizotypy*. Unpublished doctoral thesis, University of Oxford.

Beech, A. R., Baylis, G. C., Smithson, P., & Claridge, G. S. (1989). Individual differences in schizotypy as reflected in cognitive measures of inhibition. *British Journal of Clinical Psychology, 28,* 117–129.

Beech, A. R., McManus, D., Baylis, G. C., Tipper, S. P., & Agar, K. (1991). Individual differences in cognitive processes: Towards an explanation of schizophrenic symptomatology. *British Journal of Psychology, 82,* 417–426.

Beech, A. R., Baylis, G. C., Smithson, P., & Claridge, G. S. (1989). Individual differences in schizotypy as reflected in cognitive measures of inhibition. *British Journal of Clinical Psychology, 28,* 117–129.

Beech, H. R., Ciesielski, K. T., & Gordon, P. K. (1983). Further observation of evoked potentials in obsessional patients. *British Journal of Psychiatry, 142,* 605–609.

Bentall, R. P., Claridge, G. S., & Slade, P. D. (1989). The multidimensional nature of schizotypal traits: A factor analytic study with normal subjects. *British Journal of Clinical Psychology, 28,* 363–375.

Black A. (1974). The natural history of obsessional neurosis. In H. R. Beech (Ed.), *Obsessional states*. London: Methuen.

Black, D. W., & Noyes, R. (1990). Comorbidity and obsessive compulsive disorder. In J. D. Maser & C. R. Cloniger (Eds.), *Comorbidity of mood and anxiety disorders*. Washington, DC: American Psychiatric Press.

Cameron, O. G., Thyer, B. A., Nesse, R. M., & Curtis, G. C. (1986). Symptom profiles of patients with DSM-III anxiety disorders. *American Journal of Psychiatry, 143*(9), 1132–1137.

Chapman, L. J., Chapman, J. P., & Raulin, M. L. (1976). Scales for physical and social anhedonia. *Journal of Abnormal Psychology, 85*, 374–382.

Ciesielski, K. T., Beech, H. R., & Gordon, P. K. (1981). Some electrophysiological observations in obsessional states. *British Journal of Psychiatry, 138*, 479–484.

Claridge, G. S. (1967) *Personality and arousal: A psychophysiological study of psychiatric disorder*. Oxford: Pergamon Press.

Claridge, G. S. (1985). *Origins of mental illness*. Oxford: Blackwell.

Claridge, G. S. (1987). 'The schizophrenias as nervous types' revisited. *British Journal of Psychiatry, 151*, 735–743.

Claridge, G. S. (1993). A single indicator of risk for schizophrenia: Probable fact or likely myth? *Schizophrenia Bulletin,*

Claridge, G. S., & Broks, P. (1984). Schizotypy and hemisphere function: I. Theoretical considerations and the measurement of schizotypy. *Personality and Individual Differences, 5*, 633–648.

Claridge, G. S., & Hewitt, J. K. (1987). A biometric study of schizotypy in a normal population. *Personality and Individual Differences, 8*, 303–312.

Collins, A. M., & Loftus, E. (1975). A spreading activation theory of semantic processing. *Psychological Review, 82*, 407–428.

Ekblad, M., & Chapman, L. J. (1983). Magical ideation as an indicator of schizotypy. *Journal of Consulting and Clinical Psychology, 51*, 215–225.

Ekbald, M., & Chapman, L. J. (1986). Development and validation of a scale for hypomanic personality. *Journal of Abnormal Psychology, 95*, 215–225.

Enright, S. J., & Beech, A. R. (1990). Obsessional states: Anxiety disorders or schizotypes? An information processing and personality assessment. *Psychological Medicine, 20*, 621–627.

Enright, S. J., & Beech, A. R. (1993a). Further evidence of reduced inhibition in obsessive compulsive disorder. *Personality and Individual Differences 14*(3), 387–395.

Enright, S. J., & Beech, A. R. (1993b). Reduced cognitve inhibition in obsessive compulsive disorder. *British Journal of Clinical Psychology, 32*, 67–74.

Enright, S. J., Beech, A. R., & Claridge, G. S. (in press). The locus of negative priming effects in obsessive–compulsive disorder and other anxiety disorders. *Personality and Individual Differences.*

Enright, S. J., Beech, A. R., Kemp-Wheeler, S. M., & Claridge, G. S. (1995). *Suppressing thoughts of white bears: Obsessive–compulsive disorder and other anxiety disorders*. Manuscript submitted for publication.

Enright, S. J., Claridge, G. S., Beech, A. R., & Kemp-Wheeler, S. M. (1994). A questionnaire study of schizotypy in obsessional states and other anxiety disorders. *Personality and Individual Differences 16*(1), 191–194.

Eysenck, H. J. (1952). *The scientific study of personality*. London: Kegan Paul.

Eysenck, H. J., & Eysenck, S. B. G. (1975). *Manual of the Eysenck Personality Questionnaire.* London: Hodder & Stoughton.

Foa, E. B. (1979). Failure in treating obsessive–compulsives. *Behaviour Research and Therapy, 17,* 169–176.

Fenton, W. S., & McGlashan, T. H. (1986). The prognostic significance of obsessive–compulsive symptoms in schizophrenia. *American Journal of Psychiatry, 143*(4), 437–441.

Fey, E. T. (1951). The performance of young schizophrenics and young normals on the Wisconsin Card Sorting Test. *Journal of Consulting and Clinical Psychology, 15,* 311–319.

Flor-Henry, P., Yeudall, L. T., Koles, Z. J., & Howarth, B. G. (1979). Neuropsychological and power spectral EEG investigations of the obsessive–compulsive syndrome. *Biological Psychiatry, 14,* 119–130.

Foulds, G. A., & Bedford, A. (1975). Hierarchy of classes of personal illness. *Psychological Medicine, 5,* 181–192.

Fransella, F. (1974). Thinking and the obsessional. In H. R. Beech (Ed.), *Obsessional states.* London: Methuen.

Frith, C. D. (1979). Consciousness, information processing and schizophrenia. *British Journal of Psychiatry, 134,* 225–235.

Frith, C. D. (1981). Schizophrenia: An abnormality of consciousness? In G. Underwood & R. Stevens (Eds.), *Aspects of consciousness II.* London: Academic Press.

Golden, R. R., & Meehl, P. E. (1979). Detection of the schizoid taxon with MMPI indicators. *Journal of Abnormal Psychology, 84,* 217–233.

Goodwin, A. H., & Sher, K. J. (1992). Deficits in set-shifting ability in nonclinical compulsive checkers. *Journal of Psychopathology and Behavioural Assessment, 14,* 81–92.

Gorman, J. M., Liebowitz, M. R., Fyer, A. S., Dillon, D., Davies, S. O., Stein, J., & Klien, D. F., et al. (1985). Lactate infusions in obsessive–compulsive disorder. *American Journal of Psychiatry, 142,* 864–866.

Harvey, N. S. (1986). Impaired cognitive set-shifting in obsessive–compulsive neurosis. *IRCS Medical Science, 14,* 936–937.

Hathaway, S. R., & McKinley, J. C. (1943). *Manual for the Minnesota Multiphasic Personality Inventory.* New York: Psychological Corporation.

Head, D., Bolton, D., & Hymas, N. (1989). Deficits in cognitive set shifting ability in patients with obsessive–compulsive disorder. *Biological Psychiatry, 25,* 929–937.

Heaton, R. K., Baade, L. E., & Johnsen, K. L. (1978). Neuropsychological test results associated with psychiatric disorders in adults. *Psychological Bulletin, 85,* 141–162.

Hemsley, D. R. (1993). A simple (or simplistic) cognitive model for schizophrenia. *Behaviour Research and Therapy, 31*(7), 633–645.

Horowitz, M. J. (1983). *Image formation and psychotherapy.* New York: Jason Aronson.

Ingram, I. M. (1961). The obsessional personality and obsessional illness. *American Journal of Psychiatry, 117,* 1016–1019.

Ingram, R. E. (1990). Attentional nonspecificity in depressive and generalized anxious affective states. *Cognitive Therapy and Research, 14,* 25–35.

Insel, T. R., & Akiskal, H. S. (1986). Obsessive–compulsive disorder with psychotic features: A phenomenological analysis. *American Journal of Psychiatry, 143,* 530–532.

Jackson, M., & Claridge, G. S. (1991). Reliability and validity of a psychotic traits questionnaire (STQ). *British Journal of Clinical Psychology, 30*(4), 311–3224.

Jenike, M. A., Baer, L., Minichello, W. E., Schwartz, C. E., & Carey, R. J. (1986). Concomitant obsessive–compulsive disorder and schizotypal personality disorder. *American Journal of Psychiatry, 143*(4), 530–532.

Joffe, R. T., Swinson, R. P., & Regan, J. J. (1988). Personality features of obsessive–compulsive disorder. *American Journal of Psychiatry, 145,* 1127–1129.

Karno, M., Golding, J. M., Sorenson, S. B., & Burman, M. A. (1988). The epidemiology of obsessive–compulsive disorder in five US communities. *Archives of General Psychiatry, 45,* 1094–1099.

Kendler, K. S., & Hewitt, J. (1992). The structure of self report schizotypy in twins. *Journal of Personality Disorders, 6*(1), 1–17.

Laplante, L., Everett, J., & Thomas, J. (1992). Inhibition through negative priming with Stroop stimuli in schizophrenia. *British Journal of Clinical Psychology, 31,* 307–326.

Launay, G., & Slade, P. D. (1981). The measurement of hallucinatory predisposition in male and female prisoners. *Personality and Individual Differences, 2,* 221–234.

Levinson, D. F., & Mowry, B. J. (1991). Defining the schizophrenia spectrum. *Schizophrenia Bulletin, 17,* 491–514.

Lewis, A. J. (1957). Obsessional illness. *Acta Neuropsiquiatrica Argentina, 3,* 323–335.

Lindsay, D. A., & Norman, P. H. (1977). *Human information processing: An introduction to psychology* (2nd ed.). London: Academic Press.

Lowe, D. G. (1979). Strategies, context and the mechanism of response inhibition. *Memory and Cognition, 7,* 382–389.

Maher, B. A. (1972). The language of schizophrenia: A review and interpretation. *British Journal of Psychiatry, 120,* 3–17.

Malmo, H. P. (1974). On frontal lobe functions: Psychiatric patient controls. *Cortex, 10,* 231–237.

Marks, I. M. (1987). *Fears, phobias and rituals.* New York: Oxford University Press.

McCreery, C. (1993). *Schizotypy and out-of-the body experiences.* Unpublished doctoral thesis, University of Oxford.

McGuffin, P., & Thapar, A. (1991). The genetics of personality disorder. *British Journal of Psychiatry, 160,* 12–23.

Merckelbach, H., Muris, P., van den Hout, M., & de Jong, P. (1991). Rebound effects of thought suppression: Instruction dependent? *Behavioural Psychotherapy, 19,* 225–238.

Montgomery, S. A. (1990). Is obsessive–compulsive disorder diagnostically independent of both anxiety and depression? In S. A. Montgomery, W. A. Goodman, & N. Goeting (Eds.), *Current approaches: Obsessive–compulsive disorder.* London: Duphar Medical.

Morton, J. (1979). Word recognition. In J. Morton & J. C. Marshall (Eds.), *Psycholinguistics* (Vol. 2). London: Cambridge University Press.

Muntaner, C., Garcia-Sevilla, L., Fernandez, A., & Torrubia, R. (1988). Personality dimensions, schizotypal and borderline personality traits and psychosis proneness. *Personality and Individual Differences* 9(2), 257–268.

Muris, P., Merckelbach, H., & de Jong, P. (1993). Verbalization and environmental cuing in thought suppression. *Behaviour Research and Therapy, 31,* 609–612.

Neely, J. H. (1977). Semantic priming and the retrieval from lexical memory: Roles of inhibitionless spreading activation and limited capacity attention. *Journal of Experimental Psychology: General, 106,* 226–254.

Neill, W. T. (1977). Inhibitory and facilitatory processes in selective attention. *Journal of Experimental Psychology: Human Perception and Performance, 3,* 444–450.

Nielsen, T. C., & Petersen, K. E. (1976). Electrodermal correlates of extraversion, trait anxiety and schizophrenism. *Scandinavian Journal of Psychology, 17,* 73–80.

Posner, M. I., & Boies, S. J. (1971). Components of attention. *Psychological Review, 78,* 391–408.

Posner, M. I., & Snyder, C. R. R. (1975). Facilitation and inhibition in the processing of signals. In P. M. A. Rabbit (Ed.), *Attention and performance V.* New York: Academic Press.

Power, M. J. (1991). Cognitive science and behavioural psychotherapy: Where behaviour was, there shall cognition be. *Behavioural Psychotherapy, 19,* 20–41.

Rachman, S. J., & de Silva, P. (1978). Abnormal and normal obsessions. *Behaviour Research and Therapy, 16,* 233–248.

Rachman, S. J., & Hodgson, R. J. (1980). *Obsessions and compulsions.* Englewood Cliffs, NJ: Prentice-Hall.

Raine, A., & Allbutt, J. (1989). Factors of schizoid personality. *British Journal of Clinical Psychology, 28,* 31–40.

Rasmussen, S. A., Goodman, W. K., Woods, S. W., et al. (1987). Effects of yohimbine in obsessive–compulsive disorder. *Psychopharmacology, 93,* 308–313.

Robinson, S., Winnick, H. Z., & Weiss, A. A. (1976). Obsessive psychosis: Justification for a separate clinical entity. *Israeli Annals of Psychiatry, 14,* 39–48.

Roediger, H. L., & Neely, J. H. (1982). Retrieval blocks in episodic and semantic memory. *Canadian Journal of Psychology, 36,* 213–242.

Rosen, J. (1957). The clinical significance of obsessions in schizophrenia. *Journal of Mental Science, 103,* 733–785.

Rudin, E. (1953). Ein Beitrag zur frage der Zwangskrankheit, insobesondere ihrere hereditaren Beziehungen. *Archivs für Psychiatrie und Nervenkrankheiten, 191,* 14–54.

Salkovskis, P. M., & Harrison, J. (1984). Abnormal and normal obsessions: A replication. *Behaviour Research and Therapy, 22,* 549–552.

Schneider, K. (1959). *Clinical psychopathology.* Translater M. W. Hamilton. New York: Grune & Stratton.

Shakhlamov, A. V. (1988). One of the variants of schizophrenia with obsessional states. *Zhurnal Nevropatologii i Psikhiartrii, 88*(5), 87–92.

Sher, K. J., Frost, R. O., Kushner, M., Crews, T. M., & Alexander, J. (1989). Memory deficits in compulsive checkers: Replication and extension in a clinical sample. *Behaviour Research and Therapy, 27,* 65–69.

Sher, K. J., Mann, B., & Frost, R. (1984). Cognitive dysfunction in compulsive checkers: Further explorations. *Behaviour Research and Therapy, 22,* 493–502.

Solyom, L., DiNicola, V. F., & Phil, M. (1985). Is there an obsessive–compulsive psychosis? Aetiological and prognostic factors for an atypical form of obsessive–compulsive neurosis. *Canadian Journal of Psychiatry, 30,* 372–380.

Stanley, M. A., Turner, S. M., & Borden, J. W. (1990). Schizotypal features in obsessive–compulsive disorder. *Comprehensive Psychiatry, 31*(6), 551–518.

Steketee, G. S., Grayson, J. B., & Foa, E. B. (1985). Obsessive–compulsive disorder: Differences between washers and checkers. *Behaviour Research and Therapy, 23,* 197–201.

Steketee, G. S., Grayson, J. B., & Foa, E. B. (1987). A comparison of obsessive–compulsive characteristics and other anxiety disorders. *Journal of Anxiety Disorders, 1*(4), 325–335.

Stroop, J. R. (1935). Studies of interference in serial verbal reactions. *Journal of Experimental Psychology, 18,* 643–662.

Tipper, S. P. (1985). The negative priming effect: Inhibitory priming by ignored objects. *Quarterly Journal of Experimental Psychology, 37A,* 571–590.

Wegner, D. M., & Erber, R. (1991). Social foundations of mental control. In D. M. Wegner & J. W. Pennebaker (Eds.), *Handbook of mental control.* Englewood Cliffs, NJ: Prentice-Hall.

Wegner, D. M., Schneider, D. J., Carter, S. R., & White, T. L. (1987). Paradoxical effects of thought suppression. *Journal of Personality and Social Psychology, 53,* 5–13.

Wegner, D. M., Schneider, D. J., Knutson, B., & McMahon, S. (1991). Polluting the stream of consciousness: The influence of though suppression on the mind's environment. *Cognitive Therapy and Research, 15,* 141–152.

Weiss, A. A., Robinson, S., & Winnick, H. Z. (1975). Obsessive psychosis: A cross validation study. *Israeli Annals of Psychiatry, 13,* 137–141.

Westphal, K. (1978). Uber Zwangsvorstellungen. *Archivs für Psychiatrie und Nervenkrankheiten, 8,* 734–750.

Williams, J. M. G., Watts, F. N., MacLeod, C., & Matthews, A. (1988). *Cognitive psychology and emotional disorders.* Chichester, England: Wiley.

Understanding of Obsessive–Compulsive Disorder Is Not Improved by Redefining It as Something Else

Paul M. Salkovskis

THE COGNITIVE–BEHAVIORAL APPROACH provides a straightforward framework for understanding the behavior of obsessive–compulsive patients, without resorting to general deficit theories or theories proposing some pathological biochemical and/or anatomical lesion. Obsessive–compulsive disorder (OCD) is regarded as a problem in which the person's response to particular learned fears results in counterproductive attempts at coping, which have the unintended effect of maintaining and strengthening the original fears. According to this view, there may or may not be generalized vulnerabilities (such as biological or personality factors). The cognitive-behavioral approach suggests that if such vulnerabilities do exist, they are neither necessary nor sufficient to account for the origin or maintenance of OCD.

Early descriptions of obsessional disorders emphasized the importance of understanding the phenomenology of the problem (Lewis, 1936; Janet, 1903). Behavioral approaches continued this tradition by emphasizing "functional analysis" and the importance of learning history (Wolpe, 1958; Rachman & Hodgson, 1980). With the adoption of operationally defined diagnostic screenings such as DSM-IV (American Psychiatric Association, 1994), some of the clarity of the early phenomenologists appears to have been lost. Among the results of this reduced emphasis on understanding the meaning of symptoms and their interrelationship, in favor of developing endorsable symptom lists, are recurring attempts to redefine disorders such as OCD as something else. The focus on single behaviors has led to the perception of similarities where a more holistic view would clearly indicate *functional* distinctness.

A further force driving attempts at redefinition lies in the superficially inexplicable nature of the concerns, fears, and behaviors of obsessional patients. Thus it becomes easier to regard obsessional problems as stemming from some kind of neurological disease or from something akin to psychotic disorders such as schizophrenia, rather than trying to make sense of the complex phenomenology of OCD itself. I argue here that it remains more parsimonious to consider OCD as a psychologically understandable phenomenon in its own right. According to this view, similarities to other types of conditions are best understood as reflections of common psychological processes (e.g., as is seen in avoidance behavior and symptoms of autonomic arousal across a range of anxiety and other disorders). Although operationally defined criteria are useful in defining research samples, the *form* of symptoms should not be evaluated at the expense of attempts to understand the content and meaning of such symptoms to the sufferer.

The behavioral and cognitive-behavioral approaches are also *normalizing*. For treatment to be effective, the cognitive-behavioral view does not require the modification of either a neurological disease or a personality characteristic. This does not mean that helping patients to change relatively long-standing patterns of behavior and beliefs is easy, but it is nevertheless a prospect that inspires greater optimism: It offers the sufferer a real chance of being able to return to a "normal" pattern of life. Clearly, such optimism by itself is insufficient; thus this reply critically examines the data relevant to the idea of OCD as a schizotype and OCD as a brain disease.

IS OBSESSIVE–COMPULSIVE DISORDER A SCHIZOTYPE?

Enright and his colleagues have previously suggested that OCD patients suffer from what amounts to a mild form of schizophrenia; this proposal has been based on the hypothesis that schizotypy is a measure of vulnerability to schizophrenia and that OCD patients score high on measures of schizotypy. In Chapter 7, Enright sensibly moves away from this position but offers no clear alternative. Other data indicate that there is not an increased prevalence of schizophrenia among OCD patients. We also have the puzzling matter of schizophrenics scoring lower on schizotypy than high-schizotype subjects who are not schizophrenic. Schizotypy is measured by a series of questionnaires. It is unfortunate that some of these questionnaires include items on which, by definition, obsessional patients would score highly. Here are some examples:

> No matter how hard I try to concentrate, unrelated thoughts always creep into my mind.
> Have you ever felt the urge to injure yourself?
> Do you frequently have difficulty starting things?
> Do you at times have an urge to do something harmful or shocking?
> I often have difficulty in controlling my thoughts when I am thinking. (Enright, this volume, pp. 166–169)

Thus, high schizotypy scores in OCD may result from criterion contamination rather than from processes in common with schizophrenia.

The suggested reappraisal of OCD as a schizotype is also based on the suggestion that there are important differences between OCD and "other anxiety disorders" (OADs) (and corresponding similarities with schizophrenia). For example, it is argued that OCD patients differ from OADs in sex ratio, fertility, age of onset, and degree of disability. However, this only applies when OCD (one anxiety disorder) is compared with *the mean of all OCDs*. When OCD is compared to *each* OAD, the comparisons no longer suggest differences. For example, comparisons of the sex ratio in OCD and social phobia, the age of onset in OCD and panic disorder, and the level of reported disability in OCD an agoraphobia all contradict Enright's point, and simply reinforce the case for differentiation among the anxiety disorders, including OCD. Major differences exist among the different anxiety disorders, and the distinctness of OCD can be seen as an indication that it is distinct *within* the anxiety disorders group.

Suggested "biochemical" differences are even more tenuous. Contrary to Enright's suggestion, "anxiogenic" compounds (e.g., sodium lactate) show specific effects in panic, not in all OADs. Furthermore, the best current explanation for the effects of panic provocation lies in psychological, not biochemical, factors (Clark, 1993). Response to serotonergic medication is not specific to OCD (e.g., buspirone, fluoxetine). Current evidence suggests that the m-CPP challenge increases anxiety in OCD *and* in other anxiety disorders.

The "strangeness" of obsessional ideas and behavior seems to be an important factor in Enright's position on the relationship between OCD and schizophrenia. When intense, OCD beliefs are regarded by Enright as "delusional" and therefore schizophrenia-like. However, Rachman and de Silva (1978) found that clinical obsessions could not be distinguished from normal intrusive thoughts, suggesting that "bizarreness" is not key. Strongly held beliefs do not constitute delusions; indeed, most OAD patients hold intense beliefs when anxious (e.g., panic patients believe that they are going to die of a heart attack during panic). Some clinicians misdiagnose schizophrenia as OCD, but this does not support a relationship with schizophrenia, particularly given that the incidence of schizophrenia in OCD is at the level expected by chance (Black, 1974).

Enright interprets apparent similarities in negative priming scores between patients with OCD and schizophrenic patients (and the differences from normals low in schizotypy) as indicating the same failure of cognitive inhibition. The logic of this conclusion seems to run in this fashion:

> In anorexia, people consume less when they eat.
> In bulimia, people consume more when they eat.
> In cancer, people consume less when they eat.
> Anorexia is therefore wrongly classified as an eating disorder, and can be regarded as a form of cancer ("cancotype"?).

Even if one accepts that such logic can be useful, there are major problems in the experimental data itself. Enright interprets the data in Figure 7.1 as showing that OADs showed negative priming similar to that of normal (low-schizotype) to that of normal while OCD patients' scores were "closer to those exhibited by highly schizotypal and schizophrenic subjects" (p. 172). However, if one were to calculate *mean normal* scores (i.e., of high- and low-schizotype subjects), OCD subjects (and schizophrenics) are closer to normal subjects than to subjects with OADs. In conclusion, Enright's data do not indicate that OCD and schizophrenia are linked.

IS OBSESSIVE–COMPULSIVE DISORDER A BRAIN DISEASE?

Pigott, Myers, and Williams take up similar themes in Chapter 6. OCD patients and patients with neurological disorders may show some superficial similarities of behavior. Pigott et al. follow others such as Rapaport in attempting to generate a neuropsychiatric ("brain disease") model from this and other "biological" observations. The most robust observation is the specificity of serotonergic medication in treatment of OCD. It is argued that the weight of data concerning putative brain mechanisms indicates that a neurological dysfunction is involved.

It is indeed clear that OCD involves brain mechanisms. However, this does not make it a brain disease ("neurological dysfunction"). Writing this reply, for example, involves brain mechanisms that could be detected as neurophysiological, electrophysiological, and neurotransmitter changes. The observation that there are distinctive brain changes in positron emission tomoraphy (PET) scans in OCD patients, and that these are abolished by both behavioral and pharmacological treatment (Baxter et al., 1992), is essentially a statement of the obvious. For example, worry would be expected to increase blood flow in the orbito-frontal cortex of nonclinical subjects. By the same token, people who are more worried (i.e., obsessional patients) should have increased blood flow in this area relative to those who are not as worried (i.e., nonclinical subjects). When obsessionals become less worried as a consequence of effective treatment, corresponding decreases in blood flow should be observed in the orbito-frontal cortex. This is not necessarily evidence for a neurological dysfunction, nor is it necessarily evidence that these brain areas are crucial to the experience of obsessional disorder. This is just one of the problems associated with the way Pigott et al. have interpreted biological and clinical data in OCD. There is little empirical support for the notion of brain *disease*. The data may simply show neurophysiological, neuropsychological and biochemical correlates of normally functioning cognitive systems. The differences between obsessional patients and controls may or may not reflect processes that result in the *symptoms* characteristic of obsessional problems. This all raises the interesting notion that sufficiently subtle and specific modifications of biochemical "imbalances" may only be practicable by psychological means. It is difficult to foresee the development of sufficiently specific biochemical interventions to match a nonpathological psychobiological model.

The basis of the brain disease notion in animal models is even more doubtful. At first sight, Pigott et al.'s claim that "there are no current well-established animal models for OCD" (p. 146) is a little puzzling. This is an assertion frequently made in the biological literature on OCD, but it entirely ignores an important animal model based on learning theory. Solomon, Kamin, and Wynne (1954) conducted an important experiment in which a classically conditioned response to a light became associated with a shuttling response in a shuttle box. That is, with the onset of a red light that had previously heralded shock, an animal was able to avoid the shock by jumping over a low barrier to the other side of the shuttle box. Solomon et al. (1954) noted that dogs in these instances tended to develop bizarre and stereotyped variants of the shuttling response. Furthermore, once the unconditioned stimulus (electric shock) was removed, animals persisted in the shuttling response to the conditioned stimulus. The conditioned response was only extinguished when the animals were forcibly prevented from shuttling; under these circumstances, the animals demonstrated extreme agitation and the re-emergence of anxiety. This was significant because during the phase when they were allowed to shuttle freely, the avoidance response became highly practiced and appeared to be anxiety-free. This model is, of course, part of the fundamental basis for the subsequent development of exposure-based treatments. It also has the advantage of specificity, allowing for the development of highly focused anxiety reactions and responses analogous to those seen in obsessional problems (see also Chapter 5, pp. 106–109, for a discussion of specificity).

The availability of this well-validated model makes it difficult to see why canine acral lick dermatitis (as described by Pigott et al.) should be regarded as a particularly useful model for OCD. Other recent "candidates" for animal models include the rat pup ultra-sonic squeak (Olivier, 1992). In this sense, Pigott et al.'s and Enright's chapters seem to have an important component in common. It seems likely that in both instances, the superficial difficulty in understanding obsessive–compulsive thinking and behavior leads to presumption of some gross and generalized abnormality. Essentially, then, the model being sought is one that involves abnormality; from this perspective, the two-process theory (which forms the best animal model available) suffers from the "disadvantage" that it invokes the operation of normal cognitive and learning processes. It is nevertheless difficult to justify the adoption of a disease/abnormality model when there is a more parsimonious way of conceptualizing obsessive–compulsive problems, which involves the activation of normal psychological learning-based processes.

Once the assumption of abnormality is seen to be underlying the neuropsychiatric model of OCD, it becomes easier to recognize a disconnected series of biological observations in search of a lesion/disease explanation. The neuropsychiatric theory attempts to synthesize apparently disconnected observations with a common theme of biological abnormality, without considering the possibility that some of the observations may concern *normal* functioning, as in the example of the PET scan results discussed above.

The suggested link between Tourette's syndrome and OCD is another example of the problems with the neuropsychiatric model. Obsessive *symptoms* are relatively common in Tourette's. However, by definition, repetitive behavior is part of Tourette's syndrome. There seems to be some attempt to equate repetitive acts with OCD; even the briefest examination of the DSM-IV criteria shows that this is not so. There is also the problem of the relative absence of Tourette's among OCD patients.

Other evidence that is taken as indicating some sort of brain lesion includes research on "neurological soft signs." When a battery of quasi-neurological tests is conducted, it turns out that obsessional patients tend to show more "deficits" than normal controls. However, this seems less surprising when it is considered that the soft signs tap such things as muscle tone, hesitation, and so on. Indeed, the lack of any specific effects is notable; the absence of an anxious control group in any of these studies makes the results almost uninterpretable. With any tests of this kind, the possibility exists that the problem being used to select the patients (OCD) may have some direct impact on the test itself. Such effects need not be mediated by brain disease, but may be a result of being more anxious or even of being more careful. The same point may apply to the results of neuropsychological investigations. At on point in Chapter 6, Pigott et al. describe a battery of tests that identified consistent defects in patients with demonstrated basal ganglion disease. They express surprise that OCD patients did not perform significantly differently from controls in these tests. Finally, response to treatment is taken by Pigott et al. as a key piece of evidence for the neurobiological theory of OCD. They argue that OCD patients' response to drugs such as clomipramine and fluoxetine supports the validity of the serotonin hypothesis. However, it is important to consider how the serotonin hypothesis arose in the first place: It was proposed because of the effectiveness of serotonergic agents in the treatment of OCD. There is therefore little value in asserting that the serotonin hypothesis is supported by the response to serotonergic agents in the treatment of OCD. This hypothesis would be better supported by biochemical data indicating some disturbance unique to the serotonin systems of OCD patients, as opposed to those of other people suffering from mood disturbances. An extraordinarily large number of investigations of the serotonin system at rest and the response to serotonin-related challenge tests in OCD have now been carried out. Despite this investment of effort, the data indicate that the serotonergic system is probably intact in OCD (Rauch & Jenike, 1993).

The neuropsychiatric theory appears to be another example of the idea that the behavior of OCD patients is so bizarre that a gross abnormality must be present. The most problematic aspect of this primarily biological-disease-based approach is the failure to consider more normal (and, for the OCD patient, normalizing) mechanisms of OCD. Current psychological approaches are more adaptable in that a distal biological "cause" is implicit, but the more proximal psychological processes are the focus of investigation and theory. When normal brain mechanisms are better understood and some understanding of the links between biological and psychological processes is established, the biological substrate of OCD may become accessible to investigation.

IS OBSESSIVE–COMPULSIVE DISORDER OBSESSIVE–COMPULSIVE DISORDER?

OCD is characterized by a clearly identifiable pattern of thinking and behavior. The sufferer experiences thoughts that he or she finds unacceptable or repugnant (at least early in the problem), and attempts to suppress or neutralize these by engaging in some other thought or action. For most sufferers, overt compulsive behaviors (e.g., handwashing, checking, or touching rituals) are a problem. There is a clear phenomenological link between the occurrence of obsessions and subsequent compulsive behavior (e.g., thoughts of contamination lead to washing, doubts concerning an action lead to checking). Among the relatively small number of patients not troubled by overt obsessive behavior, compulsions take the form of obsession-linked "mental rituals" (Salkovskis & Westbrook, 1989). Obsessional thinking and behavior repay careful questioning (and listening) by providing rich and meaningful patterns of phenomenology. Such patterns are internally consistent and, even when firmly held, are no more "delusional" than a firmly held belief in God. It is therefore not unreasonable to regard OCD as a problem in which obsessional thinking has become the focus of concern; such thinking has resulted in responses such as selective attention, neutralizing, thought suppression, and compulsive behaviors, which maintain the condition.

Similarities between OCD and other problems can arise from two sources. The first and least interesting is superficial similarity. Repetitive behaviors such as tics fall into this category; a tic is repetitive in the same way that compulsive handwashing is repetitive. But, then, so are the casting of a fly fisherman and the joystick movements of a video game enthusiast. There may even be similar changes in brain motor areas in all of these behaviors, but few would argue that there is a common underlying cause, and fewer still that these are therefore all symptoms of a common disease. Strongly held belief is another example (see above). In a sense, the adoption by the neuropsychiatric theorists of canine acral lick dermatitis as a model for OCD illustrates the near-uselessness of this type of superficial comparison.

The second phenomenon that may lead to some degree of similarity is more interesting. When behaviors are meaningfully linked to beliefs, a certain degree of convergence may be expected; consistent links are particularly likely when the perception of threat (and therefore anxiety) is involved (Salkovskis, 1991). Good examples of this are the checking and reassurance seeking characteristically found both in OCD and in hypochondriasis. Some key processes may be similar, resulting in similar outcomes. The similarities are posited *a priori* by the cognitive hypothesis (Salkovskis & Clark, 1993). In this instance, the common underlying process is the perception that some feared catastrophe will occur at some future (and perhaps even distant future) time. This would be in sharp contrast with panic disorder, where the feared catastrophe is foreseen as occurring within the next few seconds and therefore results in quite different behavior, particularly immediate escape.

If anxiety disorders, including OCD, are not the result of some kind of lesion or brain disease but are instead the result of specific misinterpretations, then there is no need to reclassify problems such as OCD. A number of common processes across the range of conditions may be expected; also, these processes should occur in different combinations, depending on the particular focus of anxiety and discomfort. The processes involved will be such things as selective attention to stimuli believed to be threatening, physiological arousal, safety-seeking behavior, affective changes, and so on. We may then begin to speculate in a slightly different way. For example, what is the biological substrate of key psychological processes? Among such psychological processes, where are the serotonin reuptake inhibitors having their impact? Could these drugs be modifying some key maintaining factor in the problem? How can neurophysiological research into mechanisms of phenomena such as selective attention inform the understanding of psychological mechanisms and their modification (and vice versa)? The essential conclusion to all of this appears to be that OCD is still OCD.

REFERENCES

American Psychiatric Association. (1994). *Diagnostic and statistical manual of mental disorders* (4th ed.). Washington, DC: Author.

Baxter, L., Schwartz, J. M., Bergman, K. S., Szuba, M. P., Guze, B. H., Mazziotta, J. C., Alazraki, A., Selin, C. E., Ferng, H-K., Munford, P., & Phelps, M. E. (1992). Caudate Glucose Metabolic Rate Changes with Both Drug and Behaviour Therapy for Obsessive–Compulsive Disorder. *Archives of General Psychiatry, 49,* 681–689.

Black, A. (1974). The natural history of obsessional neurosis: In H. R. Beech (Ed.), *Obessional States.* London: Methuen & Co. Ltd.

Clark, D. M. (1993). Cognitive mediation of panic attacks induced by biological challenge tests. *Advances in Behaviour Research and Therapy, 15,* 75–84.

Janet, P. (1903). *Les obsessions et la psychasthenie.* (2nd ed., Vol. 1). Paris: Alcan.

Lewis, A. J. (1936). Problems of obsessional illness. *Proceedings of the Royal Society of Medicine, 29,* 325–336.

Olivier, B. (1992). Animal models in OCD. *International Clinical Psychopharmacology, 7*(Suppl. 1), 27–29.

Rachman, S. J., & de Silva, P. (1978). Abnormal and normal obsessions. *Behaviour Research and Therapy, 16,* 233–238.

Rachman, S. J., & Hodgson, R. (1980). *Obsessions and compulsions.* Englewood Cliffs, NJ: Prentice-Hall.

Rauch, S. L., & Jenike, M. A. (1993). Neurobiological models of OCD. *Psychosomatics, 34,* 20–32.

Salkovskis, P. M. (1991). The importance of behaviour in the maintenance of anxiety and panic: A cognitive account. *Behavioural Psychotherapy, 19,* 6–19.

Salkovskis, P. M., & Clark, D. M. (1993). Panic Disorder and Hypochondriasis. *Advances in Behaviour Research and Therapy, 15,* 23–48.

Salkovskis, P. M., & Westbrook, D. (1989). Behaviour therapy with obsessional ruminations: Can failure be turned into success? *Behaviour Research and Therapy, 27,* 147–160.

Solomon, & Wynne

Wolpe, J. (1958). *Psychotherapy by reciprocal inhibition.* Stanford, CA: Stanford University Press.

Obsessive–Compulsive Disorder: Beyond Cluttered Cognitions

TERESA A. PIGOTT
KAREN R. MYERS
DAVID A. WILLIAMS

REPLY TO SALKOVSKIS

In Chapter 5, Salkovskis presents a clear and often compelling theory of obsessive–compulsive disorder (OCD) as a condition that arises from a combination of cognitive and behavioral processes. In contrast, strict behavioral therapy is based upon the hypothesis that obsessional thoughts have become associated through conditioning with anxiety. This anxiety results in escape and avoidance behaviors that fail to extinguish this association. Exposure with response prevention (ERP) is focused on the uncoupling of obsessive thoughts and compulsive behaviors through habituation to anxiety-related stimuli and eventual extinction of rituals and avoidance behaviors. Unfortunately, ERP techniques are not effective in many patients with OCD. For example, the benefits of ERP are significantly reduced in OCD patients who exhibit primary obsessions without compulsions, substantial depressed mood, or overvalued ideas. Recent epidemiological studies suggest that a substantial proportion of individuals endorse only obsessional symptoms and that comorbid affective disorder is relatively common in OCD (Karno, Golding, Sorenson, & Burman, 1988; Weissman et al., 1994). In addition, the widespread use of ERP is further compromised by treatment refusal and early dropouts.

Other theories of the etiology of OCD include the cognitive deficit model and the biological model. In the cognitive deficit model, a general failure in cognitive control is posited in patients with OCD. OCD patients often report a poor general memory and impaired decision-making abilities. These reported memory and decision-making difficulties are hypothesized to represent failures of inhibition. However, OCD symptoms are highly specific (e.g., contamination worries) rather than global in content. With these issues in mind, Sher, Frost, Kushner, Crews, and Alexander (1989) compared patients with OCD and subjects who endorsed frequent checking behaviors without distress or associated obsessive thoughts. Subjects with frequent checking behaviors, as measured by elevated scores on the Checking scale of the Maudsley Obsessional–Compulsive Inventory (MOCI), had low scores on the Wechsler Memory Scale (WMS). OCD patients did not have low WMS scores or evidence of memory impairment outside of problems associated with their obsessional symptoms. Thus, OCD patients with checking compulsions may be unduly concerned about memory, so that they check even though they do not have actual memory deficits. However, OCD patients with prominent checking compulsions often experience substantial benefit after ERP therapy, but the reduction in compulsions does not appear to be correlated with improvements in real or perceived memory deficits.

The biological disease model suggests that lesions in particular brain areas or deficits in neurotransmitters (e.g., serotonin [5-HT]) result in obsessional problems. The strongest evidence for the biological etiology of OCD is the effectiveness of certain medications in treating patients with OCD. However, the biological deficit model for the etiology of OCD also has shortcomings. Salkovskis specifically cites several inconsistencies. For example, he notes that (1) the 5-HT agonist buspirone is ineffective in reducing OCD symptoms; (2) diseases such as Tourette's syndrome (TS) are commonly associated with OCD, but OCD is not frequently associated with TS; and (3) although all cognitive processes can be associated with neurophysiological activities, they do not necessarily represent a structural lesion or disease state.

However, buspirone is only a partial 5-HT agonist and therefore does not necessarily enhance 5-HT neurotransmission. Moreover, buspirone demonstrated similar and significant antiobsessive effects in comparison to clomipramine treatment in the only controlled trial that has been reported in patients with OCD (Pato et al., 1991). There is substantial comorbidity between OCD and TS. Genetic studies have suggested that relatives of OCD patients do have an elevated level of risk for exhibiting OCD symptoms, and that the family members of probands with TS have similar levels of risk for developing OCD and TS (Pauls & Leckman, 1986). In addition, a biological theory for the etiology of OCD does not have to include structural abnormalities. Indeed, structural abnormalities appear rare in patients with OCD; instead, functional differences in brain functioning are much more likely to be associated with the pathophysiology of OCD. Position emission tomography and cerebral blood flow studies conducted in patients with OCD have demonstrated evidence of significant differences in metabolism and blood perfusion from normal controls (Baxter, 1992; Machlin et al., 1991).

Regardless of these issues, Salkovskis presents an excellent model of the role of cognition in the development of OCD. OCD is theorized to represent a highly specific problem that is related to normal rather than abnormal functioning. Obsessional problems are speculated to arise from a pattern of specific responses to key stimuli, which the patient has then inexplicably linked to an affective state. The reported memory and decision-making difficulties and failures of inhibition noted in patients with OCD are felt to represent a secondary phenomenon. That is, emotional arousal and counterproductive coping strategies are thought to result from an over-control of cognitions at the expense of other competing cognitive functions. The cognitive-behavioral theory of OCD suggests that (1) intrusive thoughts are normal phenomena; (2) in OCD, these intrusive thoughts are misinterpreted; (3) distress arises from an inaccurate appraisal of the consequences of these intrusive thoughts; (4) appraisal links distress and neutralizing behaviors, which develop from neutral behaviors that are felt to combat overresponsibility; and (5) attempts to suppress the obsessive thoughts and associated overresponsibility lead to increasing overcontrol and to preoccupation with and a high frequency of obsessions.

The speculation that obsessional thinking has its origin in normal intrusive thoughts and represents a misinterpretation of these thoughts is akin to the amplification of symptoms of physiological arousal that occurs in patients with panic disorder. Evidence for this phenomenon in OCD includes studies of clinical and nonclinical checkers, which have reported that checkers *perceive* themselves to be more susceptible to failure of cognitive control, as measured by tests of inhibitory control of cognition. In addition, the diversity of OCD symptomatology can be explained by the association of neutral automatic thoughts with emotionally charged stimuli. The difference between the development of anxiety or depressive cognitions and the development of OCD symptoms is seen as dependent upon the acquisition of meaning in terms of responsibility.

The objective of cognitive-behavioral therapy in OCD is the normalization rather than the abolition of intrusive thoughts. Cognitive-behavioral therapy therefore works by modifying beliefs (1) that lead to misinterpretation of intrusive thoughts because of heightened responsibility, and (2) that are associated with the behaviors maintaining these beliefs. Salkovskis also notes that some patients with OCD endorse symptoms of "completeness." Completeness is felt to result from the development of a complicated series of behaviors that are designed to attain certainty but that instead contribute to further uncertainty. The treatment of pure obsessionals is speculated to involve the identification of covert compulsions, as well as incorporation of techniques designed to process obsessive thoughts completely and to uncouple their emotional or irrational associations.

The cognitive-behavioral theory of the etiology of OCD appears to provide a cogent and fairly believable hypothesis for the development of obsessive thoughts and associated neutralizing behaviors. However, the theory fails to clarify several issues. Many OCD patients endorse primary compulsive behaviors, with few or no eliciting obsessional thoughts or excessive concerns. For example, Mr. D. reports that he must touch the ceiling three times every time he enters a new room, and he also describes intermittent feelings of a need for symmetry. Mr. D. adamantly denies any irrational concerns or consequences associated with these behaviors, and instead endorses a generalized feeling of "discomfort" prior to the performance of these rituals. Most patients with OCD will also report that many of their behaviors are elicited by premonitory urges rather than by circumscribed fear(s). Therefore it is difficult to ascribe the misinterpretation of intrusive thoughts and inaccurate appraisals of consequences to the development of OCD symptoms in many patients with OCD. Moreover, comorbid depressions and anxiety disorders are common in OCD patients (Weissman et al., 1994; Pigott, L'Heureux, Dubbert, Bernstein, & Murphy, 1994). Yet differential responsiveness and temporal patterns in patients with OCD versus patients with depressive or anxiety symptoms are not uncommon. If anxiety or depressive symptoms arise from the same underlying phenomena of distorted cognitions, it is difficult to explain why similar pharmacological treatment modalities result in differential therapeutic effects (Mavissakalian, Turner, Michelson, & Jacob, 1985).

REPLY TO ENRIGHT

OCD is classified as an anxiety disorder. Other anxiety disorders (OADs) include generalized anxiety disorder, simple (specific) phobia, agoraphobia, social phobia, panic disorder, and posttraumatic stress disorder. Both OCD and OADs are characterized by anxiety and avoidance behaviors. Behavioral therapy or pharmacotherapy can effectively treat OCD or OADs. However, there are significant differences in age of onset and gender ratio between patients with OCD and OADs.

Patients with OCD can have some symptoms that resemble schizophrenia. In particular, overvalued ideation in patients with OCD can be similar to the delusions that are exhibited in schizophrenia. Schizophrenia and OCD also have a similar age of onset, and there is substantial comorbidity between OCD and schizophrenia. However, comparative studies of neuropsychological data in patients with OCD and with schizophrenia are sparse. There appears to be evidence suggesting that both patients with OCD and schizophrenic patients have difficulty in shifting between cognitive sets, as measured by the Wisconsin Card Sorting Test. Several personality studies conducted in OCD patients suggest that schizotypal personality disorder is common and may be related to a poor treatment outcome after behavioral or pharmacological treatment (Jenike & Raush, 1994; Black, Yates, Noyes, Pfohl, & Kelley, 1989).

In addition, dimensional theories of psychosis suggest that increased numbers of schizotypal traits are found in OCD. For example, the Eysencks' dimensional theory of psychotic disorder suggests that predisposition to psychosis exists around a continuum. Schizotypy represents healthy diversity, and schizophrenia is an aberration of otherwise normal functional processes.

As described in Chapter 7, in order to investigate the presence of schizoptypal personality traits further, Enright and his colleagues administered a battery of 18 questionnaires designed to assess potential vulnerability to psychosis and the presence of schizotypal features in OCD patients. Unusual perceptual experiences, magical thinking, paranoid ideation and suspiciousness, and impairments in mood or self-image were some of the schizotypal features that were assessed in this battery. One particular paradigm that was investigated in OCD and OAD subjects was a negative priming (NP) task. The NP paradigm presents a series of stimuli in which previously ignored information becomes the required response for the next trial. Normal control subjects delay the subsequent response when this stimuli becomes the subsequent target, since the subject must first overcome this inhibition. This NP response is felt to reflect a process of active inhibition of the ignored stimulus, which then delays the subsequent response when this stimulus becomes the target, since the subject must first overcome this inhibition. When the NP response is not negative or delayed, it is considered to be a common exhibition of reduced preattentive cognitive inhibition in the subject.

OCD patients exhibited greater evidence of schizotypal traits than OAD subjects on 13 of the 18 questionnaires. In particular, the OCD patients had elevated scores on items concerning positive psychotic symptoms and cognitive disorganization. The OCD patients also scored higher than OAD patients and similar to schizophrenic patients on the NP task. Further subdivision of the OCD subjects suggested that checkers continued to have a relative dysfunction of inhibition despite slowing of presentation of the NP task, suggesting that the more attended processes were unable to compensate as effectively for preattentive deficits. Therefore OCD patients appear to have a higher frequency of cognitive intrusions attributable to reduced preattentive cognitive inhibition. This defect is thought to arise from a misinterpretation of external stimuli. The greater failure to inhibit unwanted stimuli both preattentively and during attended processing in OCD patients is believed to result in a relatively greater cognitive load, which allows the automatic target search greater freedom to access specific unwarranted intrusive thoughts. The increased efficiency of the automatic target search is seen as contributing to the specific obsessional focus that the OCD patients are trying hardest to suppress.

Patients with elevated scores on measures of schizotypy are theorized to have the ability to compensate for a relative failure in the mechanism of inhibition with the expression of only mild symptoms. By contrast, in schizophrenia there is thought to be a complete breakdown of rational and integrated thoughts, apparently associated with a failure to cope with uninhibited stimuli.

Enright offers some data supporting the importance of abnormal information processing in the development of OCD symptoms. The information processing manifested by OCD patients is postulated to resemble the pattern exhibited by patients with schizotypal personality traits. There are several difficulties inherent in this model, however. There are few data suggesting that patients with schizotypal personality are particularly susceptible to the development of true psychotic symptoms or schizophrenia. The various personality questionnaires that Enright and colleagues used to identify schizotypal traits were biased toward identifying items suggesting "unusual" thoughts or behaviors. Unfortunately, patients with OCD often endorse such symptoms, but are also quick to identify these symptoms as distressing or "ego-alien." Their reality testing is intact, and they do not endorse the referential auditory or visual hallucinations that are described by schizophrenic patients. In addition, the "soft" paranoid ideation that is endorsed by OCD patients, such as "I think people are looking at me or are often critical," actually represents social or performance anxiety rather than self-persecutory delusions (Rasmussen & Eisen, 1992; Baer, 1994; Pigott et al., 1994).

There have been various changes in the schemes for classifying personality disorders from DSM-III to DSM-IV and from ICD-9 to ICD-10. These changing criteria have contributed to the substantial variance in diagnosis of personality disorders in patients with OCD. Therefore, assessment of the actual frequency of schizotypal personality disorder is often dependent upon the classification scheme utilized. For example, Baer and colleagues (1992) reported that schizotypal personality disorder was fairly rare in a large sample of OCD patients diagnosed by DSM-III criteria, but that this diagnosis was substantially elevated when DSM-III-R criteria were substtituted. Although the NP testing data are certainly interesting, more patients with OCD who have primary symptoms besides checking behaviors should be tested before a definitive link between the patterns of patients with OCD and with schizophrenia should be assumed.

REFERENCES

Baer, L., (1994). Subtypes of OCD. *Journal of Clinical Psychiatry, 55*(3), 18–23.

Baer, L., Jenike, M., Black, D., Treece, C., Rosenfield, R., & Greist, J. (1992). Effects of Axis II diagnosis on treatment outcome with clomipramine in 54 patients with OCD. *Archives of General Psychiatry,* 862–866.

Baxter, L. (1992). Neuroimaging studies of OCD. *Psychiatric Clinics of North America, 15*(4), 871–884.

Black, D., Yates, W., Noyes, R., Phohl, B., & Kelley, M. (1989). DSM-III personality disorder in obsessive–compulsive study volunteers: A controlled study. *Journal of Personality Disorders, 3,* 58–62.

Jenike, M. A., Baer, L., & Greist, J. H. (1990). Clomipramine versus fluoxetine in OCD: A retrospective comparison of side effects and efficacy. *Journal of Clinical Psychopharmacology, 10,* 122–124.

Jenike, M. A., Hyman, S., Baer, L., Holland, A., Minichiello, W. E., Buttolph, L., Summergrad, P., Seymour, R., & Ricciardi, J. (1990). A controlled trial of fluvoxamine in OCD: Implications for a serotonergic theory. *American Journal of Psychiatry, 147,* 1209–1215.

Karno, M., Golding, J. M., Sorenson, B., & Burnam, M. A. (1988). The epidemiology of obsessive–compulsive disorder in five US communities. *Archives of General Psychiatry, 45,* 1094–1099.

Machlin, S., Harris, G., Pearlson, G., Hoehn-Saric, R., Jeffery, P., & Camargo, E. (1991). Elevated medial–frontal cerebral blood flow in OCD patients: A SPECT study. *American Journal of Psychiatry, 148,* 1243–1245.

Mavissakalian, M., Turner, S., Michelson, L., & Jacob, R. (1985). Tricycle antidepressants in OCD: Antiobsessional or antidepressant agents? *American Journal of Psychiatry, 142,* 572.

Pato, M. T., Pigott, T. A., Hill, J. L., Grover, G. N., Bernstein, S. E., & Murphy, D. L. (1991). Controlled comparison of buspirone and clomipramine in OCD. *American Journal of Psychiatry, 148,* 127–129.

Pauls, D., & Lechman, J. (1986). The inheritance of Gilles de la Tourette's syndrome and associated behaviors: Evidence for autosomal dominant transmission. *New England Journal of Medicine, 315*(16), 993.

Pigott, T. A., L'Heureux, F., Bernstein, S., & Murphy, D. (1994). Comorbid conditions in OCD. *Journal of Clinical Psychiatry, 55*(10), 3–10.

Rasmussen, S., & Eisen, J. (1992). The epidemiology and clinical features of obsessive–compulsive disorder. *Psychiatric Clinics of North America, 15*(4), 743–758.

Sher, K. J., Frost, R. O. Kushner, M., Crews, T. M., & Alexander, J. E. (1989). Memory deficits in compulsive checkers: Replication and extension in a clinical sample. *Behaviour Research and Therapy, 27,* 65–69.

Weissman, M., Bland, R., Canino, G., Greenwald, S., Hwu, H., Lee, C., Newman, S., Oakley-Browne, M., Rubio-Stipec, M., Wickramaratne, P., Wittchen, H., & Yeh, E. (1994). The cross-national epidemiology of OCD. *Journal of Clinical Psychiatry, 55*(3), 5–10.

Forwards, Backwards, and Sideways: Progress in OCD Research

SIMON J. ENRIGHT

IT IS CLEAR that each of our three hypotheses attempting to enhance the understanding of obsessive–compulsive disorder (OCD) is related to a distinctly different level of discourse. I firmly believe that unless attempts are made to theorize about OCD at many different levels, we will never fully come to terms with this highly complex phenomenon (or phenomena). Only in this way—breaking free from narrowly focused ideology and the constraints of professional dogmatism, and allowing for theoretical cross-fertilization—will OCD be eventually understood.

I therefore have a number of concerns regarding the claim made by Salkovskis in Chapter 5 that cognitive-behavioral theories can, in and of themselves, offer an explanation for OCD. Greatest among these concerns is the apparent ongoing propensity for "black box" theorizing—an interest only in explaining the observable or what patients can tell us they are thinking or doing. Few people now believe behavioral theoretical explanations for OCD. Although bolting on "cognitive" appendages may offer greater longevity, there is clearly no panacea for OCD in cognitive-behavioral theory or treatment.

Much is made of the fact that OCD patients have an inordinate sense of responsibility for the content of their intrusive thoughts, and that they thereby seek to make reparation by overt action (compulsive behavior) or covert action (neutralizing). I am not at all convinced that the broad heterogeneity of clinical presentation in OCD can be accounted for in this

simple proposition. Many OCD patients tells us that they simply feel uncomfortable if their books are not perfectly aligned or their towels are
not always fresh. Other patients tell us that they endlessly check docu-
ments at work for swear words because they fear reprimand or dismissal.
Other patients look endlessly at bodily features in the mirror, or constantly
check useless facts, or collect all items colored red, and so on; they offer
all sorts of rationalizations for these behaviors that have apparently nothing
to do with perceived responsibility, despite the tenacity of the cognitive
therapist in trying to establish "underlying irrational beliefs."

Some OCD patients certainly do indicate increased responsibility, but
is this a cause of the ensuing rituals or an attribution to explain them?
Perhaps these patients convince themselves that they feel responsible for
their thoughts because this offers the most plausible justification for their
actions. The theory of cognitive dissonance (Festinger, 1957) would appear to be highly relevant here. If a subject has beliefs that conflict with
a behavioral tendency, the subject is motivated to reduce the dissonance
through changes in those beliefs. It therefore seems entirely likely that the
high degree of reported responsibility in some OCD patients is merely their
post hoc rationalization for their irrational neutralizing.

In the development of his theory in Chapter 5, Salkovskis states:
" 'Neutralizing' is defined as voluntarily initiated activity that is intended
to have the effect of reducing the perceived responsibility and can be overt
or covert" (p. 111). It is very difficult to imagine how the behavior of a
patient counting in threes, or reading every fourth word of a page, or recit-
ing a rhyme, or the like can be explained in this way.

Salkovskis makes much of the fact that cognitive-behavioral theory
leads us to cognitive-behavioral therapy, which can be of great benefit
to OCD sufferers. However, he admits that only 50% of patients actually benefit from behavioral therapy and that "benefit" is variously defined.
It remains a mystery why some patients can be freed from their problems
by simply being told authoritatively to stop washing, checking, or the like,
whereas others cannot apparently benefit from years of therapy. The specifically cognitive adjuncts to behavioral treatment have as yet no controlled research data to validate their utility.

Teasdale (1992) argues that cognitive-behavioral theorists in general
have made no attempt to incorporate cognitive science into their work.
They use everyday or lay concepts of "cognition" and "meaning." Ross
(1991) states; "What they do is employ some of the terminology of cognitive psychology, *schema* and *structure* for example. Such terms are usually called upon to serve as *post hoc* rationalizations when *ad hoc* clinical
procedures seemed to have worked" (p. 743). These criticism are wholly
applicable to the Salkovskis model of OCD.

Salkovskis proposes: "Other problems, such as . . . 'failures of inhibition,' are regarded as secondary to the emotional arousal and particularly to the counterproductive coping strategies deployed by the sufferer" (p. 106). However, my data propose failures of inhibition in OCD patients using neutral stimuli in the absence of emotional arousal and coping stragies. He goes on to dismiss a cognitive inhibition deficit theory in OCD by citing the work of Maki, O'Neill, and O'Neill (1994), who claimed that nonclinical checkers performed similarly to noncheckers on tests of inhibitory control of cognition involving a selective attention task. This conclusion was based upon a confusion between the concepts of "interference" and "inhibition." What Maki et al. actually found was that their two groups performed similarly on a test of cognitive interference, *not* cognitive inhibition. This finding concurs with our own in clinical checkers versus clinical nonchecking OCD subjects (Enright, Beech, & Claridge, in press). Cognitive inhibition as defined by Tipper (1985), and used in our research, was not measured in the Maki et al. study.

In conclusion, my overall impression of the Salkovskis model of OCD is that it deals with the exacerbation of one type of effect of having OCD, not with the underlying cause. It may therefore have much to offer in explaining how in *some* patients specific OCD symptoms become focused and consolidated.

Turning to Chapter 6, I am totally in agreement with Pigott, Myers, and Williams regarding the need to reconceptualize OCD as a clinical diagnosis. However, I am unconvinced by their attempt at creating subtypes of OCD. As the authors admit, their conjecture is highly speculative and almost completely unsubstantiated by any research.

Pigott et al. proposed that patients in category 1 have high levels of comorbid eating disorders; that patients in category 2 may be particularly susceptible to tics; and that many patients in category 3 will have had "brain trauma, lesions, or infections" (p. 145). These propositions simply do not fit with my clinical experience of OCD patients, where such associations are rare.

The theoretical underpinning for the creation of a separate category 2, "incompleteness/habit-spectrum disorder," appears to be that some OCD patients and most Tourette's syndrome patients report a need to perform tasks until they seem "just right." This is scant evidence.

Pigott et al.'s basic system is categorical and not dimensional; it thereby fails to recognize the continuum for a level of obsessionality that spans both normality and severe clinical presentation. Particularly in regard to their category 3, it is increasingly recognized that obsessive–compulsive ideas cannot be simply dichotomized according to patients' levels of insight; rather, a continuum of strength of beliefs is more appropriate (Kozak & Foa, 1994).

The major distinguishing characteristics among the three proposed OCD categories are relative degrees of concomitant anxiety, conviction, and perfectionism. The authors go on to state that "a patient manifesting a common OCD symptom such as repeated handwashing or cleaning rituals could be categorized in any of the three subtypes, depending upon certain characteristics" (p. 145). This raises a number of difficult questions: First, how does one make an objective assessment of these characteristics? Second, what about the fluctuations of symptom patterns common in individual OCD patients? Lastly, how does one weight each dimension in a significant number of OCD patients who express elements of all three characteristics?

I'm afraid I was staggered by Pigott et al.'s deferential references to Freudian theory—a theory that has proved singularly useless in assisting either the understanding or the treatment of OCD. In my opinion, the initial Freudian conceptualization of OCD as an anxiety disorder, and its subsequent stagnation within this same diagnostic category, have been responsible for 50 years of failure to conduct any fruitful research into this condition. Fortunately, in the last few decades this tide has turned.

Pigott et al. discuss the selectivity of serotonergic drugs whose antiobsessional action underpins the "serotonin hypothesis." My understanding is that the specificity of these drugs is something of a myth. Indeed, these authors go on to cite the dopaminergic effects of clomipramine as particularly relevant to their category 2 patients, and suggests that "neuroleptics would probably result in some symptom reduction" (p. 150) in category 3. Rauch and Jenike (1993) conclude: "The findings that 5HT uptake inhibitors also effect changes in non-5HT receptors speaks to the need for any neurochemical model of OCD to include multiple transmitter systems" (p. 29).

Pigott et al. variously point to dysfunctions at various sites within the orbito-frontal loop and basal ganglia as significant in the etiology of OCD. Many of these propositions bear a striking resemblance to the proposals of Hemsley and this colleagues to account for schizophrenia (Hemsley, 1993; Gray, Feldon, Rawlins, Hemsley, & Smith, 1991). Likewise, it is interesting that Pigott et al. emphasize dopaminergic dysregulation in OCD categories 2 and 3, and suggest that the dopamine-blocking effects of clomipramine and the use of neuroleptics may assist symptom reduction. There are obviously links here with schizophrenic etiology. As an aside, it is also noteworthy that treatment-resistant schizophrenic patients are being offered clozapine, which (among its other effects) acts as a serotonin receptor antagonist (Meltzer, 1992).

In conclusion, I believe there can be little doubt that biological theories of OCD will ultimately prove highly significant in the theory and treatment of OCD. I therefore await significant findings from the study of Pigott et al.'s different OCD categories with great interest but profound skepticism.

REFERENCES

Enright, S. J., Beech, A. R., & Claridge, G. S. (in press). The locus of negative priming effects in obsessive–compulsive disorder and other anxiety disorders. *Personality and Individual Differences.*

Festinger, L. (1957). *A theory of cognitive dissonance.* Stanford, CA: Stanford University Press.

Gray, J. A., Feldon, J., Rawlins, J. N. P., Hemsley, D. R., & Smith, A. D. (1991). The neuropsychology of schizophrenia. *Behavioral and Brain Sciences, 14,* 1–20.

Hemsley, D. R. (1993). A simple (or simplistic) cognitive model for schizophrenia. *Behaviour Research and Therapy, 31*(7), 633–645.

Kozak, M. J., & Foa, E. B. (1994). Obsessions, overvalued ideas, and delusions in obsessive–compulsive disorder. *Behaviour Research and Therapy, 32*(3), 343–353.

Maki, W. S., O'Neill, H. K., & O'Neill, G. W. (1994). Do nonclinical checkers exhibit deficits in cognitive control? Tests of an inhibitory control hypothesis. *Behaviour Research and Therapy, 32*(2), 183–192.

Meltzer, H. Y. (1992). Treatment of the neuroleptic non-responsive schizophrenic patient. *Schizophrenia Bulletin, 18,* 515–542.

Rauch, S. L., & Jenike, M. A. (1993). Neurobiological models of obsessive–compulsive disorder. *Psychosomatics, 34*(1), 20–32.

Ross, A. (1991). Growth without progress. *Contemporary Psychology, 36,* 743–744.

Teasdale, J. D. (1992). Emotion and two kinds of meaning: Cognitive therapy and applied cognitive science. *Behaviour Research and Therapy, 31*(4), 339–354.

Tipper, S. P. (1985). The negative priming effect: Inhibitory priming by ignored objects. *Quarterly Journal of Experimental Psychology, 37A,* 591–611.

8

Anxiety Sensitivity Is Distinguishable from Trait Anxiety

Richard J. McNally

PEOPLE VARY GREATLY in their anxiety proneness. Some people experience anxiety symptoms with minimal provocation, whereas others become anxious only under the most threatening circumstances. The concept of "trait anxiety" denotes these individual differences in anxiety proneness. Measures of trait anxiety include the Trait form of the State–Trait Anxiety Inventory (STAI-T; Spielberger, Gorsuch, Lushene, Vagg, & Jacobs, 1983) and the Manifest Anxiety Scale (MAS; Taylor, 1953).

Just as people vary in their proneness to experience anxiety symptoms, so may they vary in their fear of these symptoms. Whereas many people regard anxiety as merely unpleasant, others regard it with great alarm. The concept of "anxiety sensitivity" denotes these individual differences in the fear of anxiety (Reiss & McNally, 1985). More specifically, "anxiety sensitivity" refers to fears of anxiety symptoms that are based on beliefs that these symptoms have harmful consequences. A person with high anxiety sensitivity may believe that heart palpitations signify an impending heart attack, whereas a person with low anxiety sensitivity is likely to regard these sensations as merely uncomfortable. Anxiety sensitivity is measured by the Anxiety Sensitivity Index (ASI; Reiss, Peterson, Gursky, & McNally, 1986).

The relation between trait anxiety and anxiety sensitivity has been a subject of debate (Jacob & Lilienfeld, 1991; Lilienfeld, Jacob, & Turner, 1989; McNally, 1989; Reiss, 1991; Taylor, Koch, & Crockett, 1991).

In a critique of the anxiety sensitivity concept, Lilienfeld et al. (1989) argued that phenomena attributed to anxiety sensitivity can be explained by "the more parsimonious hypothesis that the ASI simply measures trait anxiety" (p. 101). I (McNally, 1989) replied that "trait anxiety" denotes a general tendency to respond fearfully to stressors, whereas "anxiety sensitivity" denotes a specific tendency to respond fearfully to anxiety symptoms themselves. Hence, persons with high trait anxiety need not have an additional fear of anxiety symptoms themselves.

Research on anxiety sensitivity has proliferated since the 1989 exchange. In this chapter, I review data pertinent to the distinction between anxiety sensitivity and trait anxiety, and demonstrate the heuristic and explanatory potential of the anxiety sensitivity concept.

THE ANXIETY SENSITIVITY INDEX

Considerable research supports the validity of the ASI as a self-report measure of the fear of anxiety (Peterson & Reiss, 1987, 1992). This questionnaire consists of 16 items that express concerns about possible consequences of anxiety (e.g., "When I notice that my heart is beating rapidly, I worry that I might have a heart attack"). Respondents indicate their degree of endorsement for each item on a 5-point Likert scale that ranges from 0 ("very little") to 4 ("very much"). Total scores range from 0 to 64. The second edition of the ASI manual reports a mean of 19.01 (SD = 9.11) for nonclinical subjects (n = 4,517; Peterson & Reiss, 1992). There is a small sex difference: Women score higher than men (19.75 vs. 17.62).

The ASI has satisfactory test–retest reliability over 2-weeks (r = .75; Reiss et al., 1986) and over 3 years (r = .71; Maller & Reiss, 1992). The ASI is characterized by a high degree of internal consistency, as revealed by alpha coefficients that range from .82 to .91 (Peterson & Reiss, 1992).

The ASI has been translated into German, Greek, Dutch, Mandarin, Spanish, Farsi, French, Catalan, and Hebrew (Peterson & Reiss, 1992). Silverman, Fleisig, Rabian, and Peterson (1991) developed the Childhood Anxiety Sensitivity Index (CASI) by adapting the ASI items for school-age children. Validation research indicates that the CASI possesses psychometric properties similar to those of the ASI.

Factor-Analytic Studies of the Anxiety Sensitivity Index

In accordance with our (Reiss & McNally, 1985) hypothesis, factor-analytic research suggests that anxiety sensitivity constitutes a unitary construct. The results of four studies favored a single-factor solution (Peterson & Heilbronner, 1987; Reiss et al., 1986; Taylor et al., 1991; Taylor, Koch, McNally, & Crockett, 1992), whereas the results of two studies favored a four-factor solution (Telch, Shermis, & Lucas, 1989; Wardle, Ahmad, & Hayward, 1990). However, researchers who reported four-factor solutions used methods that extracted an excessive number of unreliable factors; they also considered only orthogonal factor structures, which are improbable in view of the ASI's high internal consistency.

To avoid the limitations of previous studies, we (Taylor, Koch, McNally, & Crockett, 1992) used confirmatory factor analysis to examine one- and four-factor solutions. Although Telch et al.'s (1989) four-factor solution accounted for about 10% more variance than the single-factor solution, it remained viable only when we forced the factors to orthogonality. Removal of this constraint revealed highly interrcorrelated factors, implying that the four-factor solution is an artifact of the orthogonality constraint. We concluded that the ASI is unifactorial.

Anxiety Sensitivity and the Prediction of Fearfulness

To validate a measure of the fear of anxiety, one must show that it behaves differently from measures of trait anxiety in theoretically meaningful ways (Reiss et al., 1986). For example, we (Reiss et al., 1986) argued that ASI scores ought to predict the number and intensity of fears beyond what could be predicted by measures of trait anxiety. The rationale for this hypothesis was as follows. People who believe that anxiety has harmful consequences should experience episodes of anxiety as more aversive than should people who do not. Accordingly, high anxiety sensitivity ought to increase the number and intensity of acquired fears by amplifying the aversiveness of state anxiety. That is, high anxiety sensitivity ought to function like a high-magnitude unconditioned stimulus in Pavlovian conditioning. Just as highly aversive unconditioned stimuli enhance fear conditioning, elevated anxiety sensitivity ought to amplify the negative valence of each episode of anxiety, and thereby increase the number and intensity of learned fears.

Consistent with this hypothesis, we (Reiss et al., 1986) reported that the ASI predicted variance on the Fear Survey Schedule-II (Geer, 1965) beyond that predicted by the MAS and an anxiety symptom frequency checklist in a sample of college students. Similar results were obtained in an agoraphobic sample (McNally & Lorenz, 1987). Finally, Marks, Lindsay, and Al-Kubaisy (1988) reported that the ASI predicted the frequency of panic attacks in phobic patients beyond that predicted by the STAI-T.

Investigators have examined the correlations among the STAI-T, the State form of the State–Trait Anxiety Inventory (STAI-S; Spielberger et al., 1983), and the ASI in an effort to distinguish between trait anxiety and anxiety sensitivity. Reiss (1991) identified 11 data sets that included correlations among these measures. In each data set, the correlation between state and trait anxiety was greater than the correlation between trait anxiety and anxiety sensitivity. Indeed, R^2 values ranging from 0% to 36% indicated minimal overlap in the variance shared by the STAI-T and the ASI. These findings suggest that trait anxiety and anxiety sensitivity are related but distinct constructs.

Taylor et al. (1991) subjected the items of the ASI and the STAI-T to factor analysis with oblique rotation. The results revealed a two-factor solution. The STAI-T items were responsible for nearly all of the salient loadings on the first factor, whereas the ASI items were responsible for nearly all of the salient items on the second factor. The correlation between the factors was .39. Taylor et al. concluded that "the ASI is not simply a measure of trait anxiety" (1991, p. 293).

We (Taylor & McNally, 1991) examined the STAI-T and ASI scores of 142 college students fearful of spiders. We defined "elevated" STAI-T and ASI scores as those at least one standard deviation above their respective normative means, and "normal" STAI-T and ASI scores as those below these cutoffs. Among the 68 subjects with elevated STAI-T scores, 28 (41%) had normal ASI scores. Among the 54 subjects with elevated ASI scores, 14 (26%) had normal STAI-T scores. Among the 74 subjects with normal STAI-T scores, 14 (19%) had elevated ASI scores. Among the 88 subjects with normal ASI scores, 28 (32%) had elevated STAI-T scores. These data indicate that people with high trait anxiety do not necessarily have high anxiety sensitivity, and that people with high anxiety sensitivity do not necessarily have high trait anxiety.

Considered together, the aforementioned studies indicate that anxiety sensitivity and trait anxiety are related but distinguishable dispositional constructs.

THE NOSOLOGICAL SIGNIFICANCE OF ANXIETY SENSITIVITY

DSM-III-R and DSM-IV distinguish anxiety neurotics who experience spontaneous panic attacks (i.e., persons with panic disorder) from those who do not (i.e., persons with generalized anxiety disorder [GAD]; American Psychiatric Association, 1987, 1994). Nevertheless, research has revealed that spontaneous panic can occur in GAD (Barlow, 1988). Unlike patients with panic disorder, however, GAD patients usually do not worry about experiencing additional attacks (Sanderson & Barlow, 1990). Therefore, panic disorder may be distinguished from GAD as much by the *fear* of panic as by the occurrence of panic itself (McNally, 1992). Consistent with the belief that panic disorder is characterized by apprehension about subsequent attacks (Barlow, 1988), panic patients score about two standard deviations above the normative mean on the ASI (McNally & Lorenz, 1987; Rapee, Ancis, & Barlow, 1988; Taylor et al., 1991).

Subsequent findings have supported the relative diagnostic specificity of elevated anxiety sensitivity. We (Taylor, Koch, & McNally, 1992) studied the relation between trait anxiety and anxiety sensitivity across the DSM-III-R anxiety disorders. Mean STAI-T scores did not differ significantly among patients with social phobia (M = 47.9), GAD (M = 53.7), obsessive–compulsive disorder (OCD; M = 57.9), posttraumatic stress disorder (PTSD; M = 52.3), and panic disorder (M = 54.3), although all groups scored higher than a group of patients with simple phobia (M = 39.0). Patients with panic disorder, however, had significantly higher ASI scores (M = 36.6) than those with simple phobia (M = 16.1), GAD (M = 26.2), social phobia (M = 24.9), and OCD (M = 25.4), and marginally higher (p < .06) ASI scores than patients with PTSD (M = 31.6). Although panic and GAD patients scored equivalently high on a measure of trait anxiety, panic patients scored significantly higher than GAD patients on the ASI. These findings support the nosological significance of the ASI, and suggest that the fear of panic is as important as the occurrence of panic itself in distinguishing between these diagnostic entities (McNally, 1992).

Anxiety sensitivity may figure in the explanation of "nonfearful" panic attacks. Nonfearful panickers reported the full range of DSM-III-R panic symptoms; yet they experienced discomfort, not fear (Beitman et al., 1987; Kushner & Beitman, 1990). Although these people may have a biological vulnerability to experiencing sympathetic activation, they presumably have low anxiety sensitivity, and therefore do not panic in response to sudden symptoms that frighten those with high anxiety sensitivity.

IS ANXIETY SENSITIVITY A CAUSE OR CONSEQUENCE OF PANIC?

Psychopathologists have traditionally assumed that the fear of anxiety is a consequence of panic attacks (e.g., Goldstein & Chambless, 1978; Klein, 1981). This assumption is reasonable if the fear of anxiety is viewed solely as a Pavlovian interoceptive conditioned response. On the other hand, if the fear of anxiety is viewed as a dispositional variable consisting of beliefs about the harmfulness of anxiety symptoms, it could develop in ways other than through direct experience with panic. Just as other fears may arise in ways other than through Pavlovian conditioning (Rachman, 1977; Wolpe, Lande, McNally, & Schotte, 1985), so may fears of anxiety symptoms. Misinformation about heart attacks, mental illness, and anxiety may increase a person's anxiety sensitivity. Observational learning may also contribute to elevated anxiety sensitivity. Consistent with this possibility, Ehlers (1993) found that panickers reported having observed more parental modeling of "fear-of-fear" behavior than patients with other anxiety disorders reported.

If beliefs about the harmfulness of anxiety symptoms can precede the occurrence of panic attacks, then anxiety sensitivity may constitute a cognitive risk factor for developing panic disorder. One must first establish, however, that elevated levels of anxiety sensitivity can occur in the absence of a history of panic. To investigate this issue, we (Donnell & McNally, 1990) had 425 college students complete the ASI and a version of the Panic Attack Questionnaire (Norton, Dorward, & Cox, 1986). We designated as "panickers" those subjects who reported at least one DSM-III-R spontaneous panic attack during the previous 12 months, and designated as "high-ASI" those subjects who scored at least one standard deviation above the normative mean of the ASI. We found that 67% of the high-ASI subjects had never experienced a spontaneous panic attack.

Subsequent studies have confirmed that many high-ASI subjects have never panicked (Asmundson & Norton, 1993; Cox, Endler, Norton, & Swinson, 1991). Using our (Donnell & McNally, 1990) cutoff for high anxiety sensitivity, Cox et al. reported that 70% of high-ASI college students had never had a spontaneous panic attack, and that 50% had never had either a spontaneous or a cued attack. Among Asmundson and Norton's high-ASI college students, 77% had never experienced spontaneous panic, and 42% had never experienced either spontaneous or cued panic.

These studies reveal that elevated anxiety sensitivity occurs in many people who have not experienced panic attacks. Although the data suggest that fears of anxiety symptoms can be acquired in multiple ways, the subsequent occurrence of panic is likely to exacerbate anxiety sensitivity.

ANXIETY SENSITIVITY AND BIOLOGICAL CHALLENGE TESTS

Biological challenge tests provoke panic attacks under controlled laboratory conditions (Woods & Charney, 1988). They produce intense physical sensations, and trigger panic far more often in panic disorder patients than in healthy controls. Challenge tests include carbon dioxide inhalation and voluntary hyperventilation (e.g., Rapee, Brown, Antony, & Barlow, 1992).

Theorists disagree about the mechanisms underlying challenge-induced panic. Biological theorists hold that challenges directly aggravate an underlying neurochemical abnormality (e.g., Klein & Klein, 1989), whereas psychological theorists believe that challenges merely produce bodily sensations that patients are prone to fear (e.g., Margraf, Ehlers, & Roth, 1986).

In an experiment consistent with a psychological interpretation, Rapee et al. (1992) demonstrated the impact of anxiety sensitivity on response to challenge. They exposed anxiety disorder patients and normal controls to hyperventilation and 5.5% carbon dioxide challenges. Patients had DSM-III-R diagnoses of panic disorder with and without agoraphobia, simple phobia, social phobia, GAD, and OCD. As expected, panic patients reported more fear in response to both challenges than did other anxious patients, who, in turn, reported more fear than did healthy controls. Stepwise multiple regressions revealed that the ASI was the only significant predictor of either hyperventilation-induced or carbon-dioxide-induced fear. Measures of social anxiety and trait anxiety did not predict responses to either challenge.

Unfortunately, research on patients provides a problematic basis for disentangling biological and psychological determinants of challenge-induced panic. Because panic disorder is characterized by elevated anxiety sensitivity and by the presence of the putative neurochemical abnormality, one cannot unambiguously isolate the crucial variable(s) in these studies. To circumvent this interpretive impasse, investigators have challenged healthy subjects who do not have the disorder but whose ASI scores resemble those of panic patients. If elevated anxiety sensitivity is a sufficient basis for a fearful response to challenge, healthy high-ASI subjects ought to respond like panic patients to voluntary hyperventilation, carbon dioxide inhalation, and so forth.

Applying this strategy, we (Holloway & McNally, 1987) had college students who scored either high ($M = 31.5$) or low ($M = 7.9$) on the ASI hyperventilate for 5 minutes. Following hyperventilation, subjects with high anxiety sensitivity reported more intense physical symptoms and more subjective anxiety than did subjects with low anxiety sensitivity. Replicating and extending these findings, we (Donnell & McNally, 1989) found that an enhanced response to hyperventilation occured in high-ASI subjects who had never had a spontaneous panic attack. Moreover, a history of spontaneous panic was not associated with an anxious response to hyperventilation in the absence of elevated anxiety sensitivity. These results imply that anxiety sensitivity, rather than a history of panic (cf. Woods & Charney, 1988), may be the critical predictor of panic in other challenge paradigms as well.

In response to Lilienfeld et al.'s (1989) suggestion that trait anxiety might account for hyperventilation-induced anxiety in high-ASI subjects, Rapee and Medoro (1994) selected college students who scored either high ($M = 30.5$) or low ($M = 7.8$) on the ASI, and matched them on STAI-T scores. In response to 3 minutes of overbreathing, high-ASI subjects reported more fear than did low-ASI subjects. Because the two groups were equated on STAI-T scores, trait anxiety cannot explain the enhanced emotional response to challenge in the high-ASI group.

Telch and Harrington (1992) investigated the role of anxiety sensitivity and expectancy in the response to a 35% carbon dioxide challenge. Subjects were college students who had never experienced panic, and who scored either one standard deviation above or below the normative mean on the ASI. These high- and low-ASI subjects received either "expect anxiety" or "expect relaxation" instructions. All subjects received descriptions of inhalation-induced sensations that they might experience (e.g., dizziness, tingling). But the "expect anxiety" instructions described these sensations as "anxiety" responses, whereas the "expect relaxation" instructions described the same sensations as "relaxation" responses. Telch and Harrington predicted that high-ASI subjects would respond more fearfully than low-ASI subjects, especially in the "expect relaxation" condition, where their gas-induced sensations would be surprisingly frightening for subjects with high anxiety sensitivity.

The results confirmed their predictions. Blind, structured assessment for DSM-III-R panic attacks revealed that high-ASI subjects panicked more than low-ASI subjects, and that subjects who expected relaxation panicked more than those who expected anxiety. The panic rates in each group were as follows: low-ASI/"expect anxiety," (5%); low-ASI/"expect relaxation," (14%); high-ASI/"expect anxiety," (22%); and high-ASI/"expect relaxation," (57%). That high-ASI subjects in the "expect relaxation" condition showed the highest rate of panic implies that naturally occurring spontaneous panic is most pathogenic in people with pre-existing high levels of anxiety sensitivity. Telch and Harrington found that ASI scores still predicted challenge-induced panic when they statistically controlled for baseline levels of state (STAI-S) and trait (STAI-T) anxiety.

In another study, high- and low-STAI-T college students were challenged with counterbalanced inhalations of room air and 5.5% carbon dioxide (van den Bergh, Vandendriessche, de Broeck, & van de Woestijne, 1993). The authors predicted that carbon dioxide (relative to air) would provoke more anxiety in high-STAI-T subjects than in low-STAI-T subjects. The results were inconsistent with their hypothesis: High-STAI-T subjects were no more anxious than low-STAI-T subjects in the response to challenge. van den Bergh et al. concluded that an enhanced response to challenge might have occurred had they chosen high- and low-ASI subjects rather than high- and low-STAI-T subjects.

These studies indicate that anxiety sensitivity is a better predictor of a fearful response to challenge than is trait anxiety. Moreover, the findings are in accordance with research on patients. Although panic disorder and GAD are both associated with elevated trait anxiety, panic patients have higher ASI scores than GAD patients, and panic patients are more responsive to challenge than are GAD patients (e.g., Rapee et al., 1992).

ANXIETY SENSITIVITY AND ALCOHOL ABUSE

Consistent with the tension reduction theory of alcoholism, patients with panic disorder and agoraphobia are at increased risk for alcohol problems (Kushner, Sher, & Beitman, 1990). Elevated trait anxiety, however, does not necessarily increase risk for alcoholism. OCD patients, for example, score very high on measures of trait anxiety (Taylor, Koch, & McNally, 1992), yet rarely develop alcoholism (Riemann, McNally, & Cox, 1992).

Perhaps those most at risk for self-medicating with alcohol are people who have high anxiety sensitivity as well as high trait anxiety. Indeed, the mixed evidential support for the tension reduction model may be attributable to its failure to consider anxiety sensitivity.

Data are beginning to emerge concerning the relation between anxiety sensitivity and alcohol abuse. We (Kaspi & McNally, 1990) found that inpatient alcoholics with comorbid DSM-III-R agoraphobia, social phobia, or panic disorder ($n = 30$) had significantly higher ASI (33.5 vs. 26.6) and STAI-T (52.5 vs. 44.5) scores than did inpatient alcoholics without these comorbid conditions ($n = 53$). The mean ASI score of patients without a formal anxiety disorder diagnosis was nevertheless about one standard deviation above the normative mean.

Stewart, Peterson, and Pihl (in press) found that high-ASI college women had higher rates of abusive drinking than did low-ASI college women. Karp and Peterson (1993) reported that ASI scores predicted alcohol consumption as a tension reduction strategy among inpatient alcoholics, whereas STAI-T scores did not.

These preliminary findings suggest additional hypotheses for further research. For example, abusive drinking ought to be strongly predicted by the interaction of high trait anxiety and high anxiety sensitivity, and high ASI scores ought to be associated with abuse of substances that reduce arousal (e.g., benzodiazepines, alcohol) but not with substances that increase arousal (e.g., cocaine, amphetamine).

IS ANXIETY SENSITIVITY A RISK FACTOR FOR PANIC DISORDER?

Beliefs about the harmfulness of anxiety symptoms can develop in ways other than through personal experience with panic (Asmundson & Norton, 1993; Cox et al., 1991; Donnell & McNally, 1990). Accordingly, high anxiety sensitivity may constitute a cognitive risk factor for developing panic disorder (McNally & Lorenz, 1987). If so, healthy high-ASI subjects ought to exhibit information-processing biases similar to those exhibited by patients with panic disorder (McNally, 1990).

To test this hypothesis, Stewart, Achille, Dubois-Nguyen, and Pihl, (1992) had low- and high-ASI college women perform an attentional task requiring them to respond quickly to a target location in the presence of either threat or nonthreat words. As the authors predicted, threat words slowed reaction times more than nonthreat words did, but only in the high-ASI group. An intoxicating dose of alcohol abolished selective processing of threat among high-ASI subjects.

Maller and Reiss (1992) conducted a 3-year follow-up study on college students who had scored either high ($n = 23$) or low ($n = 25$) on the ASI. Relative to low-ASI subjects, those who scored high on the ASI in 1984 were five times more likely to have a DSM-III-R anxiety disorder in 1987. Three out of four subjects who experienced panic attacks for the first time during the follow-up period were from the original high-ASI group. Maller and Reiss concluded that elevated anxiety sensitivity constitutes a risk factor for anxiety disorders. A large longitudinal study is needed to establish this convincingly.

CONCLUSIONS

Psychometric (e.g., Taylor et al., 1991), nosological (Taylor, Koch, & McNally, 1992), and experimental (e.g., Telch & Harrington, 1992) studies indicate that anxiety sensitivity and trait anxiety are distinct dispositional variables (McNally, 1989). Anxiety sensitivity has demonstrated its heuristic importance by generating predictions about important phenomena that were not anticipated by trait anxiety conceptualizations. Finally, the clinical impact of the ASI is likely to grow in response to recommendations made at the National Institute of Mental Health's Consensus Conference on the Standardization of Panic Disorder Assessment. The consensus panel deemed it "essential" that pharmacological as well as psychological treatment researchers incorporate dispositional fear-of-anxiety questionnaires in treatment protocols (Shear & Maser, 1994). The panel recommended the use of the ASI, the Body Sensations Questionnaire, and the Agoraphobic Cognitions Questionnaire (Chambless, Caputo, Bright, & Gallagher, 1984) as measures of this construct.

REFERENCES

American Psychiatric Association. (1987). *Diagnostic and statistical manual of mental disorders* (3rd ed., rev.). Washington, DC: Author.

American Psychiatric Association. (1994). *Diagnostic and statistical manual of mental disorders* (4th ed.). Washington, DC: Author.

Asmundson, G. J. G., & Norton, G. R. (1993). Anxiety sensitivity and its relationship to spontaneous and cued panic attacks in college students. *Behaviour Research and Therapy, 31,* 199–201.

Barlow, D. H. (1988). *Anxiety and its disorders: The nature and treatment of anxiety and panic.* New York: Guilford Press.

Beitman, B. D., Basha, I., Flaker, G., DeRosear, L., Mukerji, V., & Lamberti, J. (1987). Non-fearful panic disorder: Panic attacks without fear. *Behaviour Research and Therapy, 25,* 487–492.

Chambless, D. L., Caputo, G. C., Bright, P., & Gallagher, R. (1984). Assessment of fear of fear in agoraphobics: The Body Sensations Questionnaire and the Agoraphobic Cognitions Questionnaire. *Journal of Consulting and Clinical Psychology, 52,* 1090–1097.

Cox, B. J., Endler, N. S., Norton, G. R., & Swinson, R. P. (1991). Anxiety sensitivity and nonclinical panic attacks. *Behaviour Research and Therapy, 29,* 367–369.

Donnell, C. D., & McNally, R. J. (1989). Anxiety sensitivity and history of panic as predictors of response to hyperventilation. *Behaviour Research and Therapy, 27,* 325–332.

Donnell, C. D., & McNally, R. J. (1990). Anxiety sensitivity and panic attacks in a nonclinical population. *Behaviour Research and Therapy, 28,* 83–85.

Ehlers, A. (1993). Somatic symptoms and panic attacks: A retrospective study of learning experiences. *Behaviour Research and Therapy, 31,* 269–278.

Geer, J. H. (1965). The development of a scale to measure fear. *Behaviour Research and Therapy, 3,* 45–53.

Goldstein, A. J., & Chambless, D. L. (1978). A reanalysis of agoraphobia. *Behavior Therapy, 9,* 47–59.

Holloway, W., & McNally, R. J. (1987). Effects of anxiety sensitivity on the response to hyperventilation. *Journal of Abnormal Psychology, 96,* 330–334.

Jacob, R. G., & Lilienfeld, S. O. (1991). Panic disorder: Diagnosis, medical assessment, and psychological assessment. In J. R. Walker, G. R. Norton, & C. A. Ross (Eds.), *Panic disorder and agoraphobia: A comprehensive guide for the practitioner* (pp. 16–102). Pacific Grove, CA: Brooks/Cole.

Karp, J., & Peterson, R. A. (1993). *The relationship between anxiety and alcohol expectancies among inpatient alcoholics.* Manuscript submitted for publication.

Klein, D. F. (1981). Anxiety reconceptualized. In D. F. Klein & J. G. Rabkin (Eds.), *Anxiety: New research and changing concepts* (pp. 235–263). New York: Raven Press.

Klein, D. F., & Klein, D. F. (1989). The nosology, genetics, and theory of spontaneous panic and phobia. In P. Tyrer (Ed.), *Psychopharmacology of anxiety* (pp. 163–195). New York: Oxford University Press.

Kushner, M. G., & Beitman, B. D. (1990). Panic attacks without fear: An overview. *Behaviour Research and Therapy, 28,* 469–479.

Kushner, M. G., Sher, K. J., & Beitman, B. D. (1990). The relation between alcohol problems and the anxiety disorders. *American Journal of Psychiatry, 147,* 685–695.

Lilienfeld, S. O., Jacob, R. G., & Turner, S. M. (1989). Comment on Holloway and McNally's (1987) "Effects of anxiety sensitivity on the response to hyperventilation." *Journal of Abnormal Psychology, 98,* 100–102.

Maller, R. G., & Reiss, S. (1992). Anxiety sensitivity in 1984 and panic attacks in 1987. *Journal of Anxiety Disorders, 6,* 241–247.

Margraf, J., Ehlers, A., & Roth, W. T. (1986). Sodium lactate infusions and panic attacks: A review and critique. *Psychosomatic Medicine, 48,* 23–51.

Marks, M., Lindsay, S. J. E., & Al-Kubaisy, T. (1988, September). *Fear of fear in different phobic groups.* Paper presented at the World Congress of Behaviour Therapy, Edinburgh.

McNally, R. J. (1989). Is anxiety sensitivity distinguishable from trait anxiety? A reply to Lilienfeld, Jacob, and Turner (1989). *Journal of Abnormal Psychology, 98,* 193–194.

McNally, R. J. (1990). Psychological approaches to panic disorder: A review. *Psychological Bulletin, 108,* 403–419.

McNally, R. J. (1992). Anxiety sensitivity distinguishes panic disorder from generalized anxiety disorder. *Journal of Nervous and Mental Disease, 180,* 737–738.

McNally, R. J., & Lorenz, M. (1987). Anxiety sensitivity in agoraphobics. *Journal of Behavior Therapy and Experimental Psychiatry, 18,* 3–11.

McNally, R. J., Riemann, B. C., & Kim, E. (1990). Selective processing of threat cues in panic disorder. *Behaviour Research and Therapy, 28,* 407–412.

Norton, G. R., Dorward, J., & Cox, B. J. (1986). Factors associated with panic attacks in nonclinical subjects. *Behavior Therapy, 17,* 239–252.

Peterson, R. A., & Heilbronner, R. L. (1987). The Anxiety Sensitivity Index: Construct validity and factor analytic structure. *Journal of Anxiety Disorders, 1,* 117–121.

Peterson, R. A., & Reiss, S. (1987). *Anxiety Sensitivity Index Manual.* Orland Park, IL: International Diagnostic Systems.

Peterson, R. A., & Reiss, S. (1992). *Anxiety Sensitivity Index Manual* (2nd ed.). Worthington, OH: International Diagnostic Systems.

Rachman, S. (1977). The conditioning theory of fear-acquisition: A critical examination. *Behaviour Research and Therapy, 15,* 375–387.

Rapee, R. M., Ancis, J. R., & Barlow, D. H. (1988). Emotional reactions to physiological sensations: Panic disorder patients and non-clinical Ss. *Behaviour Research and Therapy, 26,* 265–269.

Rapee, R. M., Brown, T. A., Antony, M. M., & Barlow, D. H. (1992). Response to hyperventilation and inhalation of 5.5% carbon dioxide-enriched air across the DSM-III-R anxiety disorders. *Journal of Abnormal Psychology, 101,* 538–552.

Rapee, R. M., & Medoro, L. (1994). Fear of physical/sensations and trait anxiety as mediators of the response to hyperventilation in nonclinical subjects. *Journal of Abnormal Psychology, 103,* 693–699.

Reiss, S. (1991). Expectancy model of fear, anxiety, and panic. *Clinical Psychology Review, 11,* 141–153.

Reiss, S., & McNally, R. J. (1985). Expectancy model of fear. In S. Reiss & R. R. Bootzin (Eds.), *Theoretical issues in behavior therapy* (pp. 107–121). San Diego, CA: Academic Press.

Reiss, S., Peterson, R. A., Gursky, D. M., & McNally, R. J. (1986). Anxiety sensitivity, anxiety frequency and the prediction of fearfulness. *Behaviour Research and Therapy, 24,* 1–8.

Riemann, B. C., McNally, R. J., & Cox, W. M. (1992). The comorbidity of obsessive-compulsive disorder and alcoholism. *Journal of Anxiety Disorders, 6,* 105–110.

Sanderson, W. C., & Barlow, D. H. (1990). A description of patients diagnosed with DSM-III-R generalized anxiety disorder. *Journal of Nervous and Mental Disease, 178,* 588–591.

Shear, M. K., & Maser, J. D. (1994). Standardized assessment for panic disorder research. A conference report. *Archives of General Psychiatry, 51,* 346–354.

Silverman, W. K., Fleisig, W., Rabian, B., & Peterson, R. A. (1991). The Childhood Anxiety Sensitivity Index. *Journal of Clinical Child Psychology, 20,* 162–168.

Spielberger, C. D., Gorsuch, R. L., Lushene, R., Vagg, P. R., & Jacobs, G. A. (1983). *Manual for the State-Trait Anxiety Inventory.* Palo Alto, CA: Consulting Psychologists Press.

Stewart, S. H., Achille, M. A., Dubois-Nguyen, I., & Pihl, R. O. (1992, June). *The effects of alcohol on the selective attentional bias for threat in anxiety sensitive women.* Paper presented at the World Congress of Cognitive Therapy, Toronto.

Stewart, S. H., Peterson, J. B., & Pihl, R. O. (in press). Anxiety sensitivity and self-reported alcohol consumption rates in university women. *Journal of Anxiety Disorders.*

Taylor, J. A. (1953). A personality scale of manifest anxiety. *Journal of Abnormal and Social Psychology, 48,* 285–290.

Taylor, S., Koch, W. J., & Crockett, D. J. (1991). Anxiety sensitivity, trait anxiety, and the anxiety disorders. *Journal of Anxiety Disorders, 5,* 293–311.

Taylor, S., Koch, W. J., & McNally, R. J. (1992). How does anxiety sensitivity vary across the anxiety disorders? *Journal of Anxiety Disorders, 6,* 249–259.

Taylor, S., Koch, W. J., McNally, R. J., & Crockett, D. J. (1992). Conceptualizations of anxiety sensitivity. *Psychological Assessment, 4,* 245–250.

Taylor, S., McNally, R. J. (1991). [Anxiety sensitivity and trait anxiety in spider-fearful subjects.]. Unpublished raw data.

Telch, M. J., & Harrington, P. J. (1992, November). *The role of anxiety sen-*

*sitivity and expectedness of arousal in mediating affective response to 35†
carbon dioxide.* Paper presented at the meeting of the Association for Advancement of Behavior Therapy, Boston.

Telch, M. J., Shermis, M. D., & Lucas, J. A. (1989). Anxiety sensitivity: Unitary personality trait or domain-specific appraisals? *Journal of Anxiety Disorders, 3,* 25–32.

van den Bergh, O., Vandendriessche, F., de Broeck, K., & van de Woestijne, K. P. (1993). Predictability and perceived control during 5.5% CO_2-enriched air inhalation in high and low anxious subjects. *Journal of Anxiety Disorders, 7,* 61–73.

Wardle, J., Ahmad, T., & Hayward, P. (1990). Anxiety sensitivity in agoraphobia. *Journal of Anxiety Disorders, 4,* 325–333.

Wolpe, J., Lande, S. D., McNally, R. J., & Schotte, D. (1985). Differentiation between classically-conditioned and cognitively based neurotic fears. *Journal of Behavior Therapy and Experimental Psychiatry, 16,* 287–293.

Woods, S. W., & Charney, D. S. (1988). Applications of the pharmacologic challenge strategy in panic disorders research. *Journal of Anxiety Disorders, 2,* 31–49.

9

Anxiety Sensitivity
Is Not Distinct
from Trait Anxiety

SCOTT O. LILIENFELD

WHY ARE SOME INDIVIDUALS more frightened of their own anxiety than are others? A number of prominent researchers have recently addressed themselves to this question (e.g., Clark, 1986; Goldstein & Chambless, 1978; McNally, 1990; Reiss, 1987). The answer to this question has important clinical implications, because the "fear of anxiety" is associated with, and may be causally related to, panic disorder, agoraphobia, and other anxiety-related syndromes (Jacob & Rapport, 1984; Ley, 1987; Reiss, 1991).

"Anxiety sensitivity" (AS) is the newest and perhaps most influential in the line of constructs that have been advanced to help explain the etiology of panic disorder and related phenomena. According to Reiss, Peterson, Gursky, and McNally (1986), AS is the extent to which individuals believe that their anxiety or anxiety symptoms have aversive consequences. Thus, individuals with elevated AS are characterized by cognitions that their anxiety or anxiety-related sensations, such as rapid heartbeat or trembling, will cause them harm or other noxious outcomes. Reiss et al. contend that AS is often present prior to panic attacks, and that it may be a risk factor for these attacks.

AS is embedded in the expectancy theory of anxiety (Reiss & McNally, 1985; Reiss, 1991), which posits that anxiety in a given situation is a joint function of two constructs: expectancy and sensitivity. "Expectancy' is the individual's subjective probability that an anxiety-provoking event will occur; anxiety expectancy, for example, is the individual's subjective probability that he or she will experience anxiety or anxiety-related symptoms (Reiss, 1991). "Sensitivity," in contrast, is the individual's *reactivity* to anxiety-provoking stimuli; AS, for example, is "the person's sensitivity to experiencing anxiety" (Reiss, 1991, p. 144). Thus, AS and other sensitivities are hypothesized to be reactive constructs that amplify or enhance anxiety responding (Reiss, 1991).

The principal operationalization of AS is the Anxiety Sensitivity Index (ASI; Reiss et al., 1986), a 16-item self-report measure designed to assess the extent to which individuals fear their anxiety and anxiety symptoms (e.g., "It scares me when I am nervous," "When I notice that my heart is beating rapidly, I worry that I might have a heart attack"). The implicit assumption behind such items appears to be that respondents who admit to these fears also harbor beliefs that their anxiety and anxiety symptoms have unpleasant consequences (Lilienfeld, Jacob, & Turner, 1989; Telch, Shermis, & Lucas, 1989). Although the ASI is highly internally consistent (Cronbach's alphas are generally in the .80 to .90 range; Reiss, 1991), there is suggestive evidence that it is multidimensional (e.g., Telch et al., 1989; cf. Taylor, Koch, McNally, & Crockett, 1992).

EVIDENCE FOR THE CONSTRUCT VALIDITY OF THE ANXIETY SENSITIVITY INDEX

There is compelling evidence that the ASI correlates in theoretically predicted directions with a variety of criteria relevant to panic disorder and other anxiety disorders (see Peterson & Reiss, 1987, and Reiss, 1991, for reviews). For example, the ASI is elevated among patients with panic disorder (Peterson & Reiss, 1987; Rapee, Ancis, & Barlow, 1988), as well as among those with posttraumatic stress disorder, social phobia, and obsessive–compulsive disorder (McNally et al., 1987; McNally, Taylor, Koch, & Louro, 1991). The ASI scores of panic disorder patients have been reported to normalize following cognitive-behavioral therapy (McNally & Lorenz, 1987). Moreover, the ASI predicts the remission rate and severity of distress among panic disorder patients over 6-month and 1-year intervals (Otto, Pollack, Sachs, & Rosenbaum, 1991). In addition, many individuals with elevated ASI scores report that they have never had a spontaneous panic attack (e.g., Donnell & McNally, 1990), apparently corroborating Reiss and his colleagues' claim that AS is not invariably a consequence of panic attacks (but see Lilienfeld, Turner, & Jacob, 1993).

Perhaps most impressively, the ASI has been found to predict increases in self-reported anxiety in response to challenge procedures, such as hyperventilation (Donnell & McNally, 1989; Holloway & McNally, 1987), mental arithmetic (Shostak & Peterson, 1990), and talking about one's anxiety-producing experiences (Maller & Reiss, 1987). These findings are consistent with the claim that AS is an amplifier of anxiety (Reiss, 1991), because AS produces differential reactivity of subjects to potentially threatening stimuli. In other words, AS has generally been found to *interact* with anxiety-inducing manipulations, in that subjects with high AS respond more intensely to these manipulations than do subjects with low AS.

THE CENTRAL CONTROVERSY: ANXIETY SENSITIVITY OR TRAIT ANXIETY?

As we have argued elsewhere (Jacob & Lilienfeld, 1991; Lilienfeld et al., 1989, 1993), one of the key claims of the developers of the AS construct is that AS is conceptually and empirically separable from trait anxiety. Thus, Reiss and his colleagues contend that AS predicts findings not derivable from trait anxiety explanations of panic disorder (e.g., Mathews & Eysenck, 1987). Moreover, Reiss (1991, p. 147) has argued that the ASI is a "unique scale" that predicts clinical phenomena not predicted by measures of trait anxiety.

The assertion that AS is distinct from trait anxiety is of considerable importance, because a number of theorists have conceptualized panic attacks as resulting from high levels of trait anxiety (see Hallam, 1991). Indeed, all anxiety disorders are characterized by an elevated rate of panic attacks (Barlow, 1988), suggesting that trait anxiety may be a nonspecific risk factor for these attacks. If the proponents of the AS construct are correct, however, trait anxiety is not sufficient to explain panic; the additional construct of AS is required.

"Trait anxiety" has generally been defined as a pervasive disposition to react anxiously to potentially anxiety-provoking stimuli (e.g., Spielberger, Gorsuch, & Luchene, 1970). Trait anxiety, in turn, loads highly on a superordinate dimension that has been termed "negative emotionality "(NE; Tellegen, 1978–1982; Watson & Clark, 1984) or "neuroticism" (Eysenck, 1981; Costa & McCrae, 1987). NE has been defined as a pervasive dimension that predisposes individuals to experience a wide variety of negative moods, including anxiety, anger, and mistrust, and to evaluate themselves and the world negatively (Watson & Clark, 1984).

Despite the claim that AS is distinct from trait anxiety, there appear to be plausible theoretical reasons for suggesting a close relation between these two constructs. Eysenck's (1979) incubation theory of anxiety posits that individuals with elevated levels of neuroticism, which overlaps considerably with trait anxiety (Watson & Clark, 1984), are highly susceptible to anxiety incubation and thus to panic attacks (but see Mineka, 1979, and Wolpe, 1979, for critiques of Eysenck's model). Indeed, Reiss (1991) has acknowledged that AS "has similarities to Eysenck's concept of neuroticism" (p. 142). In addition, Pennebaker and Watson (1991) have conjectured that individuals with elevated levels of NE are susceptible to "somatic amplification" (Barsky & Klerman, 1983), which appears to bear close affinities to the amplification posited by Reiss and his colleagues to result from elevated AS. According to Pennebaker and Watson, individuals with high NE tend to focus selectively upon internal sensations and to interpret them as dangerous, leading to an increased propensity for somatic symptoms.

Many and perhaps most of the early construct validation studies of the ASI (e.g., McNally & Lorenz, 1987) are open to the alternative explanation that their findings are attributable to trait anxiety (Lilienfeld et al., 1989). For example, panic disorder patients, as well as patients with other anxiety disorders, score high on indices of trait anxiety (Barlow, 1988). Moreover, trait anxiety indices are affected by treatments for agoraphobia (Michelson, 1987). Consequently, findings that ASI scores tend to be elevated among patients with panic disorder and several other anxiety disorders (Peterson & Reiss, 1987), and to decrease in agoraphobics following cognitive-behavioral therapy (McNally & Lorenz, 1987), are also consistent with the hypothesis that the ASI is heavily saturated with trait anxiety. In addition, measures of trait anxiety predict outcome among panic disorder patients, as does the ASI (Otto et al., 1991). Nevertheless, because many of the early ASI studies did not include trait anxiety indices (Lilienfeld et al., 1989), the possibility that the findings of these studies are attributable to trait anxiety cannot be excluded.

TRAITS AS INTERACTIVE CONSTRUCTS

It is also important to recognize that the findings of AS studies using challenge procedures can potentially be explained by trait anxiety. As discussed earlier, such studies generally demonstrate *interactions* between ASI level and threatening manipulations: Subjects with high ASI scores tend to exhibit greater increases in state anxiety following challenge procedures than subjects with low ASI scores do. Although these results are consistent with an AS explanation, they are also consistent with a trait anxiety explanation (Lilienfeld et al., 1993). Why?

Traits are inherently interactive constructs (Tellegen, 1981, 1992), because they indicate a tendency to respond in characteristic ways, given characteristic stimuli. The notion of traits as interactive constructs can be traced to Allport (1937), who asserted that "traits are often aroused in one type of situation and not in another; not all stimuli are equivalent in effectiveness" (pp. 331–332). From Allport's perspective (see Zuroff, 1986), a person with elevated trait anxiety would not be expected to exhibit elevated *state* anxiety in all situations, but only in situations he or she perceives as threatening. Thus, the findings of challenge studies are consistent with a trait anxiety explanation, because trait anxiety (Spielberger et al., 1970), like AS (Reiss, 1991), has been posited to produce differential reactivity to stimuli that are differentially anxiety-provoking.

This point appears not to have been adequately appreciated in the AS literature. Shostak and Peterson (1990), for example, in interpreting their findings on the response of subjects to a challenge procedure, stated that "as expected, trait anxiety level may prove useful in distinguishing those individuals who may experience levels of state anxiety in the *absence* of an anxiety-invoking event" (p. 519; emphasis in original). Donnell and McNally (1990) averred that the trait anxiety explanation of panic " 'explains' the tendency for people to experience anxiety attacks by invoking the tendency to experience anxiety in general (i.e., high trait anxiety)" (p. 84). Nevertheless, both of these comments neglect the interactive nature of traits, including trait anxiety.

The interactive nature of trait anxiety is illustrated in a study by Rappaport and Katkin (1972), who reported that, compared with subjects with low trait anxiety (as measured by the Taylor Manifest Anxiety Scale [MAS]; Taylor, 1953), subjects with high trait anxiety were no different in their rate of spontaneous skin conductance responses (SSCRs) at rest, but exhibited significant increases in their SSCR rate following an anxiety-provoking task (a fake "lie detector" test). The authors concluded that "scores on the Manifest Anxiety Scale reflect 'reactive' anxiety, the autonomic components of which are differentially elicited by ego-involving stress situations" (p. 219).

More recently, Larsen and Ketelaar (1989) reported that individuals with high scores on the Neuroticism scale of the Eysenck Personality Inventory, which is essentially a measure of trait anxiety (Watson & Clark, 1984), exhibited greater increases in negative mood than low scorers did following a negative mood induction technique (bogus failure feedback on a set of mental ability tasks). Others (e.g., Hodges, 1968; Parkes, 1990) have similarly reported greater anxiety reactivity among subjects high in trait anxiety, especially when the stressor is ego-threatening (Endler & Magnusson, 1976). Although some researchers have not found interactions between trait anxiety and anxiety-provoking manipulations (see Watson & Clark, 1984, pp. 475–476), both theoretical and empirical considerations suggest that the results of challenge studies are potentially consistent with a trait anxiety explanation. In other words, both trait anxiety and AS would be expected to amplify anxiety responding.

TRAITS AS ASSIMILATIVE CONSTRUCTS

Several researchers have contended that it is tautological to invoke trait anxiety as an explanation for AS findings. Donnell and McNally (1990), for instance, asserted that "the trait anxiety explanation for panic appears circular" (p. 84). They went on to say that "Although both trait anxiety and anxiety sensitivity are dispositional constructs, only the latter is embedded in a theory that explains why someone might panic in response to symptoms that are not *inherently threatening*" (p. 84; emphasis added). Thus, according to Donnell and McNally, although the construct of trait anxiety represents a propensity to react anxiously to potentially anxiety-provoking stimuli, this construct cannot explain why certain individuals react anxiously *specifically* in response to their own anxiety. McNally (1989) similarly argued that "Unless one smuggles in the concept of anxiety sensitivity under the rubric of trait anxiety, there is no theoretical basis for predicting that people who respond with excessive fear to threatening stimuli in general should also respond with excessive fear to symptoms that are not *inherently stressful*" (p. 193; emphasis added).

Such statements, however, neglect the "assimilative" character of traits (Tellegen, 1992; Wachtel, 1977). Traits can be thought of as "assimilative" because they influence how individuals construe and interpret a wide variety of stimuli. Allport's famous statement (1961, p. 347) that traits have "the capacity to render many stimuli functionally equivalent" implies that traits influence the interpretation of stimuli. Thus, individuals with high trait anxiety perceive a number of ambiguous situations (e.g., a conference, a party, a trip to a new country) as "functionally equivalent" in the sense that they tend to interpret many or all of these situations as threatening. Contrary to the statements of Donnell and McNally (1990) and McNally (1989), most anxiety-provoking stimuli are not "inherently" threatening (cf. Seligman, 1971). Instead, trait anxiety influences the degree to which ambiguous stimuli are *construed* as threatening. Beck and Emery with Greenberg (1985) have similarly pointed out that individuals with high trait anxiety tend to overestimate the probability of harm in their environment.

In a related vein, Watson and Clark (1984) have conceptualized NE as a propensity to construe minor hassles and symptoms as disastrous occurrences. Thus, one of the major ways in which NE may lead to trait anxiety is by coloring individuals' interpretations of ambiguous stimuli. From this perspective, invoking trait anxiety or NE as an explanation for AS findings is not tautological, but instead provides an explanation for why some individuals view their own anxiety and anxiety symptoms as more ominous than do others. As Pennebaker and Watson (1991) noted, "subjects with high [NE] should be more attentive to subtle sensations in their bodies . . . [and] may be more likely to interpret minor symptoms and sensations as painful or pathological" (p. 28).

In support of these assertions, there is evidence that individuals with elevated trait anxiety tend to construe ambiguous stimuli as threatening (Eysenck & Mathews, 1987). Phares (1961), for example, reported that high scorers on the MAS were more likely than low scorers to perceive threatening content in Thematic Apperception Test cards. Haney (1973) exposed subjects to a series of slides, each of which contained a semantically ambiguous sentence (e.g., "The index finger was placed on the tray"). Then, subjects were shown another slide containing two options (one threatening, the other nonthreatening), each of which would disambiguate the meaning of the sentence (e.g., "Finger: Pointing, Amputation"), and were asked to select the choice that best fit their interpretation of the word. Haney reported that subjects who were sensitizers on Byrne's (1961) Repression–Sensitization Scale, which is essentially a measure of trait anxiety (Watson & Clark, 1984), were significantly more likely to select the choices associated with threatening interpretations of the sentences.

Eysenck, MacLeod, and Mathews (1987) presented subjects with a set of homophones delivered auditorily, and asked them to write down the first spelling of each homophone that came to mind. Each homophone had both a threatening (e.g., "die") and a nonthreatening (e.g., "dye") meaning and spelling; half were relevant to physical health, and half to interpersonal problems. Eysenck et al. reported that the correlation between trait anxiety, as assessed by the Trait form of the State–Trait Anxiety Inventory (STAI; Spielberger et al., 1970), and the number of threatening homophones reported was high ($r = .60$) and statistically significant. No significant effect was found for physically versus socially threatening homophones.

Thus, there is evidence from several sources that individuals with high trait anxiety tend to interpret ambiguous stimuli as threatening, although it is conceivable that some of these findings are at least partly attributable to greater familiarity of threatening stimuli among subjects with high trait anxiety (Eysenck et al., 1987). Nevertheless, the studies reviewed in this section have important implications for the assertion that a novel construct (i.e., AS) is required to account for why certain individuals are more frightened of their own anxiety or anxiety symptoms than are others (e.g., Donnell & McNally, 1990). Specifically, individuals with elevated trait anxiety may tend to construe ambiguous physical sensations (e.g., rapid heartbeat, shortness of breath) as threatening. Thus, the findings of Phares (1961), Haney (1973), and Eysenck et al. (1987) would provide a conceptual bridge between trait anxiety and AS, because these findings indicate that subjects with elevated trait anxiety tend to interpret a variety of ambiguous stimuli, perhaps including their own anxiety and anxiety sensations, as dangerous. Moreover, these findings suggest that the additional construct of AS is not required to explain individual differences in the fear of anxiety, and that the trait anxiety explanation of AS findings is therefore not tautological.

STUDIES OF INCREMENTAL VALIDITY

Several years ago (Lilienfeld et al., 1989), we urged that "researchers include a measure of trait anxiety in all investigations of the ASI, so that the incremental validity of the latter relative to the former can be evaluated" (p. 102). Incremental validity (Meehl, 1959) is a key consideration in the AS literature, because, as noted earlier, the proponents of the AS construct assert that this construct predicts findings that cannot be accounted for by trait anxiety. Thus, the incremental validity of the ASI relative to trait anxiety measures represents an important test of both the ASI's construct validity and the verisimilitude of the expectancy theory of anxiety within which the AS construct is embedded.[1]

It is worth noting that the question of incremental validity is not equivalent to whether AS *is* trait anxiety—a point that has been a source of misunderstanding in the AS literature. Reiss (1991), for instance, presented evidence that the correlations between the ASI and trait anxiety indices are well below unity, and concluded that "These numbers are nowhere near the levels needed to support Lilienfeld et al.'s hypothesis that anxiety sensitivity is trait anxiety" (p. 146; see also McNally, 1990, p. 408). Nevertheless, this is a "straw person" argument; the distinguishability between AS and trait anxiety has never been in question. For example, we (Lilienfeld et al., 1989) pointed out that correlations between the ASI and trait anxiety measures, although positive, are generally moderate in magnitude ($r = .40$ to $.50$ in most studies). Moreover, we noted that "the ASI contains reliable variance unrelated to trait anxiety indices" (p. 101) and that the results of the study by Holloway and McNally (1987) "suggest that the ASI may be *contaminated* by trait anxiety" (p. 102; emphasis added).[2]

Instead, the key question is whether the variance shared by the ASI and trait anxiety indices is the same variance accounting for the findings of AS research; the ASI may not provide information over and above that provided by trait anxiety indices in the prediction of relevant criteria. Thus, although the ASI contains variance that is not shared with trait anxiety measures, it must be shown that this unique variance relates to the phenomena of interest to AS researchers (e.g., panic attacks, response to challenge procedures).

Because of space limitations, I do not deal here with the research on the incremental validity of the ASI in detail; suffice it to say that the ASI has generally been found to contribute information over and above that provided by trait anxiety indices for a number of criteria (Lilienfeld et al., 1993). For example, Reiss et al. (1986) found that the ASI contributes to the prediction of commonplace fears over and above the contribution of trait anxiety measures; this finding has been replicated several times (Reiss, 1991). In addition, McNally (1989) reported that in the hyperventilation challenge study by Holloway and McNally (1987), the ASI predicted posthyperventilation anxiety and hyperventilation sensations significantly better than did the Trait form of the STAI. Moreover, Maller and Reiss (1992) reported that, compared with scores on the trait form of the STAI, ASI scores were significantly more highly correlated with the occurrence of panic attacks during the previous year. Although the results of several other studies on the incremental validity of the ASI are either negative (Brown & Cash, 1990) or unclear (Cox, Endler, Norton, & Swinson, 1991; Shostak & Peterson, 1990), the overall picture suggests that at least some of the findings of AS research cannot be entirely accounted for by trait anxiety (Lilienfeld et al., 1993).

Thus, AS researchers generally appear to have successfully responded to the call (Lilienfeld et al., 1989) to demonstrate the incremental validity of the ASI relative to trait anxiety measures. These findings clearly represent a crucial step toward the construct validation of the ASI and the corroboration of Reiss's (1991) expectancy theory. At this point, however, an additional question arises: Do these findings necessarily imply that AS is qualitatively distinct from trait anxiety? As I argue in the next section, the answer to this question is no.

A REFORMULATION: A HIERARCHICAL MODEL OF ANXIETY SENSITIVITY AND TRAIT ANXIETY

It may be less profitable to ask whether AS and trait anxiety are "different" constructs than to examine how they are interrelated. We have argued that the key to resolving the AS–trait anxiety controversy may lie in distinguishing among different levels of trait specificity and generality (Lilienfeld et al., 1993). Specifically, AS may be a lower-order trait that is nested hierarchically within a higher- order dimension of trait anxiety. Trait anxiety, in turn, may covary sufficiently with other traits, such as aggressiveness and alienation, to form a still higher-order NE factor (Tellegen, 1978–1982).

As Watson and Clark (1992) have noted, a prerequisite for a hierarchical factor model is that both general and specific factors influence the traits in the hierarchy. According to the hierarchical model presented here, trait anxiety can be thought of as a tendency to react anxiously to potentially anxiety-inducing stimuli *in general,* whereas AS can be thought of as a more specific tendency to react anxiously to one's own anxiety and anxiety-related symptoms per se. AS would thus share variance with the higher-order trait anxiety factor, but would also possess unique variance that is essentially unrelated to trait anxiety. Coexisting with AS at the lower-order level may be other "sensitivities," such as the injury sensitivity and social evaluation sensitivity proposed by Reiss (1991). These sensitivities, although separable, may share sufficient variance to form a higher-order trait anxiety factor. In turn, AS may be divisible into even more specific lower-order factors, such as anxiety regarding mental incapacitation and anxiety regarding physical sensations (Telch et al., 1989). A possible hierarchical factor model encompassing the relation between AS and trait anxiety is shown in Figure 9.1.

If this hierarchical model has merit, both the trait anxiety and AS positions may contain considerable elements of truth. According to this model, AS is conceptually and empirically related to trait anxiety, but AS indices provide information that more global indices of trait anxiety do not. In a related vein, Mellstrom, Cicala, and Zuckerman (1976) reported that specific indices of fears of animals and situations, such as snakes and heights, were superior to global indices of fear in their prediction of behavior in the presence of these feared stimuli. As McNally (1989) pointed out, "if we want to predict whether someone will respond fearfully to a dog, knowing that the person is dog phobic is more useful than merely knowing the person is a phobic" (p. 193). Thus, although AS may be largely subsumable within a higher-order trait anxiety factor, AS may nevertheless possess incremental validity in the prediction of certain criteria (e.g., panic attacks), because it possesses unique variance that is especially relevant for these criteria.

This or similar hierarchical factor models could be tested through confirmatory factor analysis (Long, 1983) by positing that AS and other sensitivities load on a higher-order trait anxiety factor, but that these sensitivities also contain unique variance essentially uncorrelated with this factor. Thus, injury sensitivity might load on both a general trait anxiety factor and a harmavoidance or physical fearfulness factor (e.g., Tellegen, 1978–1982), whereas AS might load on both a general trait anxiety factor and a somatic anxiety factor (Schalling, 1978), or, more speculatively, an "absorption" factor representing a propensity to become intensely immersed in sensory experiences (Tellegen & Atkinson, 1974).

This hierarchical model may help to account for four consistent findings in the AS literature. First, the positive (although far from perfect) correlation between the ASI and trait anxiety indices is consistent with this model, because the ASI is heavily saturated with variance from the

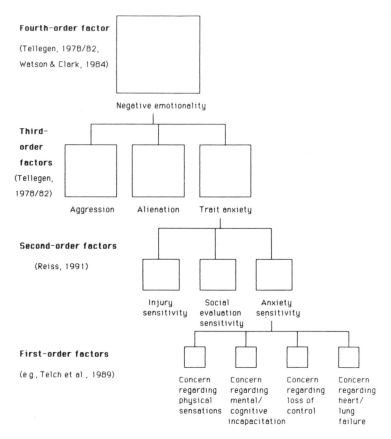

FIGURE 9.1. Proposed hierarchical factor model encompassing the relation between AS and trait anxiety. From Lilienfeld, Turner, & Jacob (1993, p. 172). Copyright 1993 by Pergamon Press, Ltd. Reprinted by permission.

higher-order trait anxiety factor, but also contains unique variance largely uncorrelated with this factor. Second, findings that the ASI possesses incremental validity relative to trait anxiety indices can similarly be explained by positing that AS contains unique variance not shared with trait anxiety. Third, the finding that some individuals possess high AS and low trait anxiety, and vice versa (Cox et al., 1991), is consistent with a hierarchical model, as only a portion of the variance of AS is shared with trait anxiety. For example, an individual could possess high trait anxiety and yet possess little of the variance specific to AS. Such an individual would probably obtain a high score on a trait anxiety index, but only a moderate or fairly low score on the ASI. Fourth and finally, this model may help to explain why panic disorder patients possess levels of trait anxiety essentially equivalent to those of generalized anxiety disorder (GAD) patients, but have higher levels of AS (McNally et al., 1991). Specifically, panic disorder patients may differ from GAD patients largely in their level of certain specific factors, such as somatic anxiety (Hoehn-Saric, 1982) or absorption (Tellegen & Atkinson, 1974).

The implications of this model can perhaps be better appreciated by examining other hierarchical models in the literature. Watson and Clark (1992), for example, found that lower-order markers of NE (such as fear/anxiety, anger/hostility, and sadness/depression) exhibited high to moderately high intercorrelations, suggesting the pervasive influence of a higher-order NE factor. At the same time, however, they found that these lower-order NE markers each possessed incremental validity relative to all other lower-order NE markers in the prediction of certain criteria, indicating that each marker possesses unique variance. Similar findings of a hierarchical structure are well known in the literature on cognitive abilities. For example, spatial visualization and clerical speed/accuracy load highly on the higher-order general intelligence factor (*g*), but possess incremental validity relative to *g* in the prediction of performance in certain occupations (Jensen, 1986). Nevertheless, it would be misleading to conclude that spatial visualization and clerical speed/accuracy are qualitatively distinct from *g* simply because the former abilities contain variance that is not shared with *g*. Similarly, it would be misleading to conclude that AS is qualitatively distinct from trait anxiety simply because AS contains variance that is not shared with trait anxiety.

Although it should be emphasized that this hierarchical model is conjectural and awaits empirical corroboration, this and similar models possess the dual advantages of being falsifiable and of providing a resolution to the AS–trait anxiety controversy. In addition, this model underscores the need to avoid a false dichotomy between AS and trait anxiety. Both constructs may contribute important information, but at different levels of explanation. As Watson and Clark (1992) noted, "evidence supporting one level of the [hierarchical] structure does not necessarily constitute a refutation of the other" (p. 499).

CONCLUDING REMARKS

Several major conclusions emerge from this discussion of the relation between AS and trait anxiety: (1) Trait anxiety, like other traits, implies interactions between individuals' trait levels and trait-relevant stimuli, and can thus account for why some individuals show greater reactivity to challenge procedures than do others; (2) trait anxiety, like other traits, has assimilative properties, and can thus explain why some individuals are more frightened of their anxiety and anxiety symptoms than are others; (3) the ASI has generally been found to possess incremental validity relative to trait anxiety indices in the prediction of certain criteria; and (4) this incremental validity does not imply that AS is qualitatively distinct from trait anxiety, because both constructs may coexist at different levels of a hierarchical structure. Researchers would do well to avoid making a false dichotomy between AS and trait anxiety, and instead to focus upon formulating and testing models of their association.

NOTES

1. It is worth noting that we disagree with McNally's (1989) argument that parsimony is an improper standard by which to judge the AS construct. As Popper (1959) noted, parsimony can be identified with "paucity of parameters" (p. 142). According to Popper, a theory (T_1) that attempts to account for the same set of data as an alternative theory (T_2), but with fewer parameters, has a *lower* prior probability and is thus more falsifiable than T_2. Thus, if T_1 is as successful as T_2 in predicting results, it will be more strongly corroborated, because it has been subjected to greater theoretical risk. In the case of the AS literature, we are faced with two theories, one of which attempts to predict findings with one parameter (trait anxiety), and the other of which attempts to predict these findings with two parameters (trait anxiety plus AS). (The latter is the case because the proponents of AS acknowledge that trait anxiety is a risk factor for panic attacks and for state anxiety following challenge procedures; e.g., McNally, 1989, p. 193.) Thus, if the trait anxiety explanation and the AS explanation were to predict these findings equally well, the former would be more strongly corroborated.

2. In fairness to both Reiss and McNally, these authors may have misinterpreted our admittedly somewhat ambiguous statement that "the results of these studies [construct validation studies of the ASI] can be equally accounted for by positing that the ASI measures trait anxiety" (Lilienfeld et al., 1989, p. 101). We certainly did not intend to imply that the ASI is a *pure measure* of trait anxiety, but only that the ASI assesses trait anxiety, *among other things*. In any case, I hope that these comments help to resolve any remaining confusion in the AS literature concerning this issue.

REFERENCES

Allport, G. W. (1937). *Personality: A psychological interpretation.* New York: Holt.

Allport, G. W. (1961). *Pattern and growth in personality.* New York: Holt, Rinehart & Winston.

Barlow, D. H. (1988). *Anxiety and its disorders: The nature and treatment of anxiety and panic.* New York: Guilford Press.

Barsky, A. J., & Klerman, G. L. (1983). Overview: Hypochondriasis, bodily complaints, and somatic styles. *American Journal of Psychiatry, 140,* 273–283.

Beck, A. T., & Emery, G., with Greenberg, R. L. (1985). *Anxiety disorders and phobias: A cognitive perspective.* New York: Basic Books.

Brown, T. A., & Cash, T. F. (1990). The phenomenon of nonclinical panic: Parameters of panic, fear, and avoidance. *Journal of Anxiety Disorders, 4,* 15–29.

Byrne, D. (1961). The Repression–Sensitization Scale: Rationale, reliability and validity. *Journal of Personality, 29,* 334–349.

Clark, D. M. (1986). A cognitive approach to panic. *Behaviour Research and Therapy, 24,* 461–470.

Costa, P. T., & McCrae, R. R. (1987). Neuroticism, somatic complaints, and disease: Is the bark worse than the bite? *Journal of Personality, 55,* 229–316.

Cox, B. J., Endler, N. S., Norton, G. R., & Swinson, R. P. (1991). Anxiety sensitivity and nonclinical panic attacks. *Behaviour Research and Therapy, 29,* 367–369.

Donnell, C. D., & McNally, R. J. (1989). Anxiety sensitivity and history of panic as predictors of response to hyperventilation. *Behaviour Research and Therapy, 27,* 325–332.

Donnell, C. D., & McNally, R. J. (1990). Anxiety sensitivity and panic attacks in a nonclinical population. *Behaviour Research and Therapy, 28,* 83–85.

Endler, N. S., & Magnusson, D. (1976). Toward an interactional psychology of personality. *Psychological Bulletin, 83,* 956–974.

Eysenck, H. J. (1979). The conditioning model of neurosis. *Behavioral and Brain Sciences, 2,* 155–199.

Eysenck, H. J. (Ed.). (1981). *A model for personality.* New York: Springer-Verlag.

Eysenck, M. W., MacLeod, C., & Mathews, A. (1987). Cognitive functioning and anxiety. *Psychological Research, 49,* 189–195.

Eysenck, M. W., & Mathews, A. (1987). Trait anxiety and cognition. In H. J. Eysenck & I. Martin (Eds.), *Theoretical foundations of behavior therapy* (pp. 197–216). New York: Plenum Press.

Goldstein, A. J., & Chambless, D. L. (1978). A reanalysis of agoraphobia. *Behavior Therapy, 9,* 47–59.

Hallam, R. (1991). A forward look: Psychosocial perspectives. In J. R. Walker, G. R. Norton, & C. A. Ross (Eds.), *Panic disorder and agoraphobia: A comprehensive guide for the practitioner* (pp. 470–503). Pacific Grove, CA: Brooks/Cole.

Haney, J. N. (1973). Approach–avoidance reactions by repressors and sensitizers to ambiguity in a structured free-association task. *Psychological Reports, 33,* 97–98.

Hodges, W. F. (1968). Effects of ego threat and threat of pain on state anxiety. *Journal of Personality and Social Psychology, 8,* 364–372.

Hoehn-Saric, R. (1982). Comparison of generalized anxiety disorder with panic disorder patients. *Psychopharmacology Bulletin, 18,* 104–108.

Holloway, W., & McNally, R. J. (1987). Effects of anxiety sensitivity on the response to hyperventilation. *Journal of Abnormal Psychology, 96,* 330–334.

Jacob, R. G., & Lilienfeld, S. O. (1991). Panic disorder: Diagnosis, medical assessment, and psychological assessment. In J. R. Walker, G. R. Norton, & C.A. Ross (Eds.), Panic disorder and agoraphobia: A comprehensive guide for the practitioner (pp. 16–102). Pacific Grove, CA: Brooks/Cole.

Jacob, R. G., & Rapport, M. D. (1984). Panic disorder. In S. M. Turner (Ed.), Behavioral theories and treatment of anxiety (pp. 187–237). New York: Plenum Press.

Jensen, A. R. (1986). g: Artifact or reality? Journal of Vocational Behavior, 29, 301–331.

Larsen, R. J., & Ketelaar, T. (1989). Extraversion, neuroticism, and susceptibility to positive and negative mood induction procedures. Personality and Individual Differences, 12, 1221–1228.

Ley, R. (1987). Panic disorder and agoraphobia: Fear of fear or fear of the symptoms produced by hyperventilation? Behaviour Research and Therapy, 18, 305–316.

Lilienfeld, S. O., Jacob, R. G., & Turner, S. M. (1989). Comment on Holloway and McNally's (1987) "Effects of anxiety sensitivity on the response to hyperventilation." Journal of Abnormal Psychology, 98, 100–102.

Lilienfeld, S. O., Turner, S. M., & Jacob, R. G. (1993). Anxiety sensitivity: An examination of theoretical and methodological issues. Advances in Behaviour Research and Therapy, 15, 147–183.

Long, J. (1983). Confirmatory factor analysis: A preface to LISREL. Beverly Hills, CA: Sage.

Maller, R. G., & Reiss, S. (1987). A behavioral validation of the Anxiety Sensitivity Index. Journal of Anxiety Disorders, 1, 265–272.

Maller, R. G., & Reiss, S. (1992). Anxiety sensitivity in 1984 and panic attacks in 1987. Journal of Anxiety Disorders, 1, 241–247.

Mathews, A., & Eysenck, A. W. (1987). Clinical anxiety and cognition. In H. J. Eysenck & I. Martin (Eds.), Theoretical foundations of behavior therapy (pp. 217–234). New York: Plenum Press.

McNally, R. J. (1989). Is anxiety sensitivity distinguishable from trait anxiety? Reply to Lilienfeld, Jacob, and Turner (1989). Journal of Abnormal Psychology, 98, 193–194.

McNally, R. J. (1990). Psychological approaches to panic disorder: A review. Psychological Bulletin, 3, 403–419.

McNally, R. J., & Lorenz, M. (1987). Anxiety sensitivity in agoraphobics. Journal of Behavior Therapy and Experimental Psychiatry, 18, 3–11.

McNally, R. J., Luedke, D. L., Besyner, J. K., Peterson, R. A., Bohm, K., & Lips, O. J. (1987). Sensitivity to stress-relevant stimuli in posttraumatic stress disorder. Journal of Anxiety Disorders, 1, 105–116.

McNally, R. J., Taylor, S., Koch, W. J., & Louro, C. E. (1991, November). Anxiety sensitivity: An overview of recent findings. Paper presented at the meeting of the Association for Advancement of Behavior Therapy, New York.

Meehl, P. E. (1959). Some ruminations on the validation of clinical procedures. Canadian Journal of Psychology, 13, 102–128.

Mellstrom, M., Jr., Cicala, G. A., & Zuckerman, M. (1976). General versus specific trait anxiety measures in the prediction of fear of snakes, heights, and darkness. *Journal of Consulting and Clinical Psychology, 44,* 83–91.

Michelson, L. (1987). Cognitive-behavioral treatment and assessment of agoraphobia. In L. Michelson & L. M. Ascher (Eds.), *Anxiety and stress disorders: Cognitive-behavioral assessment and treatment* (pp. 213–279). New York: Guilford Press.

Mineka, S. (1979). Response to Eysenck's (1979) "The conditioning model of neurosis." *Behavioral and Brain Sciences, 2,* 178.

Otto, M. W., Pollack, M. H., Sachs, G. S., & Rosenbaum, J. F. (1991, November). *Anxiety sensitivity as a diathesis for panic disorder: Results from a naturalistic, longitudinal study.* Paper presented at the meeting of the Association for Advancement of Behavior Therapy, New York.

Parkes, K. R. (1990). Coping, negative affectivity, and the work environment: Additive and interactive predictors of mental health. *Journal of Applied Psychology, 75,* 399–409.

Pennebaker, J. W., & Watson, D. (1991). The psychology of somatic symptoms. In L. J. Kirmayer & J. M. Robbins (Eds.), *Current concepts of somatization* (pp. 21–35). Washington, DC: American Psychiatric Press.

Peterson, R. A., & Reiss, S. (1987). *Test manual for the Anxiety Sensitivity Index.* Orland Park, IL: International Diagnostic Systems.

Phares, E. J. (1961). TAT performance as a function of anxiety and coping–avoiding behavior. *Journal of Consulting Psychology, 25,* 257–259.

Popper, K. R. (1959). *The logic of scientific discovery.* New York: Basic Books.

Rapee, R. M., Ancis, J. R., & Barlow, D. H. (1988). Emotional reactions to physiological sensations: Panic disorder patients and non-clinical subjects. *Behaviour Research and Therapy, 26,* 265–269.

Rappaport, H., & Katkin, E. S. (1972). Relationships among manifest anxiety, response to stress, and the perception of autonomic activity. *Journal of Consulting and Clinical Psychology, 38,* 219–224.

Reiss, S. (1987). Theoretical perspectives on the fear of anxiety. *Clinical Psychology Review, 7,* 585–596.

Reiss, S. (1991). Expectancy model of fear, anxiety, and panic. *Clinical Psychology Review, 11,* 141–153.

Reiss, S., & McNally, R. J. (1985). Expectancy model of fear. In S. Reiss & R. R. Bootzin (Eds.), *Theoretical issues in behavior therapy* (pp. 107–121). San Diego, CA: Academic Press.

Reiss, S., Peterson, R. A., Gursky, D. M., & McNally, R. J. (1986). Anxiety sensitivity, anxiety frequency, and the prediction of fearfulness. *Behaviour Research and Therapy, 24,* 1–8.

Schalling, D. (1978). Psychopathy-related personality variables and the psychophysiology of socialization. In R. D. Hare & D. Schalling (Eds.), *Psychopathic behaviour: Approaches to research* (pp. 85–106). Chichester, England: Wiley.

Seligman, M. E. P. (1971). Phobias and preparedness. *Behavior Therapy, 2,* 307–320.

Shostak, B. B., & Peterson, R. A. (1990). Effects of anxiety sensitivity on emotional response to a stress task. *Behaviour Research and Therapy, 28,* 513–521.

Spielberger, C. D., Gorsuch, R. R., & Lushene, R. E. (1970). State–Trait Anxiety Inventory: Test manual for form X. Palo Alto, CA: Consulting Psychologists Press.

Taylor, J. A. (1953). A personality scale of manifest anxiety. *Journal of Abnormal and Social Psychology, 48,* 285–290.

Taylor, S., Koch, W. J., McNally, R. J., & Crockett, D. J. (1992). Conceptualizations of anxiety sensitivity. *Psychological Assessment, 4,* 245–250.

Telch, M. J., Shermis, M. D., & Lucas, J. A. (1989). Anxiety sensitivity: Unitary personality trait or domain-specific appraisals? *Journal of Anxiety Disorders, 3,* 25–32.

Tellegen, A. (1978–1982). *Brief manual for the Multidimensional Personality Questionnaire.* Unpublished manuscript, University of Minnesota.

Tellegen, A. (1981). Practicing the two disciplines for relaxation and enlightenment: Comment on "Role of the feedback signal in electromyographic feedback: The relevance of attention" by Qualls and Sheehan. *Journal of Experimental Psychology: General, 110,* 217–226.

Tellegen, A. (1992). Personality traits: Issues of definition, evidence, and assessment. In D. Cicchetti & W. Grove (Eds.), *Thinking clearly about psychology: Essays in honor of Paul Everett Meehl* (Vol. 2, pp. 10–35). Minneapolis: University of Minnesota Press.

Tellegen, A., & Atkinson, G. (1974). Openness to absorbing and self-altering experiences ("absorption"), a trait related to hypnotic susceptibility. *Journal of Abnormal Psychology, 83,* 268–277.

Wachtel, P. (1977). *Psychoanalysis and behavior therapy: Toward an integration.* New York: Basic Books.

Watson, D., & Clark, L. A. (1984). Negative affectivity: The disposition to experience aversive emotional states. *Psychological Bulletin, 98,* 219–235.

Watson, D., & Clark, L. A. (1992). Affects separable and inseparable: On the hierarchical arrangement of the negative affects. *Journal of Personality and Social Psychology, 62,* 489–505.

Wolpe, J. (1979). Response to Eysenck's (1979) "The conditioning model of neurosis." *Behavioral and Brain Sciences, 2,* 184–185.

Zuroff, D. C. (1986). Was Gordon Allport a trait theorist? *Journal of Personality and Social Psychology, 51,* 993–1000.

Toward a Resolution
of the Anxiety Sensitivity
versus Trait Anxiety Debate

RICHARD J. McNALLY

THE RELATION BETWEEN ANXIETY sensitivity and trait anxiety is clearer today than it was in the 1980s. Clarification has arisen through conceptual refinement and through a growing body of research. These developments have counteracted theoretical polarization and have fostered rapprochement among competing perspectives on the fear of anxiety.

Among recent developments is Lilienfeld's persuasive hypothesis concerning the hierarchical relation between anxiety sensitivity and trait anxiety, which he has set forth in Chapter 9. Accommodating the relevant findings, this hypothesis provides a promising resolution to the anxiety sensitivity versus trait anxiety debate. Taylor (1995), moreover, has directly corroborated the model in a recent confirmatory factor-analytic investigation. Rather than elaborate further on points of agreement between me and Lilienfeld, I address three issues that warrant clarification.

PARSIMONY AS A BASIS FOR ADJUDICATING
THEORETICAL DISPUTES

One apparent implication of Lilienfeld, Jacob, and Turner's (1989) commentary was that the concept of anxiety sensitivity is a redundant accretion to theories of trait anxiety, and that considerations of parsimony call for abandonment of the otiose notion of anxiety sensitivity. In Chapter

9, citing Popper (1959), Lilienfeld elaborates his defense of parsimony as a basis for deciding between competing theories that account for the same data. He holds that if a theory with one parameter (e.g., trait anxiety) predicts the same results as a theory with two parameters (e.g., trait anxiety, anxiety sensitivity), the first theory ought to be preferred because of its greater parsimony and greater falsifiability.

Unfortunately, the application of this principle is often more complicated than Lilienfeld's example implies. Contrary to Popper (1959, pp. 136–155), the theory with the fewest parameters is not necessarily more falsifiable than its competitors. One need only consider the grand single-parameter theories that attribute all psychopathology to unconscious sexual conflicts, child abuse, or some other factor to realize that Popper's criterion often fails to apply in the social sciences. Moreover, it can be difficult to determine whether two theories generate precisely the same predictions; yet only under these circumstances is parsimony truly decisive in theory choice. I do not believe that parsimony is an "improper" criterion for evaluating theories, but I do believe that considerations of explanatory power, heuristic value, and so forth are more important than paucity of parameters in the adjudication of theoretical disputes. In any event, even if one did consider parsimony as important as these other guidelines, anxiety sensitivity would now seem to have passed this test.

CONTENT OVERLAP BETWEEN PANIC SYMPTOMS AND THE ANXIETY SENSITIVITY INDEX

Panic disorder is strongly related to elevated scores on the Anxiety Sensitivity Index (ASI; Reiss, Peterson, Gursky, & McNally, 1986), and ASI items directly pertaining to fears of bodily sensations readily discriminate patients with panic disorder from patients with other anxiety disorders (Taylor, Koch, & Crockett, 1991). Observing that panic attacks are defined primarily by physical sensations, Lilienfeld has suggested that "Taylor et al.'s results may be a largely tautological consequence of the tendency of panic disorder patients to endorse items assessing their own symptoms" (Lilienfeld, Turner, & Jacob, 1993, p. 167).

There are reasons for believing that the association between anxiety sensitivity and panic disorder is not simply a tautological artifact arising from content overlap between the ASI and panic attack criteria. Indeed, the ASI concerns the *fear* of certain bodily sensations, whereas panic attack criteria concern the *presence* of certain bodily sensations (Reiss et al., 1986; Taylor, 1995). The occurrence of symptoms, moreover, does not require the fear of symptoms. For example, patients with generalized anxiety disorder (GAD) experience physical symptoms, including occasional spontaneous panic attacks (Sanderson & Barlow, 1990); yet they have lower ASI scores than do patients with panic disorder (McNally, 1992). That GAD patients rarely worry about subsequent panics is consistent with their relatively low ASI scores.

TRAIT ANXIETY AND
THE INTERPRETATION OF THREAT

People with high trait anxiety tend to interpret a wide range of ambiguous stimuli as threatening. Accordingly, Lilienfeld suggests, trait anxiety may suffice to explain why some people respond fearfully to certain bodily sensations that are not inherently harmful.

But three recent experiments by Rapee and Medoro (1994) cast doubt on Lilienfeld's hypothesis. In their first experiment, Rapee and Medoro exposed two groups of college students to a hyperventilation challenge. Although both groups had similar trait anxiety scores, one group scored high on the ASI, whereas the other group scored low on the ASI. The results revealed that the high-ASI group was more responsive to challenge than was the low-ASI group. If trait anxiety were the crucial predictor of response to challenge, both groups should have responded similarly.

In their second and third experiments, Rapee and Medoro (1994) confirmed that the ASI predicted variance in the response to hyperventilation challenge in college students beyond that predicted by a measure of trait anxiety. Moreover, by forcibly entering trait anxiety first into hierarchical multiple regressions, Rapee and Medoro may have underestimated the predictive power of the ASI. Taken together, these studies suggest that unless they are also characterized by elevated anxiety sensitivity, people with high trait anxiety do not respond fearfully to bodily sensations.

CONCLUSION

During the past few years research on anxiety sensitivity has flourished, and these developments have greatly clarified issues pertaining to the anxiety sensitivity versus trait anxiety debate. Lilienfeld's hierarchical model constitutes an important proposal for resolving this debate that ought to stimulate further research on the fear of anxiety.

REFERENCES

Lilienfeld, S. O., Jacob, R. G., & Turner, S. M. (1989). Comment on Holloway and McNally's (1987) "Effects of anxiety sensitivity on the response to hyperventilation." *Journal of Abnormal Psychology, 98,* 100–102.

Lilienfeld, S. O., Turner, S. M., & Jacob, R. G. (1993). Anxiety sensitivity: An examination of theoretical and methodological issues. *Advances in Behaviour Research and Therapy, 15,* 147–183.

McNally, R. J. (1992). Anxiety sensitivity distinguishes panic disorder from generalized anxiety disorder. *Journal of Nervous and Mental Disease, 180,* 737–738.

Popper, K. R. (1959). *The logic of scientific discovery.* New York: Harper & Row.

Rapee, R. M., & Medoro, L. (1994). Fear of physical sensations and trait anxiety as mediators of the response to hyperventilation in nonclinical subjects. *Journal of Abnormal Psychology, 103,* 693–699.

Reiss, S., Peterson, R. A., Gursky, D. M., & McNally, R. J. (1986). Anxiety sensitivity, anxiety frequency and the prediction of fearfulness. *Behaviour Research and Therapy, 24,* 1–8.

Sanderson, W. C., & Barlow, D. H. (1990). A description of patients diagnosed with DSM-III-R generalized anxiety disorder. *Journal of Nervous and Mental Disease, 178,* 588–591.

Taylor, S. (1995). Issues in the conceptualization and measurement of anxiety sensitivity. *Journal of Anxiety Disorders, 9,* 163–174.

Taylor, S., Koch, W. J., & Crockett, D. J. (1991). Anxiety sensitivity, trait anxiety, and the anxiety disorders. *Journal of Anxiety Disorders, 5,* 293–311.

Another Look at the Relation between Anxiety Sensitivity and Trait Anxiety

SCOTT O. LILIENFELD

IN HIS CLEAR AND WELL-REASONED commentary in Chapter 8, Richard McNally makes a persuasive case for the distinctness of anxiety sensitivity (AS) from trait anxiety. It appears to me that the primary differences between McNally and myself are ones of emphasis. Nevertheless, sometimes emphasis matters. In my response, I outline (1) where I believe McNally and I agree, (2) where I believe McNally and I disagree, and (3) several suggestions for where to proceed next.

McNally and I agree that the AS construct has been of substantial heuristic value in the study of anxiety and anxiety disorders, and that its principal operationalization, the Anxiety Sensitivty Index (ASI), should continue to be used in research on the "fear of anxiety." McNally and I agree that AS and trait anxiety are overlapping but not identical constructs. McNally and I agree that the ASI has been demonstrated to possess incremental validity relative to trait anxiety indices for a number of important criteria (e.g., panic attacks, response to challenge procedures). Finally, McNally and I agree that AS may be an amplifier of pre-existing anxiety.

So are McNally and I fomenting a false controversy? I don't believe so. Unlike McNally, I believe that researchers are probably making a mistake by treating AS and trait anxiety at the same level of explanation. McNally states in Chapter 8 that "Just as people vary in their proneness to experience anxiety symptoms, so may they vary in their fear of these symptoms" (p. 214). Somewhat later, he asserts that " 'trait anxiety' denotes a general tendency to respond fearfully to stressors, whereas 'anxiety sensitivity' denotes a specific tendency to respond fearfully to anxiety symptoms themselves" (p. 215). But might not the fear of anxiety symptoms *stem* in part from a higher-order proneness to experience anxiety? Might not trait anxiety *lead to* AS in some individuals, such as those who have seen others experience harm in conjunction with anxiety, who are told that certain anxiety symptoms are dangerous, or who have high levels of certain personality traits (e.g., harmavoidance)?

The answers to these questions appear to depend largely upon whether one views traits as possessing "assimilative" properties (Tellegen, 1992). If one believes that all stimuli are either "inherently" threatening or "inherently" nonthreatening (e.g., McNally, 1989), then it may make sense to argue that AS and trait anxiety are distinct constructs. In contrast, if one believes (as I do) that certain personality traits, including trait anxiety, influence the degree to which stimuli are *interpreted* as threatening (Eysenck & Mathews, 1987), then the distinction between AS and trait anxiety becomes fuzzy. From this perspective, AS might better be viewed as a lower-order facet of trait anxiety, rather than as a distinct trait coexisting with trait anxiety at the same level of specificity. This implies that the relation between AS and trait anxiety is best conceived of as hierarchical — a possibility that McNally does not discuss.

One additional point regarding hierarchical factor models deserves brief mention. McNally argues that the results of factor-analytic studies (e.g., Taylor, Koch, McNally, & Crockett, 1992) suggest that the ASI is unidimensional. But even if he is correct, this implies little about the dimensionality of the AS *construct*. I suspect that McNally would agree with me that the ASI is not a perfect operationalization of the AS construct, and that the "fear of anxiety" may include a number of domains not assessed by the ASI. Thus, findings that the ASI is unidimensional do not exclude the possibility that AS is multidimensional and thus consists of lower-order traits. Measure and construct are not identical.

On a more conciliatory note, I am pleased to see that McNally had several intriguing suggestions for "risky" tests (Meehl, 1978) of Reiss's (1991) expectancy theory of anxiety. Let me highlight two of these that strike me as worth pursuing. First, I especially like McNally's suggestion to examine patients with "nonfearful" panic attacks. He conjectures that such patients do not have elevated AS, because they presumably lack the fear of anxiety symptoms typical of patients with panic disorder. If he is correct, it would seem unlikely that elevated ASI scores are simply a consequence of panic attacks, or that the relation between the ASI and panic attacks is a spurious result of content–criterion overlap (Lilienfeld, Turner, & Jacob, 1993).

Second, McNally raises the possibility that AS and trait anxiety may interact (not just combine additively) to produce certain outcomes, such as alcohol abuse. This synergistic hypothesis is intuitively appealing, because AS has been posited to amplify anxiety (Reiss, 1991). We (Orsillo, Lilienfeld, & Heimberg, 1994) have recently found suggestive support for this hypothesis by examining social phobics' response to challenge procedures. Further corroboration of this hypothesis would provide fairly impressive support for the expectancy theory of anxiety within which the AS construct is embedded.

One final comment: It seems that researchers have devoted a great deal of attention to the proposition that AS and trait anxiety are distinct constructs, but have not devoted sufficent attention to examining why they are correlated. The AS literature would be enriched by the incorporation of models of trait anxiety, such as Gray's (1982) biopsychological model of the behavioral inhibition system, that have implications for the development of AS (see Lilienfeld et al., 1993). Gray's model, for example, posits that individuals with elevated trait anxiety tend to be overly sensitive to signals of anticipated danger or harm. Because of this sensitivity, such individuals may construe a number of stimuli—including, in some cases, their own anxiety and anxiety-related sensations—as portending threat. Gray's model, as well as others, may thus provide important developmental links between trait anxiety and AS; such models may also help to explain how individual differences in trait anxiety, in conjunction with environmental experiences and perhaps other personality traits, give rise to individual differences in the fear of anxiety.

REFERENCES

Eysenck, M. W., & Mathews, A. (1987). Trait anxiety and cognition. In H. J. Eysenck & I. Martin (Eds.), *Theoretical foundations of behavior therapy* (pp. 197–216). New York: Plenum Press.

Gray, J. (1982). *The neuropsychology of anxiety.* New York: Oxford University Press.

Lilienfeld, S. O., Turner, S. M., & Jacob, R. G. (1993). Anxiety sensitivity: An examination of theoretical and methodological issues. *Advances in Behaviour Research and Therapy, 15,* 147–183.

McNally, R. J. (1989). Is anxiety sensitivity distinguishable from trait anxiety? Reply to Lilienfeld, Jacob, and Turner (1989). *Journal of Abnormal Psychology, 98,* 193–194.

Meehl, P. E. (1978). Theoretical risks and tabular asterisks: Sir Karl, Sir Ronald, and the slow progress of soft psychology. *Journal of Consulting and Clinical Psychology, 46,* 806–834.

Orsillo, S. M., Lilienfeld, S. O., & Heimberg, R. G. (1994). Social phobia and response to challenge procedures: Examining the interaction between anxiety sensitivity and trait anxiety. *Journal of Anxiety Disorders, 8,* 247–258.

Reiss, S. (1991). Expectancy model of fear, anxiety, and panic. *Clinical Psychology Review, 11,* 141–153.

Taylor, S., Koch, W. J., McNally, R. J., & Crockett, D. J. (1992). Conceptualizations of anxiety sensitivity. *Psychological Assessment, 4,* 245–250.

Tellegen, A. (1992). Personality traits: Issues of definition, evidence, and assessment. In D. Cicchetti & W. Grove (Eds.), *Thinking clearly about psychology: Essays in honor of Paul Everett Meehl* (Vol. 2, pp. 10–35). Minneapolis: University of Minnesota Press.

10

Preferential Preattentive Processing of Threat in Anxiety: Preparedness and Attentional Biases

ARNE ÖHMAN

CONSCIOUS MEDIATION IN THE CONTROL OF BEHAVIOR

Intuitive psychology gives conscious awareness a key role as a mediator between environment and action. Environmental information is held to result in perceptual experience, which is elaborated in conscious awareness before decisions about actions are taken. This view of the sequence of events between stimulus and response permeates common-sense psychology to the extent that any alternative view is met with incredulity. Freud complicated the sequence by embedding the conscious ego inside an unconscious envelope filtering both input and output in distorting ways. Yet he basically maintained a central role for conscious awareness by postulating insight as the primary vehicle for therapeutic change.

Some of the widely expressed opposition against behavior therapy can no doubt be traced to the premise of the primacy of consciousness. For intellectuals of widely different persuasions, conscious experience and insights provide not only the core of psychology, but also the raw material for their own endeavors. From this perspective, to claim that behavior can be changed most effectively by techniques focused on contingencies between actions and environmental events, rather than on cognitive change, must appear simplistic if not absurd. In this respect, cognitive therapy is closer to the psychological common sense. Here, the focus of therapeutic intervention is on maladaptive thoughts, interpretations, and expectancies, which may fail to be consciously accessed but which are at least potentially available to conscious awareness.

There is no doubt that biased expectancies (e.g., Davey, 1992; Rapee, Mattick, & Murrell, 1986; Tomarken, Mineka, & Cook, 1989), illusory beliefs about control (Sanderson, Rapee, & Barlow, 1989), and catastrophic interpretations (Clark, 1986) play important roles in anxiety and panic attacks. Thus, there is good sense in focusing therapeutic efforts on such processes in anxiety patients. Yet the central tenet of this chapter is that such efforts remain insufficient, because they miss determinants of anxiety that remain genuinely inaccessible to conscious awareness. Some of the most important psychological processes with regard to fear and anxiety remain unconscious, in the sense that they operate outside the focus of consciously controlled attention. For instance, a phobic response appears to be organized at the unconscious, preattentive level, so that components of the response are initiated before the eliciting stimulus even becomes represented in consciousness.

The theme of this chapter is related to a pervasive re-evaluation of the role of unconscious mechanisms in a range of areas of psychology (see, e.g., Bornstein & Pitman, 1992). This perspective provides a powerful challenge of the psychological common sense alluded to above. Thus, it dethrones consciousness from its central role as the main mediator where all causal links converge. Furthermore, the fact that reactions are set in motion even before the eliciting event is consciously represented, challenges the linear nature of the presumed sequence of events from a stimulus to a response. It is assumed that response processes are evoked at several stages of the processing of incoming information, including quite immediate and superficial stages of perceptual analysis. These early elicited responses, furthermore, may provide information affecting later stages of processing in an interactive fashion. For example, initially elicited physiological responses may provide perceptual cues that shape subsequent cognitive analysis of the situation's meaning (see, e.g., Mandler, 1975). Thus, the experience of autonomic arousal may intensify the fear experience evoked by perceiving a phobic stimulus.

The view of the role of unconscious processes presented in this chapter provides part of an evolutionary perspective on psychological phenomena. Thus, fear and anxiety are postulated to be part of evolved defense mechanisms that keep organisms away from life-threatening situations. This postulate entails that defenses are particularly likely to be elicited in situations related to recurrent survival threats in evolutionary history. As defense is metabolically taxing, evoking a defense response is associated with recruitment of the sympathetic branch of the autonomic nervous system to provide energy and prepare the body for vigorous and potentially hazardous action. Of course, it is of central interest that the metabolic support is immediately available, so that defensive action is not unnecessarily restrained by lack of physiological resources to act. As a consequence, it is important that the autonomic component of defense is rapidly activated, particularly as the autonomic nervous system in itself is quite sluggish. Therefore, it is assumed that perceptual systems have been evolutionarily shaped to identify potential threats easily and rapidly, in order to activate the autonomic nervous system as part of defense recruitment. However, before these postulated evolutionary mechanisms are discussed in more detail, it is necessary to consider the definition of fear and its relation to anxiety.

FEAR, ANXIETY, AND PANIC

In an evolutionary perspective, we could use a simplistic formula and argue that emotions are means devised by evolution to make organisms *want to do* what their ancestors *had to do* to survive and breed. From this point of departure, emotions may be understood as related to action sets (Lang, 1984). Some situations or stimuli are experienced as attractive, prompting approach, whereas others are aversive and thus escaped or avoided. This emotional dimension of approach and avoidance is held to define one cardinal strategic deposition of behavior, whereas the psychophysio logical arousal occasioned by autonomic recruitment provides another one (Lang, Bradley, & Cuthbert, 1990). To better allow for the complexities of our ecological niches, these simple emotional facts become, during ontogeny, embedded in complex associative networks serving the various cognitive systems. As we shall see shortly, however, such networks are not formed by arbitrary environmental coincidence, but are assumed to be channeled into some directions rather than others by evolutionary constraints.

From this perspective on emotion, "fear" is defined as an aroused, aversive state, prompting escape from and avoidance of particular situations that threaten the survival or well-being of the organism. Fear is thus postulated to result from the operation of defense systems of ancient evolutionary origin. These defense systems evolved because they helped to keep organisms away from potentially deadly contexts, such as hunting predators, dominant conspecifics, or natural threats such as fires or thunderstorms.

Fear is closely related to another emotional phenomenon, that of "anxiety." Most often, anxiety is said to differ from fear in its lack of a clear situational antecedent. Although similar to fear in experiential quality and physiological correlates, anxiety typically cannot be straightforwardly attributed to an external threat. However, Epstein (1972) provided a persuasive argument that external stimuli are insufficient to distinguish fear and anxiety. He proposed that fear is related to action, and particularly to escape and avoidance. But when the action is blocked or thwarted, so that the situation in fact becomes uncontrollable, fear is turned into anxiety. In Epstein's view, then, "fear is an avoidance motive. If there were no restraints, internal or external, fear would support the action of flight. Anxiety can be defined as unresolved fear, or, alternatively, as a state of undirected arousal following the perception of threat" (Epstein, 1972, p. 311). Hence, fear and anxiety have many similarities, so that what we learn about fear may generalize to anxiety. Most importantly, both fear and anxiety are held to originate in the same evolutionarily originated defense systems (Öhman, 1993a). In this chapter, therefore, "fear" and "anxiety" are used as equivalent terms if nothing else is said. Nevertheless, generalizing from one to the other of these two emotional phenomena is sometimes risky and must be made with caution.

Panic attacks constitute an additional emotional phenomenon that is related to both fear and anxiety. A "panic attack" is defined as a "discrete period in which there is the sudden onset of intense apprehension, fearfulness, or terror, often associated with feelings of impending doom" (American Psychiatric Association, 1994, p. 393). Physiological symptoms (e.g., dyspnea, sweating, palpitations, tachycardia, and chest pain or discomfort) figure conspicuously in the attacks, often to the extent that victims believe that they are actually suffering bodily ailments such as a heart attack. Panic is similar to fear in that it represents a sudden surge of emotional activation, and it is similar to anxiety in that it often lacks clear precipitants and escape alternatives.

AN EVOLUTIONARY ANALYSIS
OF FEAR AND ANXIETY

Evolutionary Constraints on Fear

The fear response as described here may be understood as centered on physiological mobilization for metabolically taxing flight and defense responses. In genuine fear, this mobilization is channeled into escape and avoidance behavior, whereas in panic and anxiety it is left in the system because appropriate action is ruled out for some reason (Epstein, 1972). However, as an adaptive device, the fear response must be served by perceptual and associative systems that can effectively locate threatening stimuli and use environmental contingencies to promote rapid escape. Several authors have raised the possibility that these systems have been shaped by evolution particularly to respond to threat, and that they easily associate fear with recurrent life threats in the ecology of mammalian evolution (e.g., Bolles, 1970; Marks, 1987; Mineka, 1992; Öhman, Dimberg, & Öst, 1985; Seligman, 1970, 1971). It is important to realize that the evolutionary constraints can operate at several levels of the mechanisms mediating between a fear stimulus and a fear response. In this chapter I specifically deal with constraints on associations between situations and fear, and with constraints on the perceptual processes identifying fear stimuli.

The Preparedness Theory: Constraints on Associations

Seligman (1970) developed an argument specifically claiming that the associative apparatuses of animals are constrained by evolutionary history. He argued that some types of events are more easily associated than others, because such associations were functional in an evolutionary perspective. Events that belong together because of selection pressures in the distant past are assumed to be more easily associated than arbitrarily related events. For example, Garcia and Koellig (1966) showed that rats were much quicker to associate tastes with malaise than to associate tastes with footshocks or audiovisual stimuli with malaise. In a functional perspective, it is essential to be able to relate a taste to stomach upset, if potential poisoning is to be avoided in the future. With taste aversion as the paradigmatic example, Seligman (1970) hypothesized that evolutionarily prepared learning occurs easily, is persistent, and is independent of advanced cognitive mediation.

Seligman (1971) followed up this analysis by applying it to the acquisition of fears and phobias. The nature of the distribution of human phobias with regard to the feared objects provided an important point of departure for this applied analysis. The nonrandomness of this distribution, Seligman (1971) argued, is easier to understand from a phylogenetic than from an ontogenetic perspective. Commonly feared creatures or situations, such as snakes, heights, or closed spaces, are more easily related to threats in the ecology of our ancestors than to the dangers of modern life. Conversely, common modern survival threats (e.g., cars and traffic) are seldom the sources of phobic fear. From this premise, Seligman (1971) concluded that humans have an evolutionarily originated genetic endowment to associate fear and avoidance readily with situations that have provided recurrent threats to the survival of their ancestors. In other words, humans are prepared to associate fear readily with common phobic situations, because these situations typically can be related to past selection pressures. In the evocative phrase suggested by Mineka (1992), humans may have "evolutionary memories" linking fear to particular situations.

By this analysis, Seligman (1971) was able to account for the apparently rapid learning of phobias. Furthermore, phobias, like other responses acquired through prepared learning, should be persistent and resistant to extinction. Finally, if prepared responses are not mediated by advanced cognitive mechanisms, this may promote an understanding of the "irrationality" of phobias. Typically, in phobias the fear is dissociated from the person's conscious intentions and understanding, in the sense that it is immune to rational arguments about the lack of actual danger in the situation. Even though phobics may be well aware that their fear is objectively unfounded, they may be unable to let this insight have any bearing on their avoidance behavior. My colleagues and I (Öhman et al., 1985) have developed this general perspective further by attempting to link animal phobias and social phobia to evolutionarily determined behavioral systems for predatory defense and social submissiveness, respectively.

Elsewhere (Öhman, 1993b), I have reviewed my own data as well as data from several laboratories testing various aspects of the preparedness theory. I have concluded that in general, the empirical literature supports some of the central claims of the theory. In particular, human electrodermal conditioning studies have quite consistently demonstrated enhanced resistance to extinction of responses conditioned to potentially phobic stimuli, such as pictures of snakes, spiders, and angry human faces (see McNally, 1987, for a similar conclusion).

However, there have also been a number of failures to replicate this basic effect. I have also (Öhman, 1993b) reviewed this literature and concluded that many of the alleged "failures to replicate" do not stand up to critical scrutiny. For example, claims of failed replications of the resistance-to-extinction effect have been based on data where the more important failure concerns the lack of evidence of conditioning (Merckelbach, van der Molen, & van den Hout, 1987). Without solid evidence of conditioning, there is, of course, no basis for expecting any differential effects on extinction.

However, the general supportiveness of the data notwithstanding, the mechanisms involved are still open to discussion. The basic claim of the theory—that there is a *genetically determined* preparedness to associate aversive outcomes with evolutionarily relevant threats—is inaccessible to empirical test by the type of conditioning studies reviewed earlier (Öhman, 1993b). However, examining interview-based DSM-III-R (American Psychiatric Association, 1987) diagnoses of phobias in a large sample of female twins, Kendler, Neale, Kessler, Heath, and Eaves (1992) supported this part of the hypothesis by demonstrating that genes were important but clearly insufficient to explain the etiology of phobias. In further support of evolutionary theory, model fitting showed that this genetic factor reflected additive genetic variance. Of particular significance for the present context, Kendler et al.'s data showed that specific phobias (particularly animal phobias) reflected the interaction between a genetic component common to all phobias and specific environmental influences.

Nevertheless, genetic data do not provide unique support for the preparedness hypothesis, because the mechanism mediating the environmental effect need not necessarily be Pavlovian conditioning. Lovibond, Siddle, and Bond (1993) provided ingenious experimental data to back up the assertion that the preparedness effect observed in human electrodermal conditioning studies is better understood in terms of a nonassociative, selective sensitization process than in terms of Pavlovian conditioning. Similarly, Davey (1992) presented data to support the contention that the mechanism of the human preparedness effect rests with biased expectancies to connect aversiveness with fear-relevant stimuli.

However, available nonhuman data provide more convincing demonstrations that learning to fear snake and snake-like stimuli reflects associative processes. These data concern not specifically the formation of conventional Pavlovian association, but social learning from a fearful model in rhesus monkeys. Mineka and coworkers (see, e.g., Mineka, 1992, and Mineka & Tomarken, 1989, for reviews) have demonstrated that laboratory-reared, originally nonfearful rhesus monkeys rapidly acquire fear of snakes by observing a conspecific behave fearfully in the presence of live or toy snakes. By use of videotape techniques, Mineka and coworkers could demonstrate that the same fear display in the model did not result in a learned fear response to fear-irrelevant stimuli, such as flowers (Cook & Mineka, 1989). Furthermore, snake stimuli were not more effective than other stimuli as discriminative cues for positively reinforced behavior (Cook & Mineka, 1990). From these data, Cook and Mineka (1990) concluded that learning from a fearful model reflects selective associations between snake stimuli and fear. Finally, Mineka and Cook (1993) reported data suggesting that observational learning of snake fear from a fearful model is similar to direct Pavlovian conditioning. Thus, the model's fear display appears to function as an unconditioned stimulus (US) eliciting an unconditioned fear response in the observer. This fear response is then conditioned to the snake conditioned stimulus (CS). Because the prior experiences of snakes were controlled in these studies, they provide the strongest data available suggesting a phylogenetic rather than an ontogenetic origin of the effect. Similarly, these data support the preparedness hypothesis by suggesting that the target mechanism for the evolutionary constraints is the formation of Pavlovian associations between some stimuli and fear.

EVOLUTIONARY CONSTRAINTS
ON THE PERCEPTION OF THREAT: A MODEL

Functional Considerations

Evolutionary constraints can operate at any level from the perception of a fear stimulus to the learned elicitation of a fear response. In the evolutionary perspective, the perceptual apparatus is likely to have been shaped by evolution to respond easily to potential threat. This is where the evolutionary analysis joins with the analysis focused on unconscious psychological mechanisms: It is assumed that stimuli prepared by evolution to be readily associated with fear are particularly effective in engaging unconscious perceptual mechanisms to elicit responses.

To function adequately, evolved defense responses require a perceptual system that can effectively locate threats in the surrounding world. "False negatives" (i.e., failing to elicit a defense against deadly stimuli) are more evolutionarily costly than "false positives" (i.e., eliciting a defense against a stimulus that is in effect harmless). Whereas the former failure is lethal, a false-positive response, even though distressing to the individual, merely represents wasted energy. This analysis suggests that the perceptual system is biased in the direction of a low threshold for discovering threat. This is the evolutionarily derived answer to the question of why there are anxiety disorders. To be sure that a defense is elicited when life is at stake, the system is biased to risk evoking a defense in contexts that in a further analysis turn out to be safe. When this happens, the resulting fear response looks inappropriate, unnecessary and unreasonable, and may be experienced as "irrational anxiety" by both observers and the person.

An effective defense must be quick, which puts a premium on early detection of threat. Furthermore, detection of threat stimuli must be independent of the momentary direction of selective attention. Coupled with the bias toward false-positive responses, these factors mean that the discovery of threat is better based on a quick, superficial analysis of stimuli anywhere in the perceptual field than on an effortful, detailed, and complete extraction of the meaning of one particular stimulus. Thus, from the functional evolutionary perspective, it follows that the burden for the discovery of threat should be placed on early, rapid, parallel-processing perceptual mechanisms, which define threat on the basis of relatively simple stimulus attributes.

The neural mechanisms of such a system were described by LeDoux (1990). He and his coworkers studied the neural control of auditorily elicited conditioned emotional responses in the rat. This work demonstrated a direct neural link from auditory pathway nuclei in the thalamus (the medial geniculate body) to the fear effector systems in the amygdala. This monosynaptic link was postulated to provide immediate information to the amygdala of gross features of emotionally relevant auditory stimuli. This information bypasses the traditionally emphasized thalamic–cortical pathway, giving full meaning to the stimulus, and the cortical–amygdala link, presumed to activate emotion. The thalamic–amygdaloid pathway was described as a "quick and dirty" transmission route. That is, it does not provide much information about stimulus details, but conveys information to the amygdala that the sensory receptors of a given modality have encountered a potentially significant stimulus. This information then is sufficient to start recruiting a defense response. It is explicitly stated that this system is adaptively biased toward false positives rather than false negatives, because it is less costly to abort falsely initialized defense responses than to fail to elicit a defense when life is at stake.

Automatic Information-Processing Routines to Discover Threat

My colleagues and I (Öhman, 1986, 1987, 1992, 1993a, Öhman, Dimberg, & Esteves, 1989) have developed a theoretical perspective on the generation of emotion that is consistent with this functional analysis. Originating in a model of the activation of orienting responses (Öhman, 1979), this perspective emphasizes the conventional distinction between automatic and controlled, or strategic, information processing (e.g., Posner, 1978; Schneider, Dumais, & Shiffrin, 1984; Shiffrin & Schneider, 1977) in the activation of emotion. It argues that many perceptual channels can be automatically and simultaneously monitored for emotionally relevant events. For example, when stimulus events implying threat are located by the automatic system, attention is drawn to the stimulus as the control for its further analysis is transferred to the strategic level of information processing. The switch of control from automatic to strategic information processing is associated with the activation of physiological responses, particularly the orienting response (Öhman, 1979).

Automatic processing can occur in parallel across many different sensory channels without loss in efficiency; it is involuntary, in the sense that it is hard to suppress consciously once it is activated; it is independent of focal attention; and it is typically not available for conscious introspection (Schneider et al., 1984). Controlled or strategic information processing, on the other hand, is governed by intentions; it is resource- or capacity-limited, in the sense that interference is marked between strategically controlled tasks; it works sequentially rather than in parallel; it requires effort; and it is more available to conscious awareness (Schneider et al., 1984).

This conceptualization implies that the automatic sensory monitoring processes have a capacity for sensory events exceeding that of the controlled or strategic processes. Thus, automatic perceptual processes can monitor a large number of channels, only one of which can be selected for strategic processing. In other words, sensory messages have to compete for access to the strategic processing channel for their complete analysis. Given the survival contingencies implied by potential threats in the external and internal environment, it is a natural assumption that threatening stimuli have priority to be selected for strategic processing. Thus, anxiety and fear may be activated from unconscious stimulus analysis mechanisms, as a correlate to the selection of the threatening stimulus for further conscious, controlled processing. Because threatening stimuli are located by automatic perceptual mechanisms, the person is not necessarily aware of the anxiety-eliciting stimulus. Thus, what from the inside look like "spontaneous" episodes of anxiety may in fact be the results of unconscious stimulation.

TESTS OF THE MODEL:
THE NONCONSCIOUS ORIGIN OF PHOBIAS

Responses to Masked Phobic Stimuli

The most basic assertion of the present theoretical framework is that emotional responses may be activated by preattentive processing mechanisms of which the subjects remain unaware. Empirical examination of this hypothesis requires that physiological responses can be dissociated from conscious perception of the stimulus. "Backward masking" (i.e., preventing recognition of a target stimulus by an immediately following masking stimulus) provides one method of achieving this purpose. It appears to allow quite complete analysis of the target stimulus, but prevents its conscious representation (Marcel, 1983; see also the critical discussions by Holender, 1986, and by Merikle & Reingold, 1992).

Previous work from our laboratory has explored the effect of backward masking on emotionally relevant visual stimuli. We (Esteves & Öhman, 1993) examined masking of emotional expressions in facial stimuli by an immediately following mask portraying a neutral face. We reported that a 30-millisecond (30-ms) stimulus-onset asynchrony (SOA) between the target and the mask resulted in complete masking. That is to say, the subjects both performed and felt that they performed randomly in a forced-choice recognition task, and they were only able to see one (rather than two) stimuli. Arousing the subjects by intermixing electric shocks with the masking trials did not affect these results (Esteves, Dimberg, Parra, & Öhman, 1994; Öhman & Soares, 1993). Similarly, we (Öhman & Soares, 1993) reported that a 30-ms interval between target pictures showing snakes or spiders and masks, consisting of similar pictures lacking any central object, did not result in recognition performance above chance levels. Thus, use of these temporal parameters in a backward-masking design should make it possible to evoke emotional responses without the subjects' being aware of the stimulus to which they are responding.

It is well documented that presenting pictures of phobic objects to phobics results in strong autonomic responses (e.g., Fredrikson, 1981; see Sartory, 1983, for a review). The specific question posed in a further experiment (Öhman & Soares, 1994) was whether such responses could be elicited from masked phobic stimuli. Questionnaires measuring snake and spider fears were distributed to a large pool of university students. From 800 answered questionnaires, subjects were selected so that they were either highly snake-fearful or highly spider-fearful. They had to score above the 95th percentile in one of the distributions (e.g., snake fear) and below the 50th percentile in the other (e.g., spider fear). Nonfearful control subjects, on the other hand, had to score below the 50th percentile on both questionnaires. Thus, we ended up with three groups of 16 subjects each: snake-fearful, spider-fearful, and nonfearful controls.

A pilot experiment determined that fearful and nonfearful subjects did not differ in their threshold to recognize the stimuli used (Öhman & Soares, 1994). In the subsequent main experiment, all subjects were exposed to the same stimulus sequence. It consisted of pictures of snakes, spiders, flowers, and mushrooms, with eight exemplars in each of the categories presented in random order. This series of pictures was presented twice. In the first presentations, the pictures were masked with a 30-ms SOA, which effectively prevented their conscious recognition. The procedure entailed 30-ms exposure of the target stimulus, which was immediately followed by a 100-ms mask (randomly cut and reassembled pictures of snakes, flowers, etc.). The second series consisted of unmasked stimulus presentations with 130-ms exposure time. After each of the stimulus series, examples of each stimulus type, as well as new stimuli of the same type, were rated in terms of valence, arousal, and dominance, and each subject was asked to identify the masked or nonmasked pictures and whether each had been part of the original set. The psychophysiological dependent variables were skin conductance responses to the pictures.

The results were quite dramatic and are presented in Figure 10.1. Regardless of masking conditions, the snake-fearful subjects showed elevated skin conductance responding to snake stimuli, and the spider-fearful subjects showed elevated responding to spider pictures, whereas the control subjects did not respond differentially to the four stimulus types. These results were confirmed by a highly significant interaction between groups and stimuli, with associated Tukey follow-up tests to support the elevated responding to fear stimuli in fearful subjects (see Öhman & Soares,

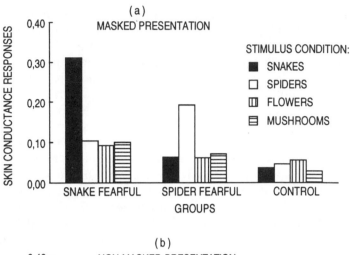

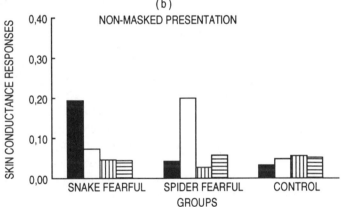

FIGURE 10.1. Skin conductance responses to backwardly masked (a) and non-masked (b) presentations of pictures of snakes, spiders, flowers, and mushrooms in snake-fearful, spider-fearful, and control subjects. From Öhman and Soares (1994, p. 236). Copyright 1994 by the American Psychological Association. Reprinted by permission.

1994, for details). The only difference between the masked and nonmasked stimulus series pertained to overall larger responses in the former series. Because of the fixed order of presentation of the series, this effect most probably reflected overall habituation from the first to the second series. Thus it was clear that the subjects differentiated as well between the feared and nonfeared stimuli when they were not able to recognize them (i.e., the masked series) as when they were clearly recognizable (i.e., the non-masked series).

The skin conductance data were exactly paralleled in the emotional ratings. Thus, snake- and spider-fearful subjects rated themselves as more disliking, more aroused, and less in control when they were exposed to their feared stimulus, even if the presentation was masked. However, the overall emotional intensity was rated as higher during nonmasked stimulus presentation.

These results give full support to the contention that phobic responses can be activated at a preattentive level of information processing. From the lack of difference between the two masking conditions, it appears that most of the emotional effect of the phobic stimulus has its basis at the preattentive level. Phobic responses therefore appear to originate at unconscious levels of information processing that are not susceptible to voluntary, intentional control. This provides an explanation for the "irrationality" of phobias (i.e., the refractoriness of the fear response to rational arguments stressing the actual inocuousness of the phobic situation).

Masked Elicitation of Conditioned Responses

If phobias are acquired through biologically prepared Pavlovian conditioning, as posited by preparedness theory, it should be possible to produce effects similar to those observed in fearful subjects in normal subjects conditioned to potentially phobic stimuli. Thus, one would expect that skin conductance responses conditioned to pictures of snakes or spiders should be elicited even when the CSs are presented during masking conditions preventing their conscious recognition. This hypothesis was tested in a series of studies (Öhman & Soares, 1993; Soares & Öhman, 1993a, 1993b; Esteves, Dimberg, & Öhman, 1994a).

We (Öhman & Soares, 1993) used a differential conditioning paradigm to condition different groups of subjects to either fear-relevant (snakes or spiders) or fear-irrelevant (flowers or mushrooms) stimuli. Subjects in the fear-relevant groups were shown two pictures portraying snakes and spiders, respectively. Subjects in the fear-irrelevant groups were shown pictures of flowers and mushrooms. After a few habituation trials, there was an acquisition phase where one of the stimuli was followed by an electric shock US, with a 500-ms interstimulus interval. This picture was designated the CS +. The other picture (e.g., a spider if the CS + was a snake) was designated the CS –. With this paradigm, the difference in skin conductance response to the CS + and the CS – reflects pure conditioning effects uncontaminated by sensitization, initial responding, or the like (see Öhman, 1983). In the extinction phase that terminated the experiment, the CS + and the CS – were presented without any USs. Half of the subjects conditioned to fear-relevant and fear-irrelevant stimuli, respectively, were extinguished with masked stimuli, and the other half

without any masks. Thus, subjects in the masked groups had both the
CS + and the CS − masked by a randomly cut and reassembled picture
with a 30-ms SOA, exactly as in the experiment on fearful subjects
described earlier Öhman & Soares, 1994).

The results were clear-cut (see Figure 10.2). Both the groups extinguished without masks showed reliable differential skin conductance
responding to the CS + and the CS − , suggesting continuing conditioning effects in both groups. In fact, these groups did not differ from each
other. This failure to obtain the standard preparedness effect may perhaps

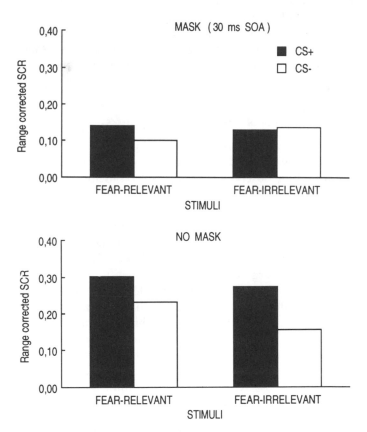

FIGURE 10.2. Mean skin conductane response (SCR) (range-corrected), square-
root-transformed) to fear-relevant (snakes and spiders) or fear-irrelevant (flowers
and mushrooms) stimuli, previously followed (CS +) or not followed (CS −) by an
electric shock US. One group of subject (left panel) had their stimuli masked by
another visual stimulus with 30-ms stimulus-onset asynchrony (SOA), which effectively precluded consiouse recognition, whereas another group (right panel) was
exposed to nonmasked stimuli. From Öhman and Soares (1993, p. 127). Copyright
1993 by the American Psychological Association. Reprinted by permission.

be attributed to the short interstimulus interval used during training (see Schell, Dawson, & Marinkovic, 1991). For the groups extinguished with masked CSs, however, fear relevance made a dramatic difference. Whereas masking completely abolished differential responding in the group conditioned to fear-irrelevant stimuli, differential responding to the CS + and the CS + remained in the group conditioned to snakes or spiders. The results for this group therefore paralleled those obtained with fearful subjects in the preceding experiment (see Figure 10.1).

This basic effect was closely replicated in two studies (Soares & Öhman, 1993a, 1993b). In both these studies, responses conditioned to fear-relevant stimuli (snakes or spiders) persisted to prompt differential skin conductance responding in spite of backward masking, whereas masking abolished differential responding to fear-irrelevant stimuli (flowers and mushrooms). Exactly parallel conditioning and extinction data were reported in experiments (Esteves et al., 1994a) using angry and happy faces as CSs + and CSs − , respectively.

This series of studies shows quite convincingly that skin conductance responses conditioned to fear-relevant stimuli (snakes, spiders, or angry faces) reliably survive backward masking, whereas differential responses to fear-irrelevant stimuli are abolished by this procedure. Most importantly from the perspective of preparedness theory, the effect appears specific to particular stimulus categories, such as snakes, spiders, or angry faces. These data strongly suggest that a perceptual mechanism of a preattentive origin contributes to the preparedness effect seen in human conditioning. It appears as if the control of responses conditioned to evolutionarily fear-relevant stimuli is easily transferred to preattentive mechanisms of response elicitation. Such a transfer of control is not seen for responses conditioned to neutral stimuli, and this difference is helpful in accounting for the differences in conditioning seen between these two stimulus classes. It is as if different types of responses were conditioned to the two types of stimuli: One, more primitive and immune to cognition, is conditioned to phobic stimuli, and the other, more advanced and cognitively governed, is conditioned to neutral stimuli (see Öhman, 1993b; Öhman, Fredrikson, & Hugdahl, 1978).

Conditioning to Masked Stimuli:
Forming Associations to Degraded Input

In the previously reported conditioning studies, subjects were conditioned to nonmasked presentations of fear-relevant or fear-irrelevant stimuli before they were tested in extinction with masked stimuli. Thus, the results demonstrate that previously conditioned responses can be *performed* without conscious awareness of the eliciting stimulus. But what about learning of new responses? Can autonomic responses be conditioned to stimuli that are prevented from reaching awareness by means of backward masking? This appears to be a possibility that is denied by contemporary learning theory. Among learning theorists dealing with both human (Dawson & Schell, 1985; Öhman, 1979, 1983) and animal (e.g., Wagner, 1976) learning, there appears to be a consensus that the forming of associations between experimental events requires the type of limited-capacity processing that is typically associated with consciousness (e.g., Posner & Boies, 1971).

However, because the preparedness theory is directed toward the ease of forming associations between specific types of events, it is consistent with this theory to expect some conditioning to masked stimuli. Seligman and Hager (1972) operationalized preparedness inversely in terms of input degradation: The more degraded the input about a contingency tolerated in the forming of associations between its elements, the more prepared the association. Masking the CS, of course, can be viewed as one method to degrade input about a contingency. Hence, if any stimulus should allow fear learning in spite of masking, it should be a prepared stimulus.

The formation of associations between anxiety responses and non-consciously perceived cues may be important for the understanding of anxiety disorder. For example, panic patients appear to be interoceptively highly sensitive, so that bodily sensations may trigger panic (e.g., Ehlers, 1993). Such triggering could be the result of Pavlovian conditioning in which an initial panic attack became associated with some bodily changes (e.g., heart rate increase, sweating) that were not within the attentional focus at the time (i.e., they were outside of the person's awareness). Such unobtrusive conditioning experiences may also prove helpful in explaining why many patients with anxiety symptoms are unable to connect their symptoms to potential traumatic conditioning experiences. Given a preattentive bias to pick out potentially threatening stimuli at an unconscious level, such unconsciously identified cues could be associated with a traumatic event or an anxiety response, even though the person remained completely unaware of the temporal juxtaposition of the cue and the trauma.

To examine these possibilities, we (Esteves, Dimberg, Parra, & Öhman, 1994b) exposed normal subjects to pictures of angry and happy faces that were effectively masked by a neutral face after a 30-ms interval. Some of the subjects had an electric shock US following the masked angry face; other subjects had the shock following the masked happy face. Different types of control subjects were either conditioned to pairs of angry and neutral or happy and neutral faces at ineffective masking intervals (> 300 ms; i.e., allowing conscious recognition) or had random presentations of shocks and masked faces. In a subsequent extinction session, the masks were removed. Across two independent experiments, the results showed evidence of conditioning to effectively masked angry faces; that is, skin conductance responses to angry faces were reliably larger to previously masked angry CSs + than to previously masked happy CSs – when they were presented without masks during extinction. This effect, in fact, was as large in groups exposed to an effective target–mask interval as in groups exposed to a long, ineffective target–mask interval. Furthermore, the effect was observed with an angry but not with a happy CS +, and no differences between angry and happy faces were observed in groups exposed to shocks and masked pictures in random order. Thus, these data clearly suggest that skin conductance responses can be conditioned to nonconsciously presented CSs, provided that they are fear-relevant (i.e., evolutionarily prepared to become associated with aversiveness and fear).

These results were replicated in an experiment (Öhman & Soares, 1995) using snakes and spiders as fear-relevant stimuli, and flowers and mushrooms as fear-irrelevant stimuli. One group of subjects was conditioned to masked snakes or spiders as CSs +, with masked spiders and snakes, respectively, serving as CSs –. Another group of subjects was conditioned to masked flowers or mushrooms in a similar differential conditioning paradigm. In this experiment, the effect of the conditioning contingency was assessed not only during nonmasked extinction, but also in a series of acquisition test trials where the masked CS + was presented without the shock US. Such test trials are necessary to assess conditioning when the CS-US interval (500 ms, in this case) is shorter than the latency of the response (approximately 1–2 seconds in the in case of skin conductance responses) (see Öhman, 1983, for a discussion of interpretational problems raised by this procedure). The results (see Figure 10.3) showed clearly larger responses to the masked CS + than to adjacent masked CSs – during the test trials provided that the stimuli were fear-relevant. Furthermore, as in the preceding study (Esteves et al, 1994), subjects conditioned to masked fear-relevant stimuli showed reliable differential response to the CS + and the CS – when they were presented nonmasked during extinction. Such differential responding was not observed in subjects conditioned to fear-irrelevant stimuli.

The results described above (Esteves et al, 1994b; Öhman & Soares, 1995) could be attributable to lowered perceptual threshold as a result of conditioning training. Thus, with repeated exposures, the subjects conceivably could have improved their recognition of the masked stimuli, and for some reason this process could have been restricted to fear-relevant stimuli. As a consequence, they may also have started to show differential skin conductance responses to shock-associated and non-shock-associated fear-relevant pictures. Another possibility is that they were able to discriminate but not necessarily recognize the CS + and the CS – when these were fear-relevant. In this case, they would be able to predict and

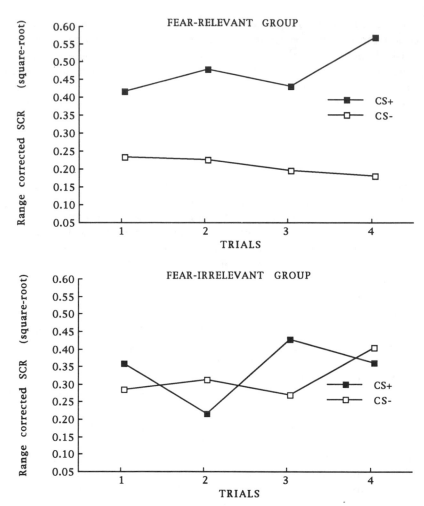

FIGURE 10.3. Mean SCR to masked fear-relevant (snakes and spiders; upper panel) or masked fear-irrelevant (flowers and mushrooms; lower panel) stimuli, followed (SC +) or not followed (CS –) by an electric shock US. The data are taken from four nonreinforced test trials interspersed among reinforced trials during an acquisition series comprising a total of 24 presentations of each of the CS + and the CS –. The CS-US interval on reinforced trials was 500 ms. From Öhman and Soares (1995). Reprinted by permission of the authors.

thus expect the shock, even though they would not be able to specify which masked CS presentation involved the snake and which the spider. Rather, they could base their expectancies on vague hunches either from some information "leaking through" the mask or, perhaps more interestingly, from bodily feedback originated in the conditioned response.

To examine these possibilities, we (Öhman & Soares, 1995) ran three groups of subjects through an identical differential conditioning paradigm. The CS + was either a masked snake or a masked spider, with a masked spider or snake, respectively, serving as the CS –. Rather than the short interstimulus interval (500 ms) used in previous studies, the interval between the CS and the shock was extended to 3.5 seconds in order to allow one of the three groups to express shock expectancy by rotating a knob from – 100 ("sure of no shock") to 0 ("shock as likely as no shock") to + 100 ("sure of shock") in the CS-US interval. A second group was simply required to guess after each trial whether the masked stimulus was a snake or a spider. The third group had no additional task, but was only exposed to the conditioning procedure.

All groups showed reliable differential responding during both the masked acquisition and the nonmasked extinction series. The groups required to guess whether a snake or a spider was presented performed randomly (50.5% correct) during the masked acquisition, but performed well (approximately 90% correct) during the nonmasked extinction. Thus, the subjects were not able to recognize the masked stimuli. The results for the expectancy rating group, finally, are presented in Figure 10.4. As shown in the figure, the subjects rated shock as equally unlikely after the masked CS + and the masked CS – during the first few habituation trials where no shocks were given. During acquisition, however, they gradually rated shock as somewhat likely after the CS + and as somewhat unlikely after the CS –, and then they rated shock as more unlikely after the CS – then after the CS + during extinction when the shock and the mask were omitted. Thus, these result do indeed show that subjects had differential expectancies during the CS + and the CS –, which may account for their differential skin conductance responses. However, the level of expectancy differentiation is quite small compared to that found in studies allowing clear perception of the CS, which typically report asymptotic performance at about + 90% and – 80% for the CS + and the CS –, respectively (e.g., Siddle, Power, Bond, & Lovibond, 1988). Nevertheless, even though the effects are comparatively small, they do indicate that negative ("catastrophic"?) expectancies can be based on vaguely perceived cues and support autonomic responses, much as appears to be the case, for example, among panic patients (e.g., Ehlers, 1993).

The results from these studies are important. They show that responses can be conditioned to masked stimuli, but only when their content is fear-relevant. Even though the subjects remain unaware of which stimulus is associated with shock, some information appears to become available to the cognitive system to support expectancies of aversive outcomes to follow masked fear-relevant stimuli. Because only stimuli that may have an evolutionary basis for becoming easily associated with fear

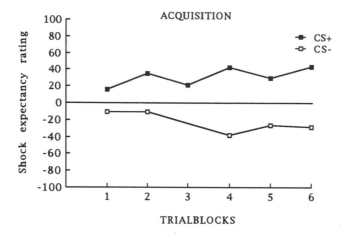

FIGURE 10.4. Mean shock expectancy ratings (– 100 = "sure of no shock"; 0 = "shock and no shock equally likely"; 100 = "sure of shock") to masked fear-relevant (snakes and spiders) stimuli followed (CD +) or not followed (CS –) or not followed (CS –) by an electric shock US. Data from 24 reinforced trials (CS-US interval, 3.5 seconds) have been averaged with four trials/blocks. From Öhman, Flykt, and Esteves (1994). Reprinted by permission of the authors.

(snakes, spiders, angry faces) appear to be able to overcome the degradation of input provided by backward masking, the data give good support for the preparedness theory.

"Beware, There Are Snakes in the Grass and Angry People in the Crowd"

Taken together, the results reviewed in this section demonstrate an important role for unconscious, preattentive mechanisms in the generation of fear and anxiety. It appears that there are perceptual systems geared to pick up potential threat from the environment at a very early stage of information processing. These data, however, have relied entirely on experimental paradigms in which there is only one stimulus input. Thus, there is no competition for attention from different inputs, and processing is limited to the preattentive level by means of backward masking. However, in the theoretical analysis it has been argued that fear-relevant stimuli should be automatically detected, regardless of the current direction of attention. Thus, with multiple stimulus inputs, attention should be drawn selectively to inputs related to biological fear relevance. This possibility has been confirmed in an independent experimental context.

Hansen and Hansen (1988) reported experiments where subjects were required to press different buttons depending on whether all pictures in a multiple-stimulus display were similar or whether a deviant picture was present. The pictures were faces arranged in 3 × 3 or 2 × 2 matrices. The main interest was in the subjects' ability to identify angry faces as deviants among happy faces, or happy faces as deviants among angry faces. The results clearly showed that it was easier to identify a deviant angry face among happy faces than vice versa. Furthermore, the time to identify deviant angry faces was independent of the size of the display (3 × 3 vs. 2 × 2 matrices), which Hansen and Hansen took to indicate a preattentive "pop-out" effect for angry but not for happy faces. These data thus appear to demonstrate that angry faces are special, in the sense that they automatically engage attention to "pop out" from a complex stimulus array.

We have recently replicated these findings with snakes and spiders as fear-relevant stimuli in our laboratory (Öhman, Flykt, & Esteves, 1995). Normal, non-fearful subjects were exposed to matrices of pictures of either snakes, spiders, flowers, or mushrooms; in half of the cases all stimuli in the matrix were the same, whereas the other half had a deviant stimulus. The subjects were quicker to find a deviant snake or spider among flowers and mushrooms than vice versa. The time to identify a fear-relevant deviant stimulus was independent of position in the display, whereas position had an effect for fear-irrelevant stimuli. Furthermore, as shown in Figure 10.5, the time to identify a deviant fear-relevant stimulus did not change with the size of the matrix. The time to identify a deviant fear-irrelevant stimulus, on the other hand, was longer in a 3 × 3 than in a 2 × 2 matrix. Thus, these results indicate that fear-relevant stimuli were picked up independently of their position in the perceptual field, in a process similar to a "pop-out" of preattentive origin. Perhaps it should be explicitly noted that the inference of a preattentive origin of this effect is based on the pattern of findings, rather than on explicit control of the time allowed for processing by means of masking. As seen in Figure 10.5, the reaction times to determine that a deviant picture was present in the display exceeded 1 second. Thus, in principle, there should have been ample time for controlled processes to enter the arena and affect the results. However, if this had been the case, one would expect size of the display and position of the target in the display to have been critical for the data.

There is one important difference between our results and those of Hansen and Hansen (1988). They reported that subjects took less time to decide that no different stimulus was present with happy than with angry stimuli. This result was used by Hampton, Purcell, Bersine, Hansen, and Hansen (1989) to argue that the faster discovery of deviant angry faces actually could be attributable to the generally faster identification of happy faces. To identify a deviant angry face, the subjects had to pass through

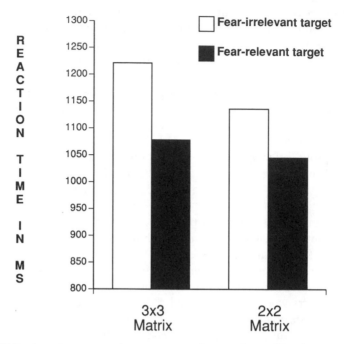

FIGURE 10.5. Mean reaction times (in milliseconds) to identify the presence of a deviant target in a matrix of pictures arranged in a 3 × 3 or a 2 × 2 pattern. The target were either fear-relevant picture (snake or spider) occuring among fear irrelevant background pictures (flowers or mushrooms), or a deviant fear-irrelevant picture occurring among fear-relevant background pictures. The subjects were reliably faster in identifying fear-relevant than fear-irrelevant targets. Furthermore, there was no significant difference between matrices of different size (3 × 3 vs. 2 × 2) for fear-relevant targets. Fear-irrelevant targets, however took significantly longer to identify a deviant stimulus in the large than in the small matrix.

a number of happy faces. To identify a deviant happy face, on the other hand, they had to identify a series of angry background faces. Because they were quicker to discard happy than angry background faces, the time to identify deviant angry and happy faces, respectively, could have been confounded by the generally quicker identification of the background happy faces. Thus, Hampton et al. (1989) questioned the pop-out interpretation advanced by Hansen and Hansen (1988). In our data, however, the subjects were faster to decide that a deviant mushroom or flower was *not* present among snake or spider background pictures than vice versa. Thus, in spite of the shorter time to identify background fear-relevant stimuli, they nevertheless were quicker to identify a deviant fear-relevant stimuli among background fear-irrelevant stimuli than vice versa. This finding, therefore, supports an automatic pop-out effect as the basis for our results.

To sum up the implications from all the studies from my laboratory reviewed in this section, there appears to be a perceptual system that automatically and preattentively focuses attention on potentially threatening stimuli, in cases where the threat has a likely origin in biological evolution. Such stimuli seem to be located by a preattentive pop-out effect, which selects them for controlled processing among complex arrays of stimuli. If the preattentively located threat stimulus is related to aversiveness because of previous conditioning, as in phobics or in our experimentally conditioned subjects, an autonomic response is recruited at this very early stage of processing. Thus, the response is elicited before the stimulus is represented in conscious awareness. This implies that the entering of the stimulus into conscious awareness may coincide with the experience of the physiological arousal. Fear is consequently experienced as immediate and inevitable, and it is likely to be perceived as completely uncontrollable by the person involved, who therefore sees few alternatives to flight.

UNCONSCIOUS ATTENTIONAL BIAS FOR THREAT IN ANXIETY DISORDER

The decisive role of nonconscious, automatic information-processing mechanisms in the control of phobic fear implied by our data has an obvious relation to data produced in recent research on perceptual biases for threat in anxiety patients (see Dalgleish & Watts, 1990, MacLeod & Mathews, 1991, and Mathews, 1990, for reviews). Basically, this research has demonstrated that individuals with high habitual levels of anxiety are more likely than controls to have their performance distracted by task-irrelevant threat words (e.g., "cancer," "disaster," "failure"). There are data to suggest, furthermore, that this interference effect is mediated at an automatic, nonconscious level of information processing.

Studies Using the Stroop Color–Word Interference Paradigm

The most frequently used paradigm in this research is the Stroop color–word interference task (see MacLeod, 1991). Mathews and MacLeod (1985) used a variety of the Stroop task in which generalized anxiety patients and controls were required to color-name lists of threat-related words and control words (matched to the threat words in length and frequency of occurrence in the language). Anxiety patients were slower in general than controls, and particularly so for the threat words, which suggests that they were unable to prevent the meaning of threat words from interfering with color naming. Enhanced interference with color naming of disorder-relevant threat words in Stroop paradigms has subsequently been demonstrated for panic patients (Ehlers, Margraf, Davies, & Roth, 1988; Hope, Rapee, Heimberg, & Dombeck, 1990; McNally, Riemann, & Kim, 1991), social phobics (Hope et al., 1990), animal phobics (Watts, McKenna, Sharrock, & Trezise, 1986), and patients with rape- and combat-related posttraumatic stress disorder (PTSD) (Foa, Festke, Murdock, Kozak, & McCarthy, 1991, and McNally, Kaspi, Riemann, & Zeitlin, 1990, respectively). In addition, studies using dichotic listening paradigms in which threat words were presented to the nonattended ear have demonstrated a processing bias for threat words among agoraphobics (Burgess, Jones, Robertson, Radcliffe, & Emerson, 1981) and obsessive–compulsives (Foa & McNally, 1986). Thus, it appears that a processing bias for threat related to anxious concerns can be documented across the whole spectrum of anxiety disorders.

To interpret these findings, Mathews (1990) suggested that all presented words are automatically processed for meaning, but that this meaning is disregarded if it is task-irrelevant. However, unlike normal subjects, anxiety patients have difficulties in rejecting the meaning as task-irrelevant if it is related to a current concern or worry; as a consequence, their color-naming performance will suffer. However, in the standard Stroop paradigm it is impossible to tie the effects specifically to the level of automatic information processing. Thus, alternative interpretations are possible, which may give the interference effect a later locus in the processing sequence.

MacLeod and Rutherford (1992) addressed this critical issue by explicitly examining whether anxiety was related to a *preattentive* bias to discover threat. They used the Stroop paradigm with backward masking of individual words flashed at a computer screen, to ensure rigorously that experimental stimuli were presented outside of awareness. Half of the color-naming trials were presented under conditions of backward masking, where colored words exposed briefly (20 ms) were replaced by a pattern mask of the same color. The other half of the trials consisted of colored words presented unmasked. The words were neutral or related to either general threat or a specific threat (examination stress). The subjects were medical students high and low in trait anxiety tested immediately before or 6 weeks after an examination period. To ensure that the subjects were unable to discriminate masked words consciously, awareness check trials were distributed across the experimental sessions. The performance on these trials was found to be random, thus supporting the effectiveness of the masking procedure.

Threat word interference with color-naming performance differed markedly for masked and nonmasked trials. On masked trials, highly trait-anxious subjects showed a reliable slowing in color naming for threatening words, particularly during examination stress. This indicates that highly trait-anxious subjects had difficulties in disregarding preattentively located threat when state anxiety was high. Subjects low in trait anxiety, on the other hand, showed the opposite pattern with less threat interference during high stress, suggesting a preattentive bias away from threat. Thus, there was a clear interactive effect of trait and state anxiety on the bias to attend to threat. However, on nonmasked trials, when the words were consciously perceived, subjects both high and low in trait anxiety showed a bias away from examination threat words when state anxiety was increased. This pattern was attributed to strategic information-processing mechanisms by MacLeod and Rutherford (1992). It was interpreted as adaptive, conscious avoidance of examination-relevant stress when the examination approached in these capable, well-adapted, normal subjects.

Studies Directly Controlling or Assessing Attention

Findings conceptually similar to those obtained with the Stroop task have been reported from several other types of paradigms allowing explicit assessment or control of attention. Mathews and MacLeod (1986) had generalized anxiety disorder patients and controls verbally "shadow" (read aloud) stories presented to one ear (the attended channel), while series of unconnected words were presented to the other ear (the rejected channel). At the same time, they were required to respond to visually presented probes by pressing a key. Some series of the words presented to the rejected channel involved threat (e.g., "injury," "disaster," "disease," "accident"), whereas others served as emotionally neutral controls. When questioned after the experiment, the subjects typically remained unaware that words had been presented in the rejected channel, and they did not perform above chance levels in forced-choice recognition tests on threat and control words. Nevertheless, anxious subjects slowed their reaction times to the probes when they occurred with threat words as compared to nonthreat words in the rejected channel, whereas the controls did not discriminate these conditions. Thus, even though the anxious subjects were unlikely to recognize consciously the threat words in the nonattended channel, they appeared to be attended at a nonconscious level that interfered with probe reaction time performance.

Similar data were reported by MacLeod, Mathews, and Tata (1986), using a visual selective attention task. In this task, the reaction time probes replaced words occurring at fixed upper or lower positions on a computer screen, and subjects were required to read the upper word aloud (thus forcing attention to this rather than to the lower word). Critical trials involved matched threat and nonthreat words, balanced for screen position, where one of the words was replaced by the probe. The results for generalized anxiety patients showed faster reaction times when the probes replaced threat rather than nonthreat words, regardless of the position on the screen. Controls, on the other hand, showed exactly the opposite bias, with faster reaction times when the probe replaced nonthreat as compared to threat words. Thus, similar to the masked Stroop data reported by MacLeod and Rutherford (1992), the attention of anxious subjects was biased toward threat words, and that of the control subjects toward nonthreat words.

MacLeod and Locke (in press) developed a modified lexical decision task to overcome some shortcomings of the Stroop test, and to constructively replicate the Stroop findings of MacLeod and Rutherford (1992). This task was constructed explicitly to assess the *encoding* of threat and nonthreat words. Thus, its results are less ambiguous than those from the Stroop task. In the latter task, subjects could show slow color naming simply because of conditioned inattention to threat words, for example. In principle, therefore, the poor performance of high-anxiety subjects on threat words in the Stroop test could as well be attributed to active rejection of these words as to an interfering bias to attend to their meaning.

In the lexical decision task used by MacLeod and Locke (in press), two words, one denoting threat and the other with a neutral content, were presented one above the other (position was counterbalanced across trials) on a computer screen. These words served as primes for a subsequent test word. The hypothesis was that anxious subjects should bias their attention toward the threat word, which thus would be preferentially encoded. Nonanxious subjects, on the other hand, were expected to encode the nonthreat word preferentially. Which word had been encoded was revealed by latencies to read aloud the following test word, which was either of the two previously presented words. On half of the trials, the test word followed immediately after the 500-ms display of the two priming words, whereas on the other half, the screen was blanked for 1500 ms before the test word was presented. To determine whether priming facilitated reading a word, comparisons were made with a nonprimed control condition in which the test word was simply preceded by two rows of asterisks. Note that preferential encoding of threat words in this paradigm, contrary to the Stroop task, would result in faster reactions to threat than to nonthreat test words.

The results presented by MacLeod and Locke (in press) showed that highly trait-anxious medical students were faster at reading threatening test words after the short priming interval (assumed to permit only automatic processing), particularly prior to an examination period. Subjects low in trait anxiety, on the other hand, showed a bias in the opposite direction with this priming interval, suggesting a preattentive bias away from threat. With the long priming interval (assumed to permit controlled processing), the data provided a nice replication of the nonmasking results reported by MacLeod and Rutherford (1992). Thus, there was no effect of trait anxiety, but both groups showed a bias away from examination-relevant threat words with impending examination stress.

The results from the studies on attentional bias show consistently across several different experimental paradigms that anxiety is associated with an unconscious bias to focus attention on, and preferentially encode, mildly threatening stimuli. These data seem to be in good agreement with Mathews's (1990) conclusion that "anxiety and worry are associated with an automatic processing bias, initiated prior to awareness, but serving to attract attention to environmental stress cues, and thus facilitating the acquisition of threatening information" (p. 462). It should be apparent that this processing bias is very similar to the preattentive picking out of fear-relevant stimuli discussed in the preceding section of this chapter. As a consequence of the preattentive bias toward processing threatening stimuli, anxiety is maintained. Thus, a vicious circle is set up in which anxiety focuses attention on threat, leading to further anxiety, and so on.

In an evolutionary perspective, however, this circle, may not be dysfunctional. If ecological threats make a person fearful and anxious, it is important to beware of further threats, as danger may not come alone or reveal itself through only one cue. It is only when the anxiety becomes chronic and unmodulated by safety signals that the circle may become dysfunctional and actually serve to maintain maladaptive anxiety.

TOWARD A THEORETICAL INTEGRATION

I have reviewed data from two different lines of research, both of which document psychological mechanisms that have been shown to influence fear and anxiety responses at a preattentive, automatic level of information processing. They both are *implicit,* in the sense that they have a nonconscious origin. First, autonomic responses to biologically fear-relevant stimuli appear to be activated by early, quick stimulus analysis mechanisms, which are invulnerable to backward masking and which thus operate prior to the entry of the stimulus into awareness. This system is limited, in the sense that it appears to work only for a restricted class of stimuli — those for which a biologically determined fear relevance is likely. A critical analysis of existing data and literature suggests that it may operate on particular stimulus characteristics, which, when encountered in a stimulus array are likely to capture attention and thus become the target of further effortful controlled processing (see Öhman, 1992). If the stimulus has been conditioned to elicit fear, autonomic responses may be elicited at this very early step in the information-processing chain.

The second type of mechanism, which is manifested as attentional bias in anxiety, also operates at a largely nonconscious level. However, it has a broader scope than the other system, because it is not limited to a class of primarily physically defined stimuli. It involves a schema-driven bias to respond to stimuli that may be construed as in some sense threatening, not in terms of human evolutionary history, but in the perspective of worries distilled in the cumulative experience of the person involved.

Of course, these two preattentive influences on the perception of threat do not rule out other, postawareness factors as determinants of fear and anxiety. The eventual response of fear or anxiety always reflects a range of influencing processes, from very early perceptual ones to late response activation processes, reflecting considerations of how to cope with the threat. Intermediate processes related to the expectancies of the individual about likely outcomes in the situation are probably pivotal in determining the resulting emotion. Even though the expectancies may be influenced by, as well as influence, the previously discussed preattentive mechanisms, the important difference is that they can be manipulated and edited at a conscious, controlled level of information processing. As such, they are critical in the final evaluation of a situation as threatening, as well as in the selection of coping responses; thus they have an important influence on the eventual fear or anxiety response. However, a more fine-grained analysis of conscious expectancies and anxiety is beyond the scope of this chapter (see Öhman, 1993a, for a review of data as well as further theoretical discussion).

Elsewhere (Öhman, 1993a), I have provided an integration of the two types of nonconscious mechanisms and the conscious, expectancy-mediated mechanism into a coherent model of fear and anxiety (see Figure 10.6). According to this model, information from the outside world (1 in the figure) is analyzed in two steps. In the first step, the information is passed through sets of feature detectors that provide a first segregation of stimuli before they are more fully analyzed in the second step (2), which involves evaluation of the significance of the stimulus. This process is based on particular feature detectors tuned to evolutionarily determined threat. If such primed features occur in the stimulus array, attention is switched to evaluate their significance more closely (2). Furthermore, if they have been previously associated with aversiveness, the arousal system is activated (3). This part of the model is directed toward the data on phobic and conditioned responses to masked fear-relevant stimuli.

Not only may the significance evaluator be primed in a bottom-up fashion from the feature detectors; it may also be biased in a top-down way (5) by the expectancy system, which contains memorial representa-

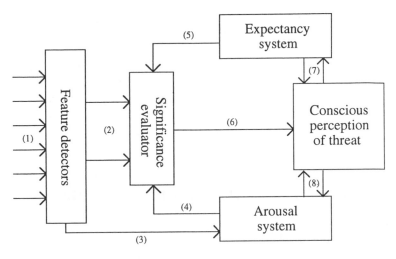

FIGURE 10.6. An information-processing model of the generation of fear and anxiety. The model suggests that stimulus input is analyzed by feature detectors and a significance evaluator. Consciously perceived threat results from the integration of information from the significance evaluator, an expectancy system, and an arousal system. The arousal system can be triggered by the feature detectors or as a result of perceived threat. The significance evaluator can be biased by the expectancy system and activated by the arousal system. From Öhman (1993a, p. 527). Copyright 1993 by The Guilford Press. Reprinted by permission.

tions of past experience with the stimuli involved, as well as of their covariations and associations with threat. This is the route addressing the data on attentional bias in anxiety reviewed above.

The significance evaluator can also be activated by the arousal system (4), which accounts for the effect of state anxiety on attentional bias for threats (e.g., MacLeod & Rutherford, 1992). However, the significance evaluator in itself has no, or only a weak, effect on the arousal system.

The conscious perception of threat provides the integration of non-consciously processed information from the significance evaluator (6) with information from the more consciously accessible expectancy (7) and arousal (8) systems.

Even though the content of the expectancy system need not be conscious, it provides the raw material for conscious expectancies of threat and for the actual perception of threat. This model therefore not only encompasses the traditional preparedness findings, but also includes data on the effect of masking of fear-relevant stimuli (Esteves, et al. , 1994a; Öhman et al., 1989; Öhman & Soares, 1993; Soares & Öhman, 1993a,

1993b) and data on the role of expectancy in responding to prepared stimuli (e.g., Davey, 1992; Tomarken et al., 1989). In addition, it provides an integration of these findings with those dealing with attentional biases in anxiety disorder. Thus, this model does a good job of integrating and of facilitating understanding of diverse sets of data. Whether it can also serve as a heuristic device to inform and stimulate new research or clinical practice is something that remains to be seen. In the concluding section of the chapter, some of its theoretical implications are discussed.

IMPLICATIONS FOR ANXIETY DISORDERS

Fear and Anxiety

The model depicted in Figure 10.6 implies that there are in effect two types of anxiety, one of a conscious and the other of an unconscious origin. Both of them, however, differ from fear. The perspective taken in this chapter views fear as an emotional response related to avoidance and escape. When escape and avoidance are impossible, fear is changed into anxiety (Epstein, 1972). However, if anxiety is construed as "unresolved fear" or "undirected arousal" related to perceived threat (Epstein, 1972), then the model implies that there is a more basic, unconscious type of anxiety than that resulting from frustrated avoidance motives. This type of anxiety results from the unconscious input to the conscious perception system from the significance evaluator and the arousal system. Because the source of this input is not necessarily available to consciousness, there are typically no escape or avoidance options available. The resulting state of undirected arousal may be experienced as anxiety. The person knows that something is wrong, but cannot pinpoint any clear reason for it. Anxiety in this sense, then, is entirely dependent on the unconscious mechanisms, whereas the anxiety resulting from interference with overt avoidance and escape responses is more readily appraised at the conscious level as originating in the external world or in personal shortcomings.

The unconsciously originated anxiety may be channeled or "resolved" into fear, if escape is selected as the action option after a complete conscious and controlled processing of the stimulus situation. Normally, of course, the eliciting stimulus is consciously perceived simultaneously with the arousal of anxiety, as attention is directed to the preattentively located threat. It is only when the attention shift fails to locate the stimulus for conscious representation that preattentively elicited unconscious anxiety is left in the system without any apparent stimulus for its explanation. This may occur when the stimulus is very faint and thus fails to be perceived, when the preattentive mechanisms falsely locates a threat that is not confirmed by controlled processing, or when several more or less simultaneous stimuli (e.g., emanating from the body) mask one another.

The Symptoms of Anxiety Disorder

In the perspective provided by the model (see Figure 10.6), phobias and panic disorder may both be taken as resulting from the automatic activation of the arousal system by specific features located by the feature detectors. This activation provides a surge of physiological arousal, cues from which become available to the conscious perception system. These two types of disorders therefore should be similar, in the sense that they both reflect increases in sympathetically mediated arousal. However, whereas the information reaching the conscious perception system from the arousal system may be quite similar, the information arriving via the significance evaluator is radically different. In the case of a phobia, the source of the physiological arousal is attributed to some factor in the external world; in the case of panic, the arousal is attributed to internal stimuli. The former situation is easier to cope with than the latter. When a phobic stimulus is consciously recognized, the resulting response is typically flight. An internal stimulus, on the other hand, cannot be fled. As there is no apparent external source suggesting ways of coping with the physiological arousal, it risks reaching overwhelming intensity. Therefore, catastrophic interpretations of the situation are readily invited. In this way, some of the similarities and the differences in symptomatology between phobias and panic disorder can be understood.

In PTSD, there is an original trauma that totally recruits the individual's defense responses, often for quite protracted periods of time and at overwhelming intensities (e.g., in combat). As a result, cues may be conditioned to activate the arousal system automatically, as in phobia and panic. In PTSD, however, there is a subsequent stage of cognitive preoccupation with the trauma. This stage is likely to be mediated through the expectancy system and the significance evaluator, which thus take on more prominent roles than in phobias and panic disorder, leading to physiological activation not only automatically but also through conscious mediation (via worries and ruminations).

Generalized anxiety disorder, finally, appears to lack arousal activation via the feature detectors; it seems to be primarily driven by the expectancy system and the bias to discover threats (Rapee, 1991). The physiological effects that are needed to turn the worry into anxiety (Mathews, 1990) are likely to be recruited through activation of the arousal system from the cognitive perception system. Thus, in this disorder the expectancy–significance–perception loop appears to play the primary role in the problem, and the nonconscious activation of arousal seems to play a secondary role.

Treatment

The model suggests that there are both "cognitive" and "noncognitive" foci for interventions with anxiety disorders. Clearly, expectancies are taken to play a key role in overt anxiety, and therefore cognitive restructuring has arguments to recommend itself. However, if (as suggested by the model) phobic responses and panic are both primarily initiated by preattentive, automatic stimulus analysis mechanisms, cognitive interventions should at least be supplemented by other procedures directed at this level. In fact, the model opens a route to the understanding of why exposure is critical to therapeutic modification of simple phobic responses (e.g., Borden, 1992; Marks, 1987), social phobia (Turner, Beidel, & Townsley, 1992), and agoraphobia and panic (Craske, Rapee, & Barlow, 1992). For the treatment of generalized anxiety disorder, the role of exposure treatment is less clear (Craske et al., 1992), as one would expect if this disorder is more dependent on expectancy than on nonconscious activation processes (as suggested by the model).

Thus, the model depicted in Figure 10.6 provides a conceptual underpinning to the commonly expressed view that exposure to the anxiety-generating cues are critical to all treatment efforts. What exposure achieves, presumably, is the dampening of the emotional response through a process of habituation (e.g., Lader & Mathews, 1968). Habituation is a ubiquitous mechanism of response inhibition through repeated exposures; it is evident at all levels of organismic organization (see, e.g., Peeke & Petrinovich, 1984). Thus, habituation may provide an "automatic procedure" to alleviate "automatically elicited" fear and anxiety. Indeed, there are data available suggesting that exposing agoraphobics subliminally to filmed agoraphobia scenes results in improvements of the phobia (Lee, Tyrer & Horn, 1983; Tyrer, Horn, & Lee, 1978). Thus, provided that effective fear-eliciting stimuli are available to evoke some anxiety when presented under conditions preventing their conscious appraisal, the view of anxiety summarized in the model suggests that therapeutic gains may be obtained from masked exposures, thus sparing the patient the anxiety of actual exposures.

ACKNOWLEDGMENT

The research reported in this chapter was supported by a series of grants from the Swedish Research Councils for the Humanities and Social Sciences.

REFERENCES

American Psychiatric Association. (1987). *Diagnostic and statistical manual of mental disorders* (3rd ed., rev.). Washington, DC: Author.

American Psychiatric Association. (1994). *Diagnostic and statistical manual of mental disorder* (4th ed.). Washington, DC; Author.

Bolles, R. C. (1970). Species-specific defense reactions and avoidance learning. *Psychological Review, 77*, 32–48.

Borden, J.W. (1992). Behavioral treatment of simple phobia. In S. M. Turner, K. S. Calhoun, & H. E. Adams (Eds.), *Handbook of clinical behavior therapy* (2nd. ed., pp. 3–12). New York: Wiley.

Bornstein, R. F., & Pittman, T. S. (Eds.). (1992). *Perception without awareness.* New York: Guilford Press.

Burgess, I. S., Jones, L. M., Robertson, S. A., Radcliffe, W. N., & Emerson, E. (1981). The degree of control exerted by phobic and non-phobic stimuli over the recognition behaviour of phobic and non-phobic subjects. *Behaviour Research and Therapy, 19*, 233–243.

Clark, D. M. (1986). A cognitive approach to panic. *Behaviour Research and Therapy, 24*, 461–470.

Cook, M., & Mineka, S. (1989). Observational conditioning of fear to fear-relevant versus fear-irrelevant stimuli in rhesus monkeys. *Journal of Abnormal Psychology, 98*, 448–459.

Cook, M., & Mineka, S. (1990). Selective associations in the observational conditioning of fear in rhesus monkeys. *Journal of Experimental Psychology: Animal Behavior Processes, 16*, 372–389.

Craske, M. G., Rapee, R. M., & Barlow, D. H. (1992). Cognitive-behavioral treatment of panic disorder, agoraphobia, and generalized anxiety disorder. In S. M. Turner, K. S. Calhoun, & H. E. Adams (Eds.), *Handbook of clinical behavior therapy* (2nd ed., pp. 39–66). New York: Wiley.

Dalgleish, T., & Watts, F. N. (1990). Biases of attention and memory in disorders of anxiety and depression. *Clinical Psychology Review, 10*, 589–604.

Davey, G. C. L. (1992). An expectancy model of laboratory preparedness effects. *Journal of Experimental Psychology: General, 121*, 24–40.

Dawson, M. E., & Schell, A. M. (1985). Information processing and human autonomic classical conditioning. *Advances in Psychophysiology, 1*, 89–165.

Ehlers, A. (1993). Interoception and panic disorder. *Advances in Behaviour Research and Therapy, 15*, 3–22.

Ehlers, A., Margraf, J., Davies, S., & Roth, W. T. (1988). Selective processing of threat cues in subjects with panic attacks. *Cognition and Emotion, 2*, 201–219.

Epstein, S. (1972). The nature of anxiety with emphasis upon its relationship to expectancy. In C. D. Spielberger (Ed.), *Anxiety: Current trends in theory and research* (Vol. 2, pp. 291–337). New York: Academic Press.

Esteves, F., Dimberg, U., & Öhman, A. (1994a). Automatically elicited fear: Conditioned skin conductance responses to masked facial expressions. *Cognition and Emotion, 3*, 393–413.

Esteves, F., Dimberg, U., Parra, C., & Öhman, A. (1994b). Nonconscious associative learning: Pavlovian conditioning of skin conductance responses to masked fear-relevant facial stimuli. *Psychophysiology. 31*. 375–385.

Esteves, F., & Öhman, A. (1993). Masking the face: Recognition of emotional facial expressions as a function of the parameters of backward masking. *Scandinavian Journal of Psychology, 34*, 1–18.

Foa, E. B., & McNally, R. J. (1986). Sensitivity to feared stimuli in obsessive–compulsives: A dichotic listening analysis. *Cognitive Therapy and Research, 10,* 477–485.

Foa, E. B., Feske, U., Murdock, T. B., Kozak, M. J., & McCarthy, P. R. (1991). Processing of threat-related information in rape victims. *Journal of Abnormal Psychology, 100,* 156–162.

Fredrikson, M. (1981). Orienting and defensive responses to phobic and conditioned stimuli in phobics and normals. *Psychophysiology, 18,* 456–465.

Garcia, J., & Koellig, R. A. (1966). Relation of cue to consequence in avoidance learning. *Psychonomic Science, 4,* 123–124.

Hampton, C., Purcell, D. G., Bersine, L., Hansen, C. H., & Hansen, R. D. (1989). Probing "pop-out": Another look at the face-in-the-crowd effect. *Bulletin of the Psychonomic Society, 27,* 563–566.

Hansen, C. H., & Hansen, R. D. (1988). Finding the face in the crowd: An anger superiority effect. *Journal of Personality and Social Psychology, 54,* 917–924.

Holender, D. (1986). Semantic activation without conscious identification in dichotic listening, parafoveal vision, and visual masking: A survey and appraisal. *Behavioral and Brain Sciences, 9,* 1–66.

Hope, D. A., Rapee, R. M., Heimberg, R. G., & Dombeck, M. J. (1990). Representations of the self in social phobia: Vulnerability to social threat. *Cognitive Therapy and Research, 14,* 177–189.

Kendler, K. S., Neale, M. C., Kessler, R. C., Heath, A. C., & Eaves, L. J. (1992). The genetic epidemiology of phobias in women: The interrelationship of agoraphobia, social phobia, situational phobia and simple phobia. *Archives of General Psychiatry, 49,* 273–281.

Lader, M. H., & Mathews, A. M. (1968). A physiological model for phobic anxiety and desensitization. *Behaviour Research and Therapy, 6,* 411–421.

Lang, P. J. (1984). Cognition in emotion: Concept and action. In C. E. Izard, J. Kagan, & R. B. Zajonc (Eds.), *Emotion, cognition, and behavior* (pp. 192–266). New York: Cambridge University Press.

Lang, P. J., Bradley, M. M., & Cuthbert, B. N. (1990). Emotion, attention, and the startle reflex. *Psychological Review, 97,* 377–395.

LeDoux, J. E. (1990). Information flow from sensation to emotion: Plasticity in the neural computation of stimulus value. In M. Gabriel & J. Moore (Eds.), *Learning and computational neuroscience: Foundations of adaptive networks* (pp. 3–51). Cambridge, MA: MIT Press.

Lee, I., Tyrer, P., & Horn, S. (1983). A comparison of subliminal, supraliminal and faded phobic cine-films in the treatment of agoraphobia. *British Journal of Psychiatry, 143,* 356–361.

Lovibond, P. F., Siddle, D. A. T., & Bond, N. W. (1993). Resistance to extinction of fear-relevant stimuli: Preparedness or selective sensitization? *Journal of Experimental Psychology: General, 122,* 449–461.

MacLeod, C. (1991). Half a century of research on the Stroop effect: An integrative review. *Psychological Bulletin, 109,* 163–203.

MacLeod, C., & Locke, V. (in press). Differentiating automatic from strategic patterns of anxiety-linked encoding selectivity using a dual priming methodology. *Behaviour Research and Therapy.*

MacLeod, C., & Mathews, A. (1991). Cognitive-experimental approaches to the emotional disorders. In P. R. Martin (Ed.), *Handbook of behavior therapy and psychological science: An integrative approach* (pp. 116–150). Elmsford, NY: Pergamon Press.

MacLeod, C., Mathews, A., & Tata, P. (1986). Attentional bias in emotional disorders. *Journal of Abnormal Psychology, 95,* 15–20.

MacLeod, C., & Rutherford, E. M. (1992). Anxiety and the selective processing of emotional information: Mediating roles of awareness, trait and state variables, and personal relevance of stimulus materials. *Behaviour Research and Therapy, 30,* 479–491.

Mandler, G. (1975). *Mind and emotion.* New York: Wiley.

Marcel, A. (1983). Conscious and unconscious perception: An approach to the relations between phenomenal experience and perceptual processes. *Cognitive Psychology, 15,* 238–300.

Marks, I. M. (1987). *Fears, phobias, and rituals: Panic, anxiety, and their disorders.* New York: Oxford University Press.

Mathews, A. (1990). Why worry? The cognitive function of anxiety. *Behaviour Research and Therapy, 28,* 455–468.

Mathews, A., & MacLeod, C. (1985). Selective processing of threat cues in anxiety states. *Behaviour Research and Therapy, 23,* 563–569.

Mathews, A., & MacLeod, C. (1986). Discrimination of threat cues without awareness in anxiety states. *Journal of Abnormal Psychology, 95,* 131–138.

McNally, R. J. (1987). Preparedness and phobias: A review. *Psychological Bulletin, 101,* 283–303.

McNally, R. J., Kaspi, S. P., Riemann, B. C., & Zeitlin, S. B. (1990). Selective processing of threat cues in posttraumatic stress disorder. *Journal of Abnormal Psychology, 99,* 398–402.

McNally, R. J., Riemann, B. C., & Kim, E. (1990). Selective processing of threat cues in panic disorder. *Behaviour Research and Therapy, 28,* 407–412.

Merckelbach, H., van der Molen, G. M., & van den Hout, M. A. (1987). Electrodermal conditioning to stimuli of evolutionary significance: Failure to replicate the preparedness effect. *Journal of Psychopathology and Behavioral Assessment, 9,* 131–326.

Merikle, P. M., & Reingold, E. M. (1992). Measuring unconscious perceptual processes. In R. F. Bornstein & T. S. Pittman (Eds.), *Perception without awareness* (pp. 55–80). New York: Guilford Press.

Mineka, S. (1992). Evolutionary memories, emotional processing, and the emotional disorders. In D. Medin (Ed.), *The psychology of learning and motivation* (Vol. 28, pp. 161–206). New York: Academic Press.

Mineka, S., & Cook, M. (1992). Mechanisms involved in the observational conditioning of fear. *Journal of Experimental Psychology: General, 122,* 23–38.

Mineka, S., & Tomarken, A. J. (1989). The role of cognitive biases in the origin and maintenance of fear and anxiety disorders. In T. Archer & L.-G. Nilsson (Eds.), *Aversion, avoidance and anxiety* (pp. 195–221). Hillsdale, NJ: Erlbaum.

Öhman, A. (1979). The orienting response, attention, and learning: An information processing perspective. In H. D. Kimmel, E. H. van Olst, & J. F. Orlebeke (Eds.), *The orienting reflex in humans* (pp. 443–472). Hillsdale, NJ: Erlbaum.

Öhman, A. (1983). The orienting response during Pavlovian conditioning. In D. A. T. Siddle (Ed.), *Orienting and habituation: Perspectives in human research* (pp. 315–369). Chichester, England: Wiley.

Öhman, A. (1986). Face the beast and fear the face: Animal and social fears as prototypes for evolutionary analyses of emotion. *Psychophysiology, 23,* 123–145.

Öhman, A. (1987). The psychophysiology of emotion: An evolutionary–cognitive perspective. *Advances in Psychophysiology, 2,* 79–127.

Öhman, A. (1992). Orienting and attention: Preferred preattentive processing of potentially phobic stimuli. In B. A. Campbell, H. Haynes, & R. Richardson (Eds.), *Attention and information processing in infants and adults: Perspectives from human and animal research* (pp. 263–295). Hillsdale, NJ: Erlbaum.

Öhman, A. (1993a). Fear and anxiety as emotional phenomena: Clinical phenomenology, evolutionary perspectives, and information-processing mechanisms. In M. Lewis & J. M. Haviland (Eds.), *Handbook of emotions* (pp. 511–536). New York: Guilford Press.

Öhman, A. (1993b). Stimulus prepotency and fear: Data and theory. In N. Birbaumer & A. Öhman (Eds.), *The organization of emotion: Cognitive, clinical and psychophysiological perspectives* (pp. 218–239). Toronto: Hogrefe.

Öhman, A., Dimberg, U., & Esteves, F. (1989). Preattentive activation of aversive emotions. In T. Archer & L.-G. Nilsson (Eds.), *Aversion, avoidance, and anxiety* (pp. 169–193). Hillsdale, NJ: Erlbaum.

Öhman, A., Dimberg, U., & Öst, L.-G. (1985). Animal and social phobias: Biological constraints on learned fear responses. In S. Reiss & R. R. Bootzin (Eds.), *Theoretical issues in behavior therapy* (pp. 123–178). New York: Academic Press.

Öhman, A., Flykt, A., & Esteve, F. (1994). [The snake in the grass effect]. Unpublished raw data.

Öhman, A., Fredrikson, M., & Hugdahl, K. (1978). Orienting and defensive responding in the electrodermal system: Palmar–dorsal differences and recovery rate during conditioning to potentially phobic stimuli. *Psychophysiology, 15,* 93–101.

Öhman, A., & Soares, J. J. F. (1993). On the automaticity of phobic fear: Conditioned skin conductance responses to masked phobic stimuli. *Journal of Abnormal Psychology, 102,* 121–132.

Öhman, A., & Soares, J. J. F. (1994). Unconscious anxiety: Phobic responses to masked stimuli. *Journal of Abnormal Psychology, 103,* 231–240.

Öhman, A., & Soares, J. J. F. (1995). *Unconscious emotional learning: Conditioning of skin conductance responses to masked phobic stimuli.* Manuscript submitted for publication.

Peeke, H. V. S., & Petrinovich, L. (Eds.). (1984). *Habituation, sensitization, and behavior.* New York: Academic Press.

Posner, M. I. (1978). *Chronometric explorations of mind.* Hillsdale, NJ: Erlbaum.

Posner, M. I., & Boies, S. J. (1971). Components of attention. *Psychological Review, 78,* 391–408.

Rapee, R. M. (1991). Generalized anxiety disorder: A review of clinical features and theoretical concepts. *Clinical Psychology Review, 11,* 419–440.

Rapee, R., Mattick, R., & Murrell, E. (1986). Cognitive mediation in the affective component of spontaneous panic attacks. *Journal of Behavior Therapy and Experimental Psychiatry, 17,* 245–253.

Sanderson, W. C., Rapee, R.M., & Barlow, D.H. (1989). The influence of an illusion of control on panic attacks induced via inhalation of 5.5% carbon dioxide-enriched air. *Archives of General Psychiatry, 46,* 157–162.

Sartory, G. (1983). The orienting response and psychopathology: Anxiety and phobias. In D. A. T. Siddle (Ed.), *Orienting and habituation: Perspectives in human research* (pp. 449–474). Chichester, England: Wiley.

Schell, A. M., Dawson, M. E., & Marinkovic, K. (1991). Effects of the use of potentially phobic CSs on retention, reinstatement, and extinction of the conditioned skin conductance response. *Psychophysiology, 28,* 140–153.

Schneider, W., Dumais, S. T., & Shiffrin, R. M. (1984). Automatic and control processing and attention. In R. Parasuraman & D. R. Davies (Eds.), *Varieties of attention* (pp. 1–28). Orlando, FL: Academic Press.

Seligman, M. E. P. (1970). On the generality of the laws of learning. *Psychological Review, 77,* 406–418.

Seligman, M. E. P. (1971). Phobias and preparedness. *Behavior Therapy, 2,* 307–320.

Seligman, M. E. P., & Hager, J. E. (Eds.). (1972). *Biological boundaries of learning.* New York: Appleton-Century-Crofts.

Shiffrin, R. M., & Schneider, W. (1977). Controlled and automatic human information processing: II. Perceptual learning, automatic attending, and a general theory. *Psychological Review, 84,* 127–190.

Siddle, D. A. T., Power, K., Bond, N. W., & Lovibond, P. F. (1988). Effects of stimulus content and devaluation of the unconditioned stimulus on retention of human electrodermal conditioning. *Australian Journal of Psychology, 40,* 179–193.

Soares, J. J. F., & Öhman, A. (1993a). Backward masking and skin conductance responses after conditioning to non-feared but fear-relevant stimuli in fearful subjects. *Psychophysiology, 30,* 460–466.

Soares, J. J. F., & Öhman, A. (1993b). Preattentive processing, preparedness, and phobias: Effects of instruction on conditioned electrodermal responses to masked and non-masked fear-relevant stimuli. *Behaviour Research and Therapy, 31,* 87–95.

Tomarken, A. J., Mineka, S., & Cook, M. (1989). Fear-relevant selective associations and covariation bias. *Journal of Abnormal Psychology, 98,* 381–394.

Turner, S. M., Beidel, D. C., & Townsley, R. M., (1992). Behavioral treatment of social phobia. In S. M. Turner, K. S. Calhoun, & H. E. Adams (Eds.), *Handbook of clinical behavior therapy* (2nd ed., pp. 13–37). New York: Wiley.

Tyrer, P. J., Horn, S., & Lee, I. (1978). Treatment of agoraphobia by subliminal and supraliminal exposure to phobic cine film. *Lancet, i,* 358–360.

Wagner, A. R. (1976). Priming in STM: An information-processing mechanism for self-generated or retrieval-generated depression in performance. In T. J. Tighe & R. N. Leaton (Eds.), *Habituation: Perspectives from child development, animal behavior, and neurophysiology* (pp. 95–128). Hillsdale, NJ: Erlbaum.

Watts, F. N., McKenna, F. P., Sharrock, R., & Trezise, L. (1986). Colour naming of phobia-related words. *British Journal of Psychology, 77,* 97–108.

11

The Preparedness Account of Social Phobia: Some Data and Alternative Explanations

NIGEL W. BOND
DAVID A. T. SIDDLE

THE CONDITIONING MODEL of the acquisition and maintenance of phobias has had a checkered history since it was first proposed by Watson (1924). His early work with Rayner that purported to demonstrate the acquisition of a rat phobia in an 11-month-old boy, "Little Albert," appeared promising. Briefly, Watson and Rayner (1920) demonstrated that prior to conditioning, Albert, like many children of his age, was not afraid of a white rat. Watson then exposed Albert to a series of trials in which Albert was placed in a room with the white rat. As soon as Albert looked at or reached toward the rat, Watson, who stood out of sight, would hit an iron bar with a hammer. The loud noise frightened Albert, who cried and showed other signs of distress. Following a number of pairings of the white rat (the conditioned stimulus, or CS) with the loud noise (the unconditioned stimulus, or US), which produced crying and distress in Albert (the unconditioned response, or UR), Watson and Rayner stated that Albert began to show fear (the conditioned response, or CR) upon seeing the white rat. Furthermore, Watson reported that the fear generalized to similar objects, such as a white rabbit, white fur mittens, and even Watson's white beard. However, a number of attempts to replicate this classic study have produced little in the way of confirmatory evidence (Harris, 1979).

As conceived by Watson, the conditioning account of the acquisition and maintenance of phobias was both popular and influential, particularly as a paradigmatic application of learning theory to psychopathology. However, the theory has also been subjected to robust criticism from both outside and within the field of learning. Some of these arguments have been discussed in detail by Rachman (1977) and by ourselves (Siddle & Bond, 1988; Bond & Siddle, 1988).

One of the major arguments advanced by Rachman (1977) was that the assertion that any CS paired with an effective US produces a robust CR is patently false. This issue was addressed by Seligman (1970), who revived the view first expressed by Thorndike (1911) that the associations formed during conditioning are not arbitrary, but rather that some stimuli and responses "belong" together. Seligman has updated Thorndike's view and attempted to operationalize the concept of "belongingness," which he terms "preparedness." Briefly, all associations, whether between stimuli or between responses and reinforcers, are said to lie along a continuum of preparedness. Prepared associations are said to be acquired rapidly under normal circumstances, to be acquired even under impoverished conditions, and to be difficult to extinguish once acquired. In contrast, "unprepared" associations are said to be difficult to acquire, to be acquired only under optimal conditions, and to be extinguished rapidly. The classic example of a prepared association is taste aversion learning in the rat. A thirsty rat given access to a novel flavor such as saccharin, and then made ill for a brief period by an injection of lithium chloride, will subsequently avoid drinking saccharin-flavored fluid (Garcia & Koelling, 1966). This aversion is acquired following only one pairing of the novel flavor with the illness, and despite delays of up to 24 hours between the first presentation of the fluid and the rat's experience of illness (Smith & Roll, 1967). Moreover, such an aversion is difficult to extinguish. Possibly the most famous example of an "unprepared" association is the difficulty apes have in acquiring human language (Terrace, 1979).

Seligman (1971) applied his theorizing to psychopathology and offered an account of phobias based upon the concept of "preparedness." Although there are problems with the original theory (see Schwartz, 1974), Öhman and his colleagues have developed a sophisticated account of the acquisition and maintenance of phobias that takes as its starting point the possibility that many phobias are examples of prepared associations. Briefly, Öhman, Dimberg, and Öst (1985) have argued that the stimuli that are the focus of many current phobias are "prepared" with respect to their ability to be associated with aversive events. This preparedness is said to have arisen as a result of the importance of these stimuli in our evolutionary past. Thus, Öhman et al. have argued that an ability to learn quickly that snakes are dangerous would have been of considerable survival value to those protomammals who were our ancestors. However, the theory is much more sophisticated than the typical "just so" story and requires some elaboration.

First, Öhman et al. have drawn upon Mayr's (1974) distinction between communicative and noncommunicative behaviors. Within the former category, Mayr distinguished between interspecific and intraspecific communicative behaviors. In the present context, these distinctions fit neatly with the three general categories of phobias—namely, "nature" fears, "animal" fears, and "social" fears (Marks, 1969; Torgersen, 1979). Importantly, the fears represented by these categories are not arbitrary. Thus, the frequency with which people seek treatment for various phobias and the incidence of various fears in the general population all point to the selective nature of human fears (Agras, Sylvester, & Oliveau, 1969; Costello, 1982; Torgersen, 1979). Thus, most investigators have reported that animal fears are the most frequent. Within this category, people are most likely to report a fear of snakes. Note that many of these surveys have been carried out in situations where there are few if any poisonous snakes (e.g., Torgersen, 1979). In contrast, we assessed the degree to which young adults feared snakes in an Australian population. Nine of the 10 most poisonous snakes in the world are found in Australia, and a number of poisonous species can be found in suburban gardens during the summer months. Despite the obvious difference in exposure to dangerous snakes, we found that the level of reported fear in Australian subjects was very similar to that observed in North American and Swedish samples (Packer, Bond, & Siddle, 1987).

Öhman et al. (1985) have also argued that learning plays a crucial role in the acquisition of such fears. Mineka's (1987) work with rhesus monkeys provides an excellent example of this crucial role. Almost all wild-reared rhesus monkeys show a considerable fear of snakes. However, their fear is not innate, because almost no laboratory-reared rhesus monkeys display a fear of snakes during their initial exposure to them. Nonetheless, Mineka has demonstrated that laboratory-reared monkeys learn to fear snakes very quickly if they see a conspecific acting fearfully in the presence of a snake. The fact that the fear is acquired vicariously rather than through direct aversive conditioning echoes Bolles's (1970) point that predator avoidance is too important to leave solely to the vagaries of conditioning[1] An animal cannot learn to avoid predation on the basis of repeated aversive experiences in the presence of a predator. Such an animal would have provided the predator with a meal long before it learned to avoid that predator.

Finally, it is clear from twin studies that there is some genetic component associated with these common fears. Thus, Torgersen (1979) reported that there was a heredity index of approximately .50 for both the focus and the intensity of fear.

The evidence described thus far indicates that human fears are selective, that they have some genetic basis, and that there is a role for learning in their acquisition. However, the theory proposed by Öhman et al. (1985) is much more sophisticated than the simple assertion that there is a biological constraint on human fears and phobias. Perhaps the most impressive aspect of the theory is its detailed analysis of the evolutionary origins of various classes of fear, which enables precise predictions concerning the outcomes of laboratory investigations of the theory to be made.[2] In the next section, we discuss in detail research that has been stimulated by Öhman with respect to one class of phobia—namely, social phobia.

SOCIAL PHOBIA

Öhman et al. (1985) have argued that social phobias originate as a result of social conflict. This conflict is a natural outcome of the fact that humans, like other primates,[3] form dominance hierarchies. Furthermore, they have argued that humans, like other primates, form separate hierarchies based upon gender, with the male hierarchy dominating the female hierarchy.[4] The advantages of being nearer the top than the bottom of a hierarchy are manifold and need not concern us here. However, even those who occupy the lower rungs of a hierarchy gain advantages from living within a social group; therefore, these individuals are better off remaining in the group, despite their lowly status. Nevertheless, this does mean that such individuals are placed in a position where they must interact with those higher in the hierarchy. This is the quintessential aspect of social phobia: Despite the fact that an individual is made anxious by social encounters, they cannot be avoided.

Öhman et al. (1985) have made the reasonable assumption that the formation of dominance hierarchies begins during adolescence. Unlike interspecific communication, however, intraspecific communication has to account for the fact that there will be many such contests and that it is important for injuries arising from them to be kept to a minimum. Such circumstances are ripe for the formation of ritualized contests that are settled by a display of strength, rather than by its use (Lorenz, 1966). In the case of most primates, the ritualization has led to the evolution of specific facial expressions of emotion. Dominance contests involve threat and fear. In humans, threat is portrayed by an angry facial expression of emotion, and fear is displayed by a fearful facial expression of emotion. There may be bodily postures associated with these facial expressions, as there are in other primates, but they are of little consequence for the present argument.

A number of predictions follow from the theory of social phobia outlined by Öhman et al. (1985). First, all of us will show some readiness to make an association between an individual who directs an angry facial expression toward us and an aversive outcome. However, we might expect some individual differences; people with social phobia might be expected to be especially sensitive, given their history. Second, we might expect such differences to be especially noticeable in interactions involving strangers, presumably because we have to sort out our dominance relationships with them, particularly in the context of interactions that involve food and sex. Certainly, these are the situations that people who exhibit social phobia report to be the most difficult (Marks, 1987).

Third, social phobia may involve more cognitive appraisal of fear-eliciting situations than does animal phobia. Thus, if we are afraid of a particular animal and we encounter the animal, we will remove ourselves from the situation. The need for a rapid escape results in sympathetic arousal and relatively automatic processing of the situation. In contrast, social encounters require a different strategy. We cannot simply escape from the situation if we lose a dominance encounter. Because of our need to stay within the social group, we have to signal that loss and then make the best of it. Thus, there will be some sympathetic activation. However, because our response must be more subtle, we need to appraise the situation; as a consequence, there will be less reflexive sympathetic activation than that associated with animal phobias. Furthermore, our need to appraise the situation and to choose from a number of possible responses means that there will be a greater reliance on controlled processing (Shiffrin & Schneider, 1977).

Fourth, because of the pervasive nature of social interaction in humans, social phobia will be far more debilitating than will animal phobia. As Öhman et al. (1985) have pointed out, the animals that are the focus of the latter are specific, and it is possible to construct one's daily movements in such a way that even the most profound phobia can be circumvented. In contrast, a person who suffers from social phobia must continually place himself or herself in the very situation that elicits fear and anxiety, because these situations are the ones that provide the benefits associated with group living.

Finally, social and animal phobias will differ with respect to their onset. Öhman et al. (1985) have argued that animal phobias will arise when humans become independent and explore their environment, because this is the appropriate time at which to learn the characteristics of a predator. Thus, animal phobias will show an onset during childhood. In contrast, social phobia arises as a result of the outcomes of dominance encounters. Because these begin during adolescence, social phobia will begin during this time.

EMPIRICAL INVESTIGATIONS

It is not our intention to review all of the literature that speaks to the predictions set out above. Rather, we focus upon the various studies conducted by others in the context of our own work.

Effects of Gender of the Conditioned Stimulus

Öhman et al. (1985) have argued that humans form male–male and female–female hierarchies, with the male hierarchy being dominant over the female hierarchy. If this is the case, then one can predict that the associations between both male and female angry faces and aversive outcomes will be "prepared" in females. For males, however, the association between angry male faces, but not female faces, and aversive outcomes will be "prepared." In their second study, Ohman and Dimberg (1978) reported that for angry faces, a male depicting anger (CS +) led to significant resistance to extinction, whereas a female face did not. This result held for both male and female subjects. Importantly, there was no effect of gender when happy male and female faces were employed as the CS + . However, Öhman and Dimberg pointed out that this pattern of results is also consistent with the view that the male pictures were better depicters of anger than were the female pictures.

We examined the effects of the gender of the CS in a study in which male and female subjects were exposed to pictures of males or females who exhibited angry and neutral facial expressions of emotion. In addition, half of the subjects were tested by a female experimenter and half by a male. The study employed a differential conditioning procedure, in which a picture of an individual who displayed an angry face was always followed by shocks[5] and a picture of a second individual was not. Both the skin conductance response (SCR) and a measure of US expectancy were employed as the dependent variables.[6]

The skin conductance measure provided the results of most interest. Figure 11.1 shows first-interval response (FIR) SCR magnitude during the habituation, acquisition, and extinction phases. There were no differences during the habituation phase. During acquisition, both male and female subjects acquired the discrimination. However, male subjects responded more strongly to slides of males who displayed anger than they did to females who displayed anger. Although female subjects exhibited greater differential responding than did males, this was not affected by the sex of the picture. There were no between-group differences during extinction.

These results are exactly as predicted by Öhman et al. (1985). Males appear to be more ready to associate an angry expression with an aversive outcome if the expression is displayed by a male rather than by a fe-

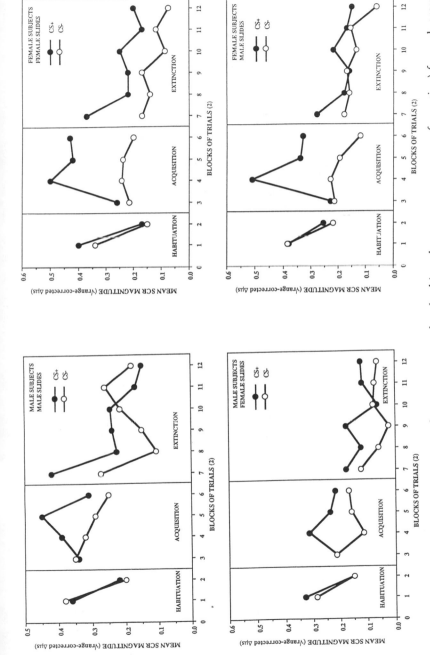

FIGURE 11.1 Mean SCR (FIR) magnitude (range-corrected and subjected to a square-root transformation) for each group during each phase. For all groups, a picture of a person displaying an angry face served as the CS +, and a picture of a different person displaying a neutral face served as the CS − .

male; females appear to be equally ready to associate angry faces displayed by both males and females with aversive outcomes. Note that these findings cannot be attributed to differences in encoding or decoding skills on the part of the sexes. First, the results cannot be attributed to differences in the ability of the two sexes to *encode* the facial expressions depicted, because male subjects differentiated between the male and female pictures, whereas female subjects did not. If the difference were in the pictures as exemplars of the emotions, the findings would have been the same for both sexes. Furthermore, the usual finding is that females are better encoders than males (Hall, 1978; Rosenthal, Hal, DiMatteo, Rogers, & Archer, 1979), and thus the encoding hypothesis would predict that responding would be greater to the female slides. Second, the results cannot be attributed to differences in *decoding* skills, in that females have been shown to be better decoders of facial expressions of emotion than males (Hall, 1978; Rosenthal et al., 1979). In the present case, the decoding hypothesis would predict a pattern of results opposite to that obtained.

Effects of Age of the Conditioned Stimulus

Öhman et al. (1985) have argued that social phobia originates as a result of dominance conflicts and that these conflicts begin in earnest during adolescence. If this is the case, it can be predicted that an association between the angry face of a prepubertal child and an aversive outcome will not be prepared in adult subjects. Although a child can certainly produce an angry facial expression of emotion, a child cannot engage in dominance encounters of the type envisaged by Öhman et al. Thus, an angry face shown by a child will not be seen by an adult as depicting a threat.

To test this prediction, we again employed a differential conditioning procedure. Male and female subjects were exposed to pictures of either male adults or prepubertal children exhibiting either angry or happy facial expressions of emotion. During the acquisition phase, a picture of one individual who displayed either an angry or a happy expression was followed by shock, and the picture of a second individual who displayed the other facial expression was not. Again, the SCR and a measure of US expectancy were employed as the dependent variables. Two of the groups viewed adults' faces, and two viewed children's faces. Within each of these, the angry face was paired with shock during acquisition in one group, and the happy face was paired with shock in another.

The SCR provided the data of most interest, and the mean FIR magnitude for the various groups are displayed for each phase of the experiment in Figure 11.2. There were no differences during the habituation phase as a function of the age of the individual who depicted the expres-

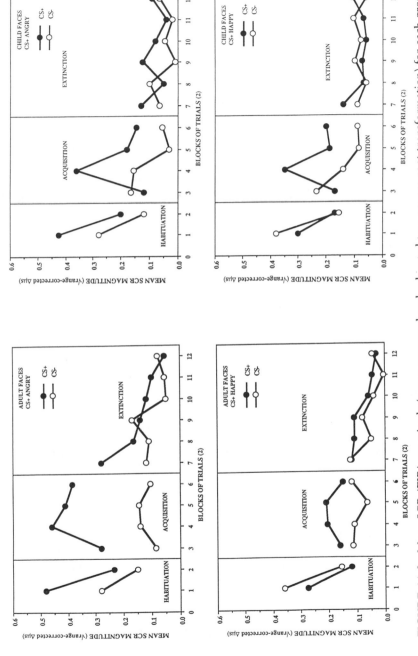

FIGURE 11.2. Mean SCR (FIR) magnitude (range-corrected and subjected to a square-root transformation) for each group during each phase. All groups observed pictures of one individual displaying an angry face and of a second displaying a happy face. For some subjects the angry face served as the CS+, and for others the happy face served as the CS+.

sion. When the angry picture was the CS + during acquisition, however, responses were significantly larger to the adults' than to the children's angry faces. There were no differences in the strength of discrimination when an adult male or a male child displaying a happy face was the CS +. Finally, subjects responded more vigorously to the CS + when it was an angry face than when it was a happy face. There were no between-group differences during extinction.

Again, the findings confirm predictions derived from Öhman et al.'s (1985) theorizing. Subjects exhibited larger SCRs to the CS + when it was an angry face than when it was a happy face. There were no differences in responding to the angry and happy CSs –. Importantly, the discrimination between CS + and CS – was stronger when the CS + was a male adult who displayed an angry face than when it was a male child who displayed an angry face. There were no differences as a function of age when a happy face was the CS +.

Our initial studies thus bear out predictions derived from Öhman et al.'s theorizing (1985) with respect to the gender and age of the individuals exhibiting the facial expressions of emotion that we employed as CSs. Furthermore, we have confirmed the basic finding that conditioning with an angry face as the CS + is more robust than is conditioning with a happy face as the CS +. Interestingly, we observed this effect as greater differentiation in responding to CS + and CS – during acquisition. Typically, Öhman and Dimberg (1978; Dimberg & Öhman, 1985) have reported greater resistance to extinction following conditioning with angry faces than with happy faces. They have not reported differences during acquisition.

Conditioning to the Individual or the Expression Exhibited

According to Dimberg and Öhman (Dimberg, 1986; Dimberg & Öhman, 1983), conditioning with facial expressions of emotion is not to the expression per se, but rather to the individual who displays the expression. They have argued that responding is then modulated by the facial expression exhibited. Given that the model is based on the role played by facial expressions of emotion in the formation of dominance hierarchies, this has to be the case. If a dominance hierarchy is to function properly, then individuals within the hierarchy have to know which individuals they are dominant over and to whom they should submit. The skill necessary for the formation of dominance hierarchies is therefore the ability to recognize individuals (Brown, 1975). Responding to these individuals is then modulated according to the facial expressions they exhibit at the time.

Dimberg (1986) examined the effects of changing the person who exhibited the expression from acquisition to extinction. He observed that a group that was switched from one individual who displayed an angry face in acquisition, to a different individual who displayed an angry face in extinction, exhibited little resistance to extinction. These data seem to suggest that subjects learned the characteristics of the individual through conditioning. If the subjects were changed from acquisition to extinction, then conditioning was lost.

There is a problem, however, with the experiments that examined the effects of changing the individual who exhibited the expression from acquisition to extinction. When subjects saw the same individual during both acquisition and extinction, they saw exactly the same picture. When subjects saw two different individuals who depicted the expressions, they necessarily saw two different pictures. It is standard practice in work on face recognition to employ different pictures of the same individual during training and test phases, in order to avoid the problem of "picture" rather than "face" learning (Bruce, 1988). A more appropriate control is to examine the effects of switching during extinction to a different individual who displays the same facial expression, in comparison with observing a different picture of the same person.

We carried out a pair of differential conditioning studies, in which three groups of subjects saw an individual who displayed an angry facial expression of emotion as the CS + and a second individual who displayed a happy facial expression of emotion as the CS –. During extinction, Group Same saw the same pictures of the two individuals displaying the same facial expressions; Group Different saw different pictures of the same individuals displaying the same facial expressions of emotion; and Group New saw pictures of two new individuals displaying anger or happiness. Dimberg and Öhman's theory would predict that Group Same would show the most resistance to extinction, followed by Group Different, and that these two groups would show significantly more resistance to extinction than Group New. As noted, we carried out two studies—one that employed the SCR and the measure of US expectancy as dependent variables, and a second that employed only the SCR. The SCR results were the same across the two studies; thus, only the FIR data from the first study are shown in Figure 11.3.

All three groups acquired differential conditioning, responding more to the angry CS + than to the happy CS-. However, there were no between-group differences either during acquisition or, more importantly, during extinction. Thus, Group New, which saw two new individuals displaying the facial expressions during extinction, displayed as much resistance to extinction as did Groups Same and Different, which saw the same individuals displaying the emotions during acquisition and extinction. If conditioning were to the individual depicting the expression, then Groups Same

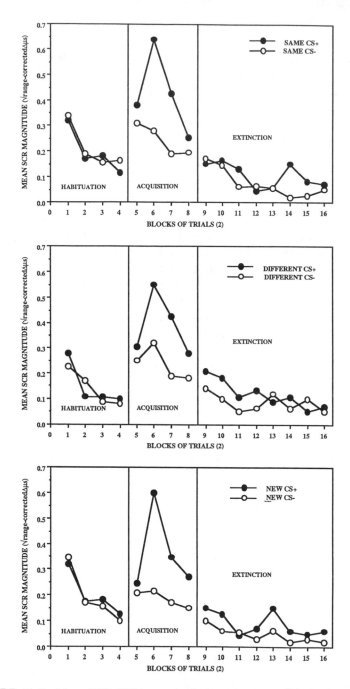

FIGURE 11.3. Mean SCR (FIR) magnitude (range-corrected and subected to a square-root transformation) for each group during each phase. For all groups, a picture of a person displaying an angry face served as the CS +, and a different person displaying a happy face served as the CS − . Group Same saw the same two pictures in acquisition and extinction; Group Different saw different pictures of the same individuals; Group New saw different individuals.

and Different should have displayed greater resistance to extinction than Group New. The fact that the three groups exhibited the same resistance to extinction suggests that conditioning is not to the person depicting the expression; rather, it is to the expression itself.

The work of Lanzetta and Orr (Lanzetta & Orr, 1980, 1981; Orr & Lanzetta, 1980, 1984) presents a further problem for the hypothesis that conditioning with facial expressions of emotion is to the individual who displays the expression[7] In their studies, Öhman and his colleagues have used a procedure in which a subject sees the same individual depicting the CS +, and a second individual depicting the CS −. In many studies, the expressions displayed by the two individuals are the same in order to control for sensitization. Thus, for any subject, the individual depicting the CS + and not the expression is the best predictor of the US. The Lanzetta and Orr (Lanzetta & Orr, 1980, 1981; Orr & Lanzetta, 1980, 1984) studies, however, employed pictures of several different individuals with each subject. Thus, the common element and the best predictor of the US was the expression. Despite this, they obtained more robust conditioning with facial expressions of fear than with neutral or happy facial expressions. In view of these findings, it is surely more parsimonious to conclude that the cue that best predicts the US is the one that acquires associative strength.

The Nature of the Unconditioned Stimulus

Öhman et al. (1985) have argued that the association between anger and an aversive outcome is prepared because of the association's pivotal role in the formation of dominance hierarchies. One way to test this assertion is to examine conditioning with facial expressions of emotion with aversive and nonaversive USs. Thus, Dimberg (1986) has argued that conditioning with an angry face and a nonaversive US will be less robust than conditioning with an angry face and an aversive US, because the former is a "contraprepared" association, whereas the latter is a "prepared" association. We (Packer, Clark, Bond, & Siddle, 1991) tested this assertion by examining conditioning with either angry or happy facial expressions of emotion and either an aversive US (electric shock) or a nonaversive US (reaction time to an imperative stimulus).

A differential conditioning procedure, in which half the subjects saw two pictures of adult males who displayed angry faces, was used. Half the subjects saw two pictures of adult males who displayed happy faces. Within each of these conditions, half the subjects were exposed to a shock US; for the other half, the US was a 1-second tone that served as a stimulus for a speeded motor response. The SCR served as the dependent variable.

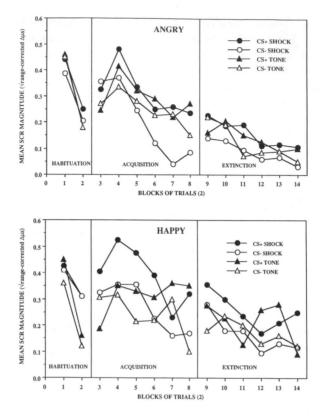

FIGURE 11.4. Mean SCR (SIR) magnitude (range-corrected and subjected to a square-root trannsformation) to the CS + and CS − during each phase of the experiment. The top half of the figure summarizes the data for those groups exposed to the angry facial expressions as the CSs; the bottom half summarizes the data for those groups exposed to the happy facial expressions. Reprinted from Packer et al. (1989). Journal of Psychophysiology, with permission.

In this particular study, the data from the second-interval response (SIR) provided a clearer picture of the outcome[8] As illustrated in Figure 11.4, all four groups acquired the discrimination, responding more to the CS + than to CS − . They also exhibited an orderly decline in responding during extinction, when the CS + was no longer followed by the US. However, there were no differences between the groups during either acquisition or extinction. Note that robust differential conditioning was obtained in the two groups that received the nonaversive US. Thus, any failure to obtain differences between the groups cannot be attributed to a failure of the nonaversive US to maintain responding.

ALTERNATIVE ACCOUNTS
OF THE "PREPAREDNESS" EFFECT

Latent Inhibition

We have described a number of studies that examined the preparedness account of social phobia. We obtained evidence consistent with the theory from studies that investigated the effects of the gender and age of the individuals who displayed the facial expressions of emotion employed as the CSs. In other studies, however, we obtained evidence appearing to be inconsistent with preparedness theory. Thus, we observed that resistance to extinction of the SCR was the same regardless of whether subjects saw the same pictures, different pictures of the same individuals, or pictures of different individuals. Contrary to a preparedness account, this implies that conditioning is to the expression and not to the individual. Moreover, we found that conditioning with angry and happy facial expressions of emotion was equally robust with an aversive US (shock) or a nonaversive US (reaction time to an imperative stimulus). Again, this result is at odds with preparedness theory, which predicts more robust conditioning when an angry expression is paired with shock than when an angry expression is paired with a nonaversive US.

Classical conditioning studies with human subjects have often employed pictures of geometric shapes as the conditioned stimuli. Although subjects are likely to have seen such shapes before taking part in an experiment, there is no particular reason why they should have seen one more than the other. However, the same cannot be said of facial expressions of emotion. Consider this: Is it likely that we see anger, fear, sadness, surprise, happiness, and disgust equally often? What if we are more likely to see happy faces than angry faces? If this is the case, we will have greater difficulty in associating a happy face with any stimulus, not just electric shock. The phenomenon whereby prior exposure to a stimulus retards subsequent conditioning is called "latent inhibition" (Lubow, 1973). Thus, the pattern of results reported by Öhman and Dimberg (1978; Dimberg & Öhman, 1983) and said to support the preparedness account of social phobia might well be attributable to differences in prior exposure to angry and happy faces.

Can these competing explanations be tested? First we need to determine whether there are differences in the frequency with which people see different facial expressions of emotion. To answer this question, we utilized methods derived from the social psychology literature. It is difficult to argue that any one of these methods indicates the "true" situation. However, the ordering of the various expressions was quite similar from one method to another, enabling us to make sensible choices about which stimuli to use for a conditioning study. Data were obtained in six different ways:

1. Subjects were asked to indicate the last time that they had seen each of Ekman and Friesen's (1975) primary facial expressions of emotion.
2. Subjects were asked to indicate which facial expression of emotion they thought was the most frequently displayed, and so on down the list.
3. Subjects were asked to take a scoring sheet, go to a shopping center, observe each time an emotion was displayed, and tally the emotions displayed over a 30-minute period. Subjects were instructed not to intrude in any way.
4. Subjects were asked to take a scoring sheet, go to the University Union, observe each time an emotion was displayed, and tally the emotions displayed over a 30-minute period.
5. Subjects were asked to take a scoring sheet and carry out the exercise at home (e.g., during a meal, observing each time an emotion was displayed and tallying the emotions displayed over a 30-minute period).
6. We asked subjects to go through a newspaper each day for a week and to note the number of times each expression appeared, including advertisements.

The results (see Table 11.1) indicated that happy facial expressions were seen more frequently than expressions of any other emotion, regardless of the way the data were acquired. Most importantly, these were seen more frequently than were angry expressions. Thus, the latent-inhibition hypothesis provides a viable explanation of the results obtained by Öhman and Dimberg (1979; Dimberg & Öhman, 1983). However, a crucial test of the preparedness and latent-inhibition hypotheses is to select an expression that is seen even less frequently than anger and to employ that expression in a conditioning study. If the preparedness hypothesis is correct, anger will show greater resistance to extinction following conditioning with an aversive stimulus such as electric shock. In contrast, if the latent-inhibition hypothesis is correct, then the expression seen less frequently than anger will show the greatest resistance to extinction. What expression should one choose? The obvious one is fear. However, we have already seen that there are studies indicating that conditioning with fear exhibits greater resistance to extinction than does conditioning with a happy face. Thus, it seemed appropriate to choose a different emotion for this test. Furthermore, we decided to employ an emotion that was not obviously negative in the way that fear, sadness, and disgust are so per-

TABLE 11.1. Rank Order of Frequency of Occurrence of Different Facial Expressions of Emotion across Different Sampling Situations

Situation	Emotion					
	Happiness	Anger	Surprise	Sadness	Disgust	Fear
Last seen	1	2	3	4	5	6
Expected	1	2	4	3	5	6
Shops	1	3	5	2	4	6
Home	1	2	3	4	5	6
Campus	1	4	2.5	2.5	5	6
Magazines	1	3	4	2	6	5

ceived. Thus, we chose surprise as the facial expression that is seen less frequently than anger.[9]

There were three groups of subjects in this differential conditioning study. During the conditioning phase, one group saw an angry face followed by shock; a second group saw a happy face followed by shock; and the third group saw a face displaying surprise followed by the shock. All three groups also saw a neutral face that was not followed by shock. The SCR and the measure of US expectancy were employed as the dependent variables. At the end of the experiment, we checked that each subject was able to state the emotion depicted in the slides he or she had viewed during the study. All were able to do so correctly.

The results for the FIR are shown in Figure 11.5a. All three groups acquired the discrimination, responding more to the CS + than to CS − . Most importantly, there were no differences among them. The extinction phase was the most important phase of the experiment. It was here that Öhman and Dimberg (1978; Dimberg & Öhman, 1983) normally observed the effects of preparedness. Inspection of Figure 11.5a indicates that there was little resistance to extinction in the group for whom the CS + was a happy face. There appeared to be somewhat more in the group for whom the CS + was an angry face. However, the greatest resistance to extinction was seen in the group for whom the CS + was a surprised face. Indeed, this effect was significantly greater than that observed in the angry group. Thus, the skin conductance data clearly indicate that the greatest resistance to extinction is associated with the stimulus that is seen least frequently in everyday situations. The results are consistent with the latent-inhibition hypothesis and are contrary to predictions derived from the preparedness hypothesis.

The expectancy data are illustrated in Figure 11.5b. Note that the vertical axis ranges from − 20 ("certain that shock will not occur") to + 20 ("certain that shock is about to occur"). During acquisition, subjects in each of the three groups displayed an increase in the expectancy that the

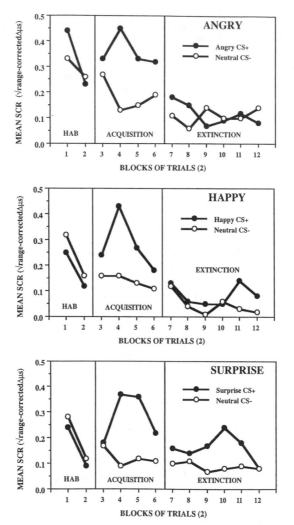

FIGURE 11.5(a). Mean SCR (FIR) magnitude (range-corrected and subjected to a square-root tranformation) to the CS + and CS − during each phase of the experiment. Responding to the CS + is indicated by the filled circles, and responding to the CS − by the open circles. (b) Mean US expectancy scores to the CS + and CS − during both acquisition and extinction. Responding to the CS + is indicated by the filled circles, and responding to the CS − by the open circles.

CS + was followed by shock and an increase in the expectancy that the CS − , the neutral face, would not be followed by shock. Importantly, there were no differences among the three groups in the acquisition of these expectancies.

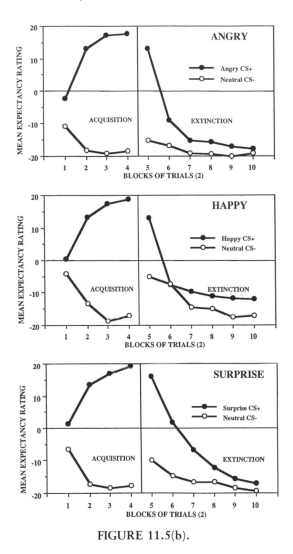

FIGURE 11.5(b).

Again, the most important data came from the extinction phase. Ex-amination of Figure 11.5b reveals that all three groups showed a decline in the expectancy that the CS + would be followed by shock. Important-ly, however, there were differences among the groups in the rate at which the expectancy declined. As shown in Figure 11.5b, the group that saw the surprised face showed the slowest decline (or, to put it another way, the greatest resistance to extinction of the expectancy), with the group seeing the angry face second, and the one seeing the happy face third. Like the skin conductance data, the expectancy data support the latent-inhibition view. The emotion that is viewed least frequently in everyday situations (surprise) is the one that shows the greatest resistance to extinction; the emotion that is seen most frequently in everyday situations (happiness) shows the least resistance to extinction.

Thus, both the autonomic measure and the expectancy measure provided data supporting the latent-inhibition hypothesis. Indeed, the basic preparedness effect can be accounted for parsimoniously by the latent-inhibition hypothesis, together with other well-established principles of associative learning. For example, the latent-inhibition account argues that because of less prior exposure, an angry facial expression is a more salient CS + than a happy facial expression, and thus leads to more rapid conditioning (Rescorla & Wagner, 1972). Similarly, Lanzetta and Orr, (Lanzetta & Orr, 1980, 1981; Orr & Lanzetta, 1980, 1984) have reported faster acquisition and greater resistance to extinction after conditioning with a picture of a face depicting fear. Öhman and his colleagues (Öhman et al., 1985) mention these data as supporting preparedness theory, although it is not clear why. In contrast, the latent-inhibition hypothesis predicts that fear will condition readily and exhibit greater resistance to extinction, because it is the emotion that is seen least frequently in everyday situations (see Table 11.1.)

A number of authors have suggested that the preparedness effects reported by Öhman and his colleagues may have resulted from subjects' prior experiences with the stimuli employed (Carr, 1979; Delprato, 1980). The latent-inhibition hypothesis provides an explicit account of the effects of such experiences on subsequent conditioning.

Selective Sensitization

We (Lovibond, Siddle, & Bond, 1993) have investigated another explanation of the preparedness effect — selective sensitization. We took as our starting point an observation by Öhman, Eriksson, Fredriksson, Hugdahl, and Ölofsson (1974) that fear-relevant stimuli elicited larger electrodermal responses than did fear-irrelevant stimuli prior to conditioning. Responding to all stimuli increased with the threat of shock, but increased more with fear-relevant events. The increase in responding is termed "sensitization" and the differential increase "selective sensitization." In our first experiment, we demonstrated that selective sensitization to a fear-relevant stimulus was attenuated when that stimulus served as a CS − . The results of the second study showed that selective sensitization was maintained to a fear-relevant stimulus that served as a CS + , and failed to demonstrate any evidence for greater resistance to extinction for the fear-relevant CS + . The effects in Experiment 2 were shown in both electrodermal and

US expectancy measures, whereas only the skin conductance data revealed the effects in Experiment 1.

In discussing these data, we (Lovibond et al., 1993) considered two possible accounts. The first was couched in terms of covariation bias (Alloy & Tabachnik, 1984; Davey, 1992) and Davey's expectancy model of fear, based on an integration of covariation bias and current concepts of human conditioning. Essentially, the argument is that prior learning leads subjects to overestimate the association between fear-relevant stimuli and aversive outcomes, leading to stronger expectancy judgments in the case of fear-relevant stimuli (Lovibond et al., 1993, Experiment 2). However, covariation bias may be overridden when subjects learn that a fear-relevant stimulus is relatively safe (Lovibond et al., 1993, Experiment 1). The second approach we discussed attributes selective sensitization to a property of fear-relevant stimuli that does not involve anticipation of an aversive outcome. In this case, selective sensitization occurs when the latent properties of fear relevant stimuli are activated by a state of fear. In order to account for the effects of fear relevance on US expectancy ratings, we argued that the increment in expectancy associated with fear-relevant stimuli derives not from heightened appraisal of the aversive outcome, but from heightened experience of fear during the stimulus. In this connection, Öhman (Chapter 10, this volume) and Öhman and Soares (1993) have reported data from studies in which conscious identification of stimuli was prevented by backward masking. The data indicate that even under masked conditions, responding to fear-relevant stimuli was elevated during extinction.

How might the explanations we offered (Lovibond et al., 1993) be integrated with the explanation offered earlier in terms of prior exposure? These two accounts leave open the reasons for covariation bias and/or the fear-eliciting properties of the stimulus. As noted previously, there is considerable evidence indicating that novel stimuli are more likely to elicit fear than familiar stimuli are (Carr, 1979). Given that this is the case, then subjects come to the typical conditioning experiment with the knowledge that one type of stimulus has been encountered frequently (e.g., the typical "nonprepared" stimulus, such as a picture of a flower or a house). In contrast, the second type of stimulus has been encountered only rarely (e.g., the typical "prepared" stimulus, such as a picture of a snake or a spider). Thus, the pairing of the "prepared" stimulus with an aversive outcome is likely to be of greater moment to the subject than the pairing of the "nonprepared" stimulus with the aversive outcome, because subjects have fewer expectations about the former stimulus than the latter (Alloy & Tabachnik, 1984).

A similar explanation can be provided for the selective sensitization effect we reported (Lovibond et al., 1993). As indicated above, novelty is associated with fear. If two novel stimuli (e.g., a spider and a snake) are presented as in the typical differential conditioning study (one paired with an aversive outcome and one unpaired), then selective sensitization occurs to the stimulus paired with the aversive outcome, because the fear based upon novelty of the stimulus is prevented from declining by its pairing with the aversive outcome and summates with the conditioned fear that results from the pairing. In contrast, subjects exhibit a decline in fear to the stimulus that is unpaired because of continued exposure and the lack of an aversive outcome. If "nonprepared" stimuli are used, then there is no novelty-based fear to such stimuli, and thus any effects are attributable solely to conditioned fear.

The focus of the present chapter has been on the preparedness theory of social phobia. However, the latent-inhibition hypothesis can account for many of the data supporting the preparedness account of small-animal phobias. Furthermore, the phenomenon of latent inhibition provides a technique for "immunizing" individuals against the adverse effects of conditioning episodes (e.g., visits to the dentist; Siddle & Remington, 1987). Importantly, in the present context, a knowledge of conditioning remains important to our understanding of the acquisition and removal of both social and small-animal phobias.

NOTES

1. The Mineka (1987) data may need to be re-evaluated. Recently, Masataka (1993) reported a study in which three groups of female squirrel monkeys were exposed to real, toy, and model snakes. One of the groups had been captured from the wild; the other two were laboratory-reared. The latter two groups differed in that one group was fed live grasshoppers in addition to fruit and monkey chow, whereas the second group was fed only fruit and monkey chow. The wild-reared group displayed an intense fear response to the snake-like stimuli, whereas the laboratory monkeys reared only on fruit and chow showed no fear, replicating the Mineka (1987) data. However, the laboratory-bred group that received live grasshoppers in its diet, in addition to fruit and monkey chow, displayed as strong a fear reaction to the snake-like stimuli as the wild-bred monkeys did. This outcome suggests that experience with live prey leads laboratory-bred monkeys to fear snakes, despite the fact that they have had no previous experience with them.

2. In fact, Öhman (e.g., Öhman, 1986, 1992, 1993; Öhman & Soares, 1993) has extended his theorizing to combine notions of biological preparedness with recent conceptions of human information processing. The essentials of this functional evolutionary approach is that threat- or fear-relevant stimuli are capable of activating emotional structures after only preattentive analysis, the output of which is not available in consciousness. We do not analyze this theoretical development here, as it is covered extensively by Öhman in Chapter 10 of this volume.

3. Öhman et al. (1985) used gorillas and chimpanzees as their model for the formation of hierarchies in humans, presumably on the basis of close genetic relationship. However, most ethologists would argue that similarity of ecological context is a better predictor of similarities in behavior (Krebs & Davies, 1987). Interestingly, such an approach would actually strengthen the argument. Thus, of modern-day primates, baboons are regarded as occupying an ecological niche similar to that of early hominids (Barash, 1982). Baboons form hierarchies of the sort that Öhman et al. argue is found in modern humans, whereas chimpanzees and gorillas do not (Goodall, 1985).

4. This is a sweeping generalization. In fact, the respective status of male and female hierarchies is determined by the nature of the group structure, which is determined in turn by ecological context. Nevertheless, this is an explicit prediction of the theory and one that we have tested.

5. In all of the experiments where electric shock was employed as the US, there was a work-up procedure during which subjects indicated the level at which the shock first became "uncomfortable, but not painful." This level was then employed throughout the rest of the study, unless a subject requested that it be turned down while the study was in progress.

6. Expectancy of shock was measured by the use of a dial fitted on the right arm of the subject's chair. The dial moved across 180 degrees from the extreme left ("certain no shock") through "uncertain" to the extreme right ("certain shock"). Expectancy was recorded on each trial in terms of pen position (-20 to $+20$) 500 milliseconds prior to US onset (Siddle, Power, Bond, & Lovibond, 1988).

7. Öhman and Dimberg have focused upon neutral, angry, or happy facial expressions of emotion. However, Lanzetta and Orr (Lanzetta & Orr, 1980, 1981; Orr & Lanzetta, 1980, 1984) have reported that conditioning with facial expressions of fear and a shock US is acquired more quickly and is more resistant to extinction than conditioning with a neutral stimulus (e.g., a tone) or with another facial expression of emotion (e.g., happy or neutral). Öhman et al. (1985) have taken these findings as providing support for the "preparedness" account of social phobia. However, if an angry face directed at the subject is perceived as a threat and is therefore associated with greater resistance to extinction, why should a fearful face directed at the subject lead to more robust acquisition and greater resistance to extinction? In the latter case, it might be argued that the fearful face is an indication not of threat, but of victory on the part of the subject. If this is the case, it is difficult to see why such robust conditioning should be obtained with a fearful facial expression.

8. The outcomes for the FIR and SIR were the same. However, the latter were clearer pictorially.

9. Of course, a surprise can be positive or negative. One can be happily surprised by a letter from a friend, or fearfully surprised by an intruder on a dark night. For the present purposes, this ambiguity was deemed better than the obviously negative concomitants of the other possibilities.

REFERENCES

Agras, W. S., Sylvester, D., & Oliveau, D. (1969). The epidemiology of common fears and phobias. *Comprehensive Psychiatry, 10,* 151–156.

Alloy, L. G., & Tabachnik, N. (1984). Assessment of covariation by humans and animals: The joint influence of prior expectations and current situational information. *Psychological Review, 91,* 112–149.

Barash, D. P. (1982). *Sociobiology and behavior.* New York: Elsevier.

Bolles, R. C. (1970). Species-specific avoidance reactions and avoidance learning. *Psychological Review, 77,* 32–48.

Bond, N. W., & Siddle, D. A. T. (1988). Human Pavlovian conditioning: Commentaries. *Biological Psychology, 27,* 185–191.

Brown, J. L. (1975). *The Evolution of Behavior.* New York: Norton.

Bruce, V. (1988). *Recognizing Faces.* Hillsdale, NJ: Erlbaum.

Carr, A. T. (1979). The psychopathology of fear. In W. Sluckin (Ed.), *Fear in animals and man* (pp. 199–235). New York: Van Nostrand Reinhold.

Costello, C. G. (1982). Fears and phobias in women: A community study. *Journal of Abnormal Psychology, 91,* 280–286.

Davey, G. C. L. (1992). An expectancy model of laboratory preparedness effects. *Journal of Experimental Psychology: General, 121,* 24–40.

Delprato, D. J. (1980). Hereditary determinants of fears and phobias: A critical review. *Behavior Therapy, 11,* 79–103.

Dimberg, U. (1986). Facial expressions as excitatory and inhibitory stimuli for conditioned autonomic responses. *Biological Psychology, 22,* 37–57.

Dimberg, U., & Öhman, A. (1983). The effects of directional facial cues on electrodermal conditioning to facial stimuli. *Psychophysiology, 20,* 160–167.

Ekman, P., & Friesen, W. V. (1975). *Unmasking the Face.* Englewood Cliffs, NJ: Prentice-Hall.

Garcia, J., & Koelling, R. A. (1966). Relation of cue to consequence in avoidance learning. *Psychonomic Science, 4,* 123–124.

Goodall, J. (1985). *The chimpanzees of Gombe: Patterns of behavior.* Cambridge, MA: Harvard University Press.

Hall, J. (1978). Gender effects in decoding nonverbal cues. *Psychological Bulletin, 85,* 845–857.

Harris, B. (1979). Whatever happened to little Albert? *American Psychologist, 34,* 151–160.

Krebs, J. R., & Davies, N. B. (1987). *An introduction to behavioral ecology.* Sunderland, MA: Sinauer.

Lanzetta, J. T., & Orr, S. P. (1980). Influence of facial expressions on the classical conditioning of fear. *Journal of Personality and Social Psychology, 39,* 1081–1087.

Lanzetta, J. T., & Orr, S. P. (1981). Stimulus properties of facial expressions on the classical conditioning of fear. *Motivation and Emotion, 5,* 225–234.

Lorenz, K. Z. (1966). *On aggression.* New York: Harcourt, Brace & World.

Lovibond, P. F., Siddle, D. A. T., & Bond, N. W. (1993). Resistance to extinction of fear-relevant stimuli: Preparedness or selective sensitization? *Journal of Experimental Psychology: General, 122,* 449–461.

Lubow, R. E. (1973). Latent inhibition. *Psychological Bulletin, 79,* 398–407.

Marks, I. M. (1969). *Fears and phobias.* New York: Academic Press.

Marks, I. M. (1987). *Fears, phobias, and rituals: Panic, anxiety, and their disorders.* New York: Oxford University Press.

Masataka, N. (1993). Effects of experience with live insects on the development of fear of snakes in squirrel monkeys, *Saimiri sciureus*. *Animal Behaviour, 46*, 741–746.

Mayr, E. (1974). Behavior programs and evolutionary strategies. *American Scientist, 62*, 650–659.

Mineka, S. (1987). A primate model of phobic fears. In H. J. Eysenck & I. Martin (Eds.), *Theoretical Foundations of Behavior Therapy* (pp. 81–111). New York: Plenum Press.

Öhman, A. (1986). Face the beast and fear the face: Animal and social fears as prototypes for evolutionary analyses of emotion. *Psychophysiology, 23*, 123–145.

Öhman, A. (1992). Orienting and attention: Preferred preattentive processing of potentially phobic stimuli. In B. A. Campbell, H. Hayne, & R. Richardson (Eds.), *Attention and information processing in infants and adults: Perspectives from human and animal research* (pp. 263–295). Hillsdale, NJ: Erlbaum.

Öhman, A. (1993). Fear and anxiety as emotional phenomena: Clinical phenomenology, evolutionary perspectives, and information-processing mechanisms. In M. Lewis & J. M. Haviland (Eds.), *Handbook of emotions* (pp. 511–536). New York: Guilford Press.

Öhman, A., & Dimberg, U. (1978). Facial expressions as conditioned stimuli for electrodermal responses: A case of "preparedness"? *Journal of Personality and Social Psychology, 36*, 1251–1258.

Öhman, A., Dimberg, U., & Öst, L.-G. (1985). Animal and social phobias: Biological constraints on learned fear responses. In S. Reiss & R. R. Bootzin (Eds.), *Theoretical issues in behavior therapy* (pp. 123–175). New York: Academic Press.

Öhman, A. Eriksson, A., Fredrikson, M., Hugdahl, K., & Olofsson, C. (1974). Habituation of the electrodermal orienting reaction to potentially phobic and supposedly neutral stimuli in normal human subjects. *Biological Psychology, 2*, 85–93.

Öhman, A., & Soares, J. J. F. (1993). On the automaticity of fear: Conditioned skin conductance responses to masked phobic stimuli. *Journal of Abnormal Psychology, 102*, 121–132.

Orr, S. P., & Lanzetta, J. T. (1980). Facial expressions of emotion as conditioned stimuli for human autonomic responses. *Journal of Personality and Social Psychology, 38*, 278–282.

Orr, S. P., & Lanzetta, J. T. (1984). Extinction of an emotional response in the presence of facial expressions of emotion. *Motivation and Emotion, 8*, 55–66.

Packer, J. S., Bond, N. W., & Siddle, D. A. T. (1987). Animal fears in the Antipodes: Normative data from an Australian sample. *Scandinavian Journal of Psychology, 28*, 150–156.

Packer, J. S., Clark, B. M., Bond, N. W., & Siddle, D. A. T. (1991). Conditioning with facial expressions of emotion: A comparison of aversive and nonaversive unconditioned stimuli. *Journal of Psychophysiology, 5*, 79–88.

Rachman, S. (1977). The conditioning theory of fear-acquisition: A critical examination. *Behaviour Research and Therapy, 15,* 375–387.

Rescorla, R. W., & Wagner, A. R. (1972). A theory of Pavlovian conditioning: Variations in the effectiveness of reinforcement and non-reinforcement. In A. H. Black & W. F. Prokasy (Eds.), *Classical Conditioning II: Current research and theory.* New York: Appleton-Century-Crofts.

Rosenthal, R., Hall, J. A., Di Matteo, M. R., Rogers, P. L., & Archer, D. (1979). *Sensitivity to non-verbal communications: The PONS test.* Baltimore, MD: The Johns Hopkins University Press.

Schwartz, B. (1974). On going back to nature: A review of Seligman and Hager's "Biological boundaries of learning". *Journal of the Experimental Analysis of Behavior, 21,* 183–198.

Seligman, M. E. P. (1970). On the generality of the laws of learning. *Psychological Review, 77,* 406–418.

Seligman, M. E. P. (1971). Phobias and preparedness. *Behavior Therapy, 2,* 307–320.

Shiffrin, R. M., & Schneider, W. (1977). Controlled and automatic human information processing: II. Perceptual learning, automatic attending, and a general theory. *Psychological Review, 84,* 127–190.

Siddle, D. A. T., & Bond, N. W. (1988). Avoidance learning, Pavlovian conditioning, and the development of phobias. *Biological Psychology, 27,* 167–183.

Siddle, D. A. T., Power, K., Bond, N. W., & Lovibund, P. (1988). Effects of stimulus content and postacquisition devaluation of the unconditioned stimulus on retention of human electrodermal conditioning. *Australian Journal of Psychology, 40,* 179–193.

Siddle, D. A. T., & Remington, R. E. (1987). Latent inhibition and human Pavlovian conditioning: Research and relevance. In G. Davey (Ed.), *Cognitive processes and Pavlovian conditioning in humans* (pp. 115–146). Chichester, England: Wiley.

Smith, J. C., & Roll, D. L. (1967). Trace conditioning with X-rays as an aversive stimulus. *Psychonomic Science, 9,* 11–12.

Terrace, H. S. (1979). *Nim.* New York: Knopf.

Thorndike, E. L. (1911). *Animal intelligence: Experimental studies.* New York: Macmillan.

Torgersen, S. (1979). The nature and origin of common phobic fears. *British Journal of Psychiatry, 134,* 343–351.

Watson, J. B. (1924). *Behaviorism.* New York: Norton.

Watson, J. B. & Rayner, R. (1920). Conditioned emotional reactions. *Journal of Experimental Psychology, 3,* 1–14.

Outcome and Mechanisms in the Evolution of Phobias: Surprise, Latent Inhibition, and the Status of the Preparedness Hypothesis

Arne Öhman

THERE IS AN IMPORTANT DISTINCTION between "outcome" and "mechanism" in evolutionary biology. "Outcome" refers to an adaptive relation between environment and organism that evolution has selected for (e.g., with regard to a particular functional response, given a specific stimulus context). The evolutionary pressures resulting in the adaptive outcome provides the *ultimate* explanation for the particular behavior under interest. This outcome, however, can be achieved by diverse underlying mechanisms that provide its *proximate* explanation. A given outcome does not necessarily imply a unitary and specific underlying mechanism.

The distinction between outcome and mechanisms has often been overlooked in the subsequent discussion of Seligman's (1971) preparedness theory of phobias. At the basic level, the theory actually involved two partly independent propositions. First, it suggested that human phobias reflect evolutionary constraints, with avoidance as the important adaptive outcome. Phobias, therefore, were viewed as vehicles for keeping persons away from potentially lethal circumstances. Second, Seligman suggested that these constraints operate through one exclusive mechanism, that of selective associations or prepared Pavlovian conditioning (Seligman, 1970). It is important to recognize that these two propositions are partly independent. For example, fears and phobias may be constrained by evolution, but the constraints may operate through other mechanisms than, or mechanisms in addition to, associative learning. In this case, the first proposition is correct but the second proposition is false.

Indeed, evolution is likely to be opportunistic rather than exclusive. It may be adaptive to achieve the evolutionarily desired outcome, avoidance, through different and not mutually exclusive mechanisms. Thus, showing that alternative mechanisms such as latent inhibition (Bond & Siddle, Chapter 11, this volume) or selective sensitization (Lovibond, Siddle, & Bond, 1993) contribute to enhanced responding to biologically fear-relevant stimuli does not necessarily exclude prepared Pavlovian conditioning as another contributor. Moreover, even if it could be conclusively demonstrated that enhanced resistance to extinction to fear-relevant stimuli is *not* attributable to prepared associations, this does not exclude an important role for evolutionary constraints in human phobias.

Bond and Siddle's chapter provides one set of data that is broadly consistent with the first proposition of Seligman's (1971) preparedness theory as my colleagues and I have elaborated it (Öhman, Dimberg, & Öst, 1985). Thus, the demonstrations that the gender and the age of the stimulus person are important for conditioning to facial stimuli support the evolutionary speculations we have offered (Öhman et al., 1985). The other set of data presented by Bond and Siddle, however, challenges the second assumption of Seligman's preparedness theory—namely, that the effect of stimulus content is mediated exclusively through prepared Pavlovian conditioning. To account for their findings, Bond and Siddle propose that differential latent inhibition (i.e., prior nonreinforced exposure to the conditioned stimulus [CS]) is the critical factor explaining the potency of biologically fear-relevant stimuli for human aversive conditioning. Thus, they acknowledge no role for phylogenetic factors in the enhanced associability between, for instance, angry faces and aversive outcomes, which I have documented in Chapter 10 of this volume. Rather, they claim that the effect can be attributed to an ontogenetic effect in terms of differential prior exposure to different types of stimuli.

I have previously argued that latent inhibition and learned irrelevance—that is, random prior exposure to potentially phobic and aversive stimuli (e.g., Baker, 1976)—may be instrumental in immunizing people to phobias (Öhman, 1987). Bond and Siddle take this argument a significant step further by examining both the prevalence of potentially phobic stimuli in the natural environment, and laboratory conditioning to environmentally more or less prevalent stimuli.

Bond and Siddle have employed several methods to assess the relative prevalence of various facial expressions in the environment of the population they have used for their experiments: college students. They find comfort in the convergence of all these different methods in suggesting that angry faces are encountered more seldom than happy faces. However, all these methods suffer from the same flaw: Relative prevalence of a stimulus is a conceptually invalid measure of latent inhibition. Laboratory demonstrations of latent inhibition make sure that prior exposure to the CS-to-be is not confounded with differences in prior exposures to the unconditioned stimulus (US) or with contingent CS-US presentations. However, this requirement is hard to deal with in the natural environment. Indeed, one could argue that aversive outcomes (angry interactions, guilt, fear, etc.) are "significantly unlikely" following facial expressions of happiness, and "significantly likely" following expressions of anger. Thus, there is reason to suspect that the measure of latent inhibition used by Bond and Siddle can be reduced to the familiar formula of "prior conditioning experience" (e.g., Delprato, 1980). This version of the prior-exposure hypothesis, however, is conclusively refuted by Mineka's (1993) data on vicarious conditioning in monkeys. The hypothesis of differential prior conditioning suggests that human subjects enter the preparedness research laboratory with happy faces as conditioned inhibitors, and with angry faces as excitatory CSs with regard to fear and aversiveness. This is the primary reason to require discrimination between two angry faces as compared to discrimination between two happy faces in the standard facial version of the preparedness paradigm (e.g., Öhman & Dimberg, 1978). Nevertheless, subjects typically acquire a stronger (Bond & Siddle, Chapter 11, this volume), more persistent (see reviews by Öhman, 1993; Öhman & Dimberg, 1984), and less cognitively controlled (Pitman & Orr, 1986) differential skin conductance response to angry than to happy faces, in spite of the predicted lower efficacy of an expected as compared to an unexpected US (Rescorla & Wagner, 1972).

But what about surprised faces? Indeed, Bond and Siddle report an exciting and potentially crucial observation from the experiment where aversive skin conductance conditioning was compared among groups having happy, angry and surprised faces as CSs. Surprised faces, it appears, are undecided with regard to outcome aversiveness. Basically, surprise follows from violated expectancies. Violated expectancies are intimately connected to the disruption of plans, which has been regarded as the primary antecedent condition for anxiety (Mandler, 1975). On the other hand, violated expectancy is an important ingredient in humour and the elicitation of laughter. Surprise, therefore, is a transient state that can be channelled into emotions of widely different valence. According to the data presented by Bond and Siddle, surprised faces appear to be highly effective stimuli for aversive skin conductance conditioning. This is certainly in agreement with the latent-inhibition hypothesis, but alternative interpretations spring readily to mind.

From a functional evolutionary perspective, surprise can be interpreted as an alert-and-alarm response to interrupt ongoing activity and focus attention on an unexpected event, much like the orienting response (e.g., Donchin, 1981; Öhman, 1979). Surprise has been described as a "channel-clearing emotion" (Tomkins, 1962), the primary function of which "is to help prepare the individual to deal effectively with the new or sudden event and with the consequences of this event" (Izard, 1991, p. 180). From this perspective, it is not surprising (sic!) that a facial expression of surprise is an effective CS, particularly for the skin conductance response, which is especially sensitive to violated expectancies (e.g., Grings, 1960).

Thus, the latent-inhibition hypothesis appears to be hampered by conceptual obscurity, and the data presented in its favor are open to alternative interpretations. Similar things can be said about other recently presented alternatives to the preparedness theory, such as Davey's (1992, 1995) biased-expectancy account (Öhman, 1995). Nevertheless, these accounts all point to a crucial weakness that the preparedness hypothesis shares with many other evolutionarily based hypotheses: the lack of a tight conceptual specification that allows crucial empirical tests. As shown in this commentary, the evolutionary framework is rich in generating new and alternative hypotheses, but it is often hard to narrow them down to strong formulations that can be confronted with critical data. In this respect, the development of preparedness theory into the realm of unconscious information processing as described in Chapter 10 provides an important additional step. The set of data reported there suggest that biologically fear-relevant stimuli have some peculiar and consistent effects that make sense in a functional-evolutionary perspective. Furthermore, the masking methodology will allow crucial tests of the evolutionary perspective — for example, by examining the resilience to masking of responses conditioned to ontogenetically fear-relevant stimuli such as pointed guns (e.g., Hugdahl & Johnsen, 1989).

REFERENCES

Baker, A. G. (1976). Learned irrelevance and learned helplessness: Rats learn that stimuli, reinforcers, and responses are uncorrelated. *Journal of Experimental Psychology: Animal Behavior Processes, 2,* 130–141.

Davey, G. C. L. (1992). An expectancy model of laboratory preparedness effects. *Journal of Experimental Psychology: General, 121,* 24–40.

Davey, G. C. L. (1995). Preparedness and phobias: Specific evolved associations or a generalized expectancy bias? *Behavioral and Brain Sciences.*

Delprato, D. J. (1980). Hereditary determinants of fears and phobias: A critical review. *Behavior Therapy, 11,* 79–103.

Donchin, E. (1981). Surprise! . . . Surprise? *Psychophysiology, 18,* 493–513.

Grings, W. W. (1960). Preparatory set variables related to classical conditioning of autonomic responses. *Psychological Review, 67,* 243–252.

Hugdahl, K., & Johnsen, B. H. (1989). Preparedness and electrodermal fear-conditioning: Ontogenetic vs. phylogenetic explanations. *Behaviour Research and Therapy, 27,* 269–278.

Izard, C. E. (1991). *The psychology of emotions.* New York: Plenum Press.

Lovibond, P. F., Siddle, D. A. T., & Bond, N. W. (1993). Resistance to extinction of fear-relevant stimuli: Preparedness or selective sensitization? *Journal of Experimental Psychology: General, 122,* 449–461.

Mandler, G. (1975). *Mind and emotion.* New York: Wiley.

Mineka, S. (1992). Evolutionary memories, emotional processing, and the emotional disorders. In D. Medin (Ed.), *The psychology of learning and motivation* (Vol. 28, pp. 161–206). New York: Academic Press.

Öhman, A. (1979). The orienting response, attention, and learning: An information processing perspective. In H. D. Kimmel, E. H. van Olst, & J. F. Orlebeke (Eds.), *The orienting reflex in humans* (pp. 443–472). Hillsdale, NJ: Erlbaum.

Öhman, A. (1987). Evolution, learning, and phobias: An interactional analysis. In D. Magnusson & A. Öhman (Eds.), *Psychopathology: An interactional perspective* (pp. 143–158). Orlando, FL: Academic Press.

Öhman, A. (1993). Stimulus prepotency and fear: Data and theory. In N. Birbaumer & A. Öhman (Eds.), *The organization of emotion: Cognitive, clinical and psychophysiological perspectives* (pp. 218–239). Toronto: Hogrefe.

Öhman, A. (1995). Eggs in more than one basket: Mediating mechanisms between evolution and phobias. *Behavioral and Brain Sciences.*

Öhman, A., & Dimberg, U. (1978). Facial expressions as conditioned stimuli for electrodermal responses: A case of preparedness? *Journal of Personality and Social Psychology, 36,* 1251–1258.

Öhman, A., Dimberg, U. (1984). An evolutionary perspective on human social behavior. In W. M. Waid (Ed.), *Sociophysiology* (pp. 47–86). New York: Springer-Verlag.

Öhman, A., Dimberg, U., & Öst, L.-G. (1985). Animal and social phobias: Biological constraints on learned fear responses. In S. Reiss & R. R. Bootzin (Eds.), *Theoretical issues in behavior therapy* (pp. 123–178). New York: Academic Press.

Pitman, R. K., & Orr, S. P. (1986). Test of a conditioning model of neurosis: Differential aversive conditioning of angry and neutral facial expressions in anxiety disorder patients. *Journal of Abnormal Psychology, 95,* 208–213.

Rescorla, R. A., & Wagner, A. R. (1972). A theory of Pavlovian conditioning: Variations in the effectiveness of reinforcement and nonreinforcement. In A. H. Black & W. F. Prokasy (Eds.), *Classical conditioning II: Current research and theory* (pp. 64–99). New York: Appleton-Century-Crofts.

Seligman, M. E. P. (1970). On the generality of the laws of learning. *Psychological Review, 77,* 406–418.

Seligman, M. E. P. (1971). Phobias and preparedness. *Behavior Therapy, 2,* 307–320.

Tomkins, S. S. (1962). *Affect, imagery, consciousness: Vol. 1. The positive affects.* New York: Springer.

Is Attentional Bias Due to "Preparedness" or Preexposure?

NIGEL W. BOND
DAVID A. T. SIDDLE

ÖHMAN HAS PRODUCED a chapter that is rich both in terms of theoretical conjecture and in its description of his empirical program. In offering comment, we should not lose sight of the fact that this entire area of research and its acceptance into the wider psychological literature stem from the work by Öhman and his colleagues. Nevertheless, we attempt here to demonstrate weaknesses in Öhman's theoretical analysis in Chapter 10, and suggest some empirical studies that provide critical tests of our own and Öhman's position.

Öhman has described a series of studies, conducted with his colleagues, that employed the backward-masking technique to prevent subjects' awareness of certain stimuli (see Chapter 10 for references). Öhman has argued that these studies demonstrate that subjects can acquire conditioned responding to masked fear-relevant stimuli, or display greater resistance to extinction to such stimuli. Furthermore, he has argued that these data indicate that subjects are processing fear-relevant stimuli in an automatic, unconscious fashion. He has elaborated a theory suggesting that humans are especially sensitive to threatening stimuli (e.g., snakes, spiders, or angry faces) and provided an account of how such stimuli can be processed outside of awareness. The theory holds that the physiological responding associated with fear can be aroused under conditions in which the subject has not consciously registered the presence of a dangerous stimulus.

Öhman has argued in Chapter 10 that the ability to process stimuli automatically and outside of conscious awareness is evidence in favor of a preparedness account of social and animal phobias. However, some of his own data suggest that this conclusion lacks parsimony. In one study, subjects were preselected on the basis of a prior fear of spiders, snakes, or neither of these animals. Subjects received backwardly masked presentations of the stimuli, followed by unmasked presentations. Subjects who were fearful of spiders responded more to spiders than to snakes, flowers, or mushrooms, in both the masked and unmasked conditions. Similarly, subjects who were fearful of snakes responded more to snakes than to the other stimuli. Unafraid subjects were equally unresponsive to all stimuli. These data suggest that a subject's ability to process a stimulus unconsciously is determined by his or her prior fear of that stimulus, presumably acquired through experience. If this is the case, then parsimony suggests that this apparently unconscious bias toward threatening stimuli is not the result of biological preparedness, but rather the result of prior experience with the stimulus. In this respect, the data are consistent with those of Mathews and MacLeod (1985, 1986), who have demonstrated in a number of studies that subjects show an unconscious bias toward stimuli that from a clinical perspective are an important aspect of their anxiety.

We have argued that many of the outcomes of studies on preparedness can be explained by examining subjects' prior experience with the stimuli employed. The same may be true for the stimuli employed by Öhman in the backward-masking studies. Again, snakes and spiders are usually compared with flowers and mushrooms, and angry faces are compared with happy faces. One way to test our prior-experience hypothesis and the preparedness hypothesis would be to carry out a backward-masking study of either acquisition or extinction, comparing an expression of anger to an even rarer facial expression of emotion (e.g., surprise). Our position predicts that a surprised face will condition and show greater resistance to extinction than will a happy face under backwardly masked conditions, and that these effects might even be more robust than those obtained with an angry expression.

The same argument applies with respect to spiders and snakes when compared to flowers and mushrooms. Prior to a conditioning experiment, one might expect subjects to have had greater experience with flowers and mushrooms than with snakes and spiders. Again, one could test whether backwardly masked conditioning and greater resistance to extinction are unique to spiders and snakes by using comparison stimuli that are also rare in comparison with flowers and mushrooms. Again, we would predict that a lack of prior exposure to a stimulus will lead to conditioning and greater resistance to extinction under conditions of backward masking.

A similar argument applies to the "pop-out" studies, which have been taken to indicate a special sensitivity to angry faces compared to happy faces, and to snakes and spiders compared to flowers and mushrooms. Even if we accept Öhman's argument that his data confirm that fear-relevant stimuli "pop out" when presented in a group of fear-irrelevant stimuli, we would argue that it is not fear relevance that is the important factor, but lack of prior exposure. Again, our hypothesis could be tested by examining whether a face that depicts surprise "pops out" from a group of happy faces, and, more importantly, whether such a face "pops out" from a group of angry faces.

We have argued that it is a lack of prior exposure that leads to the preparedness effects reported by Öhman and others. Indeed, our hypothesis subsumes most of the alternative explanations of the preparedness effects, such as the "expectancy" model of Davey (1992), our own model of "selective sensitization" (Lovibond, Siddle, & Bond, 1993), and the "covariation bias" model of Tomarken, Mineka, and Cook (1989). None of these models explains why it is that subjects enter a study with a particular expectancy that certain stimuli are more likely to be followed by shock, or are selectively sensitized by fear. Our hypothesis suggests that these effects arise because subjects have had considerable experience of some of these stimuli in the past (e.g., happy faces, flowers, and mushrooms) and relatively fewer experiences with other stimuli (e.g., angry faces, spiders, and snakes). The differing levels of exposure can then be converted into expectancies, covariation bias, or likelihood of selective sensitization, according to the general principles of learning and cognition.

For example, Alloy and Tabachnik (1984) have indicated that when a subject has considerable prior experience of a stimulus, this experience will override any covariation with another event to which the subject is exposed during an experiment. In contrast, when a subject encounters an experimental stimulus to which he or she has little prior exposure, then the covariation experienced during the study will guide the subject's behavior. In the present case, this suggests that happy faces will be difficult to condition in comparison with faces that depict either anger or surprise, as we have reported.

Similarly, one might explain the backward-masking studies on the basis that preattentive processing is more likely to occur when stimuli that are rare or significant are presented. If subjects have had considerable experience of a stimulus in the past, in the absence of any deleterious consequences, then that stimulus does not recruit preattentive processing. It would also be the case that rare and significant stimuli would also be more likely to recruit subsequent controlled processing, although the data reported by Öhman in Chapter 10, and previously by Mathews and MacLeod (1985, 1986), indicate that this may not always be the case.

Öhman and we agree that the stimuli employed in conditioning studies have some meaning for the subjects taking part in such studies. We differ in how that meaning comes to be established. Öhman takes a phylogenetic perspective and argues that meaning arises as a result of natural selection and its product, evolution. In contrast, we take an ontogenetic perspective and argue that the meaningfulness of stimuli arises from the differing experiences that subjects have had with these stimuli. In our chapter and in the present commentary, we have attempted to set out ways in which these two approaches might be examined empirically. Indeed, it is one of the strengths of the position set out by Öhman that it leads to such eminently testable predictions. That such a position can be distilled from a rich and complex literature highlights the importance of Öhman's contribution to our understanding of human fears and phobias.

REFERENCES

Alloy, L. G., & Tabachnik, N. (1984). Assessment of covariation by humans and animals: The joint influence of prior expectations and current situational information. *Psychological Review, 91,* 11–149.

Davey, G. C. L. (1992). An expectancy model of laboratory preparedness effects. *Journal of Experimental Psychology: General, 121,* 24–40.

Lovibond, P. F., Siddle, D. A. T., & Bond, N. W. (1993). Resistance to extinction of fear-relevant stimuli: Preparedness or selective sensitization? *Journal of Experimental Psychology: General, 122,* 449–461.

Mathews, A., & MacLeod, C. (1985). Selective processing of threat cues in anxiety states. *Behaviour Research and Therapy, 23,* 563–569.

Mathews, A., & MacLeod, C. (1986). Discrimination of threat cues without awareness in anxiety states. *Journal of Abnormal Psychology, 95,* 131–138.

Tomarken, A. J., Mineka, S., & Cook, M. (1989). Fear-relevant selective associations and covariation bias. *Journal of Abnormal Psychology, 98,* 381–394.

III

Treatment

12

Mechanisms of Change in Exposure Therapy

EDNA B. FOA
RICHARD J. McNALLY

MORE THAN TWO DECADES of controlled treatment research have demonstrated that systematic exposure to frightening stimuli reduces pathological fear markedly (e.g., Barlow, 1988; Foa & Kozak, 1986). Although the efficacy of exposure therapy is unquestioned, the mechanisms underlying its effectiveness remain controversial. Early theories conceptualized pathological fear in terms of stimulus–response (S-R) associations, and viewed treatment as entailing the severing of these associations. Eradication of pathological associations was thought to be accomplished either by replacing the fear response to the evocative stimulus with an incompatible response (e.g., relaxation), presumably through the mechanism of reciprocal inhibition (Wolpe, 1958), or by weakening associations through extinction procedures (Stampfl & Levis, 1967).

The S-R conditioning theories that provided the original explanation for how exposure therapy reduces fear encountered empirical (e.g., Kazdin & Wilcoxin, 1976) and theoretical (e.g., Rachman, 1976, 1977) difficulties. Not only did this S-R framework fail to account for the effects of exposure therapy; it also could not explain important phenomena in animal learning, and thus was abandoned by the very experimental psychologists who once advocated it (e.g., Kamin, 1969; Rescorla & Wagner, 1972). To replace the discarded S-R paradigm, these animal learning theorists developed stimulus–stimulus (S-S) informational theories of conditioning.

Proponents of exposure therapy responded in two ways to the collapse of the S-R paradigm. Some concentrated on pragmatically identifying parameters of treatment while eschewing the elucidation of mechanisms of change (e.g., Marks, 1987). Others adopted the information-processing approach that had already gained currency in both animal and human experimental psychology. Lang (1977), for example, formulated a bioinformational model of pathological fear. In the tradition of Lang, we provide an information-processing analysis of the mechanisms underlying fear reduction through exposure therapy. We describe how pathological fear can be construed within this framework, and suggest how exposure alters impairments that underlie symptoms.

THE COGNITIVE STRUCTURE OF FEAR

Adopting Pylyshyn's (1973) construal of a propositional network as an organization of interrelated concepts, Lang (1977, 1979) proposed that fear is represented in memory as a structure consisting of (1) information about feared stimuli; (2) information about verbal, physiological, and motor responses; and (3) interpretive information about their meanings. He suggested that this "fear structure" constitutes a program for escape from threat.

If the fear structure is indeed a program to escape threat, it must involve information that stimuli, responses, or both are dangerous, in addition to information about physiological mobilization for escape. As noted by Foa and Kozak (1986), the programs for running ahead of a baton-carrying competitor in a race and for running ahead of a club-carrying assailant on a racetrack involve similar stimulus and response information. But what distinguishes the fear structure is the meaning of the stimuli and responses: Only the fear structure involves running to escape threat.

THE STRUCTURE OF PATHOLOGICAL FEAR

Normal fear is evoked by the perception of real threat, and it dissipates when danger passes. Occasionally fear occurs when a person evaluates a safe situation as dangerous, but recognition of the error decreases the fear. Fear becomes pathological when it is disruptively intense, or when it persists despite information indicating safety. That is, pathological fear structures contain representations of excessive responses (e.g., avoidance, physiological activity) and are resistant to change. A fear is unrealistic when its underlying memory structure contains S-S associations that do not accurately represent relations in the world. For example, for many obsessive–compulsives, floors are strongly associated with urine (and are therefore contaminated), whereas in reality urine is rarely found on floors. Pathological fear structures also contain unrealistic S-R associations between harmless stimuli and fear responses, such as escape or avoidance. Avoiding floors does not enhance safety, and therefore it unnecessarily hampers the person's ability to function normally. Embedded in these dysfunctional S-S and S-R associations is some of the erroneous meaning of the pathological fear structure. Additional erroneous meaning can be represented by interpretive elements in the structure.

Individuals with pathological fear commit several evaluative errors. First, they commonly believe that anxiety, once activated, will persist unless they escape the feared situation. Second, they overestimate the probability that their feared stimuli and fear responses will cause physical (e.g., dying, being ill) or psychological harm (e.g., going crazy, losing control). Third, their feared consequences have an especially high negative valence. That is, they regard these consequences as more aversive than do people without pathological fear.

According to Foa and Kozak (1986), different anxiety disorders are characterized by different fear structures. For example, both agoraphobia and obsessive–compulsive disorder (OCD) reflect pathological S-S and S-R associations, but what distinguishes the agoraphobic structure from that of OCD is erroneous meaning associated with the fear responses themselves. Relative to OCD and other anxiety disorders, agoraphobics regard anxiety itself as dangerous because of their belief that it is likely to lead to either physical harm (e.g., suffocation) or psychological harm (e.g., going crazy). Stimuli (e.g., tunnels) are not evaluated as intrinsically dangerous; the danger is perceived to lie in the anxiety that they evoke. Likewise, the motivation for avoiding flying on airplanes in specific phobics is very different from the motivation for airplane avoidance in agoraphobics (McNally & Louro, 1992). Whereas people with specific phobias of flying in airplanes are characterized by inflated probabilities of plane crashes, agoraphobics do not fear plane crashes, rather, they fear the occurrence of panic and its imagined consequences during flight.

Unlike agoraphobics who fear their own responses, obsessive–compulsive washers and specific phobics mistakenly interpret certain harmless stimuli as harmful. For example, the fear structures of washers who fear infection from even indirect contact with feces and urine represent three types of conceptual errors: S-S associations (e.g., floor–urine), S-R associations (e.g., floor–fear response), and associations between meaning elements and stimulus elements (e.g., "Floors are dangerous").

Although fear is represented in consciousness, the underlying information structures that generate fear are not themselves accessible to introspection. But some elements of the structure may be reflected in consciousness, insofar as people are often aware of the stimuli that frighten them, their evaluations of these stimuli and their responses to them.

EXPOSURE TREATMENT:
MODIFICATION OF THE FEAR STRUCTURE

Foa and Kozak (1986) suggested that treatment for pathological fear entails modification of the underlying fear structure, and that this modification is the essence of what Lang (1977) and Rachman (1980) called "emotional processing." Foa and Kozak further proposed that two conditions are required for emotional processing. First, therapists must activate the fear structure by providing information that matches information represented in the structure. Just as one needs to access a computer program to debug it, one must also access the relevant cognitive structure to correct it. Second, the information provided during therapy must also be incompatible with the pathological elements in the structure. If a perfect match occurred between information provided in therapy and information represented in the structure, either no change would occur or the dysfunctional associations would be strengthened rather than weakened. For example, therapists often take airplane phobics to the airport and have them go on short flights, in an effort to disconfirm inflated probabilities of harm associated with air travel. However, if a patient, during exposure at an airport, were to witness the crash of a plane, it would confirm rather than disconfirm information incorporated in the structure; this would result in exacerbation of the phobia.

Three indicators of emotional processing predict successful outcome of exposure therapy (Foa & Kozak, 1986). First, patients who improve exhibit physiological arousal and self-reported fear during exposure sessions. Second, their fear responses diminish gradually during exposure to feared objects or situations; that is, they exhibit within-session habituation of anxiety. Third, initial fear responses at each session decline across sessions (i.e., between-session habituation). Data supporting these indicators are summarized by Foa and Kozak (1986).

Further research has partly confirmed the validity of these indicators (Kozak, Foa, & Steketee, 1988). Studying obsessive–compulsives, Kozak et al. found that activation of fear, as measured by self-report and physiological indices, predicted successful outcome following exposure and response prevention. Although within-session habituation occurred, it failed to predict outcome, perhaps because most patients exhibited marked improvement. Habituation across sessions in heart rate and self-report predicted successful outcome.

Treating speech-anxious volunteers with imaginal exposure, Schwartz and Kaloupek (1987) also obtained support for the validity of these indicators of emotional processing. Outcome measures included self-reported fear, observations of speech performance, and cardiac and electrodermal activity. Both within-session and between-session habituation on self-report and physiological measures of fear during exposure predicted successful outcome.

Treating assault victims with posttraumatic stress disorder (PTSD), Foa, Riggs, Massie, and Yarczower (in press) measured activation by coding facial fear expression during reliving of a traumatic event (e.g., of sexual assault). Patients were asked to report their level of distress at 10-minute intervals during their recounting of the trauma. Facial expressions were coded during the 15-second period prior to each patient's highest rating of distress in the first therapy session. Foa et al. found that intensity of facial fear expression and self-reported distress during this first session predicted improvement on a composite measure of PTSD and anxiety symptoms. Regression analyses revealed that facial fear expressions, relative to other variables, overwhelmingly accounted for variance in outcome. Interestingly, pretreatment levels of self-reported anger were negatively related to facial fear expression and to improvement. This suggests that therapists ought to discourage activation of anger during exposure.

How does exposure alter fear structures and thereby promote emotional processing? As noted earlier, a fear structure is accessed when a fearful individual confronts information that matches some of the information represented in the structure (Lang, 1977). Matching information may concern feared stimuli, fear responses, or their meanings. Lang suggested that some critical number of information units must be matched for sufficient activation, and that some elements may be more important than others. For example, input information that activates representations of feared responses as well as feared stimuli promotes greater fear evocation than information that activates only stimulus representations (Lang, Kozak, Miller, Levin, & McLean, 1980). These findings underscore the importance of activating representations of fear responses.

Especially coherent fear structures, such as those in specific phobia, can be evoked with minimal matching input. For example, the mere sight of a coiled garden hose may elicit intense fear in a snake phobic. Likewise, a warm sensation may evoke a panic attack in the agoraphobic who fears certain physiological sensations.

Although input information can be embodied in a variety of media (e.g., imagery scripts, videotapes), an obvious way to access a fear structure is confrontation with an *in vivo* feared situation. But as Borkovec (1985) emphasized, not all exposures are functional. That is, not all exposures to feared stimuli match the structure sufficiently so that fear occurs. For example, an agoraphobic patient who fears entering shopping malls alone will not benefit by entering them accompanied by her husband; indeed, she will not experience fear under these circumstances. Although "shopping mall plus husband" partly matches the relevant information embodied in the structure, the crucial match entails "being in the shopping mall alone." Likewise, a speech phobic who fears criticism is unlikely to benefit from speaking to a nonevaluative audience. Only speaking before an evaluative audience constitutes an appropriate match.

Researchers have identified several variables that facilitate the effectiveness of exposure. One such variable is the medium of exposure. From the foregoing discussion, one would expect that the effectiveness of a medium will depend on how well it provides a match with crucial elements in the fear structure, as well as on the person's willingness or ability to access the structure. For example, in specific phobics, real-life (in vivo) confrontation with a feared situation is more likely to evoke a fear response than is imaginal exposure. Indeed, Watson, Gaind, and Marks (1972) found that for specific phobics, the average initial heart rate response during fear-relevant images was 8 beats per minute, whereas the average response during in vivo exposure to these same stimuli was 28 beats per minute. Watson et al.'s results suggest that the pathology of specific phobia lies largely in excessive responsiveness; therefore, in vivo exposure that promotes activation and habituation ought to be sufficient for recovery. This interpretation is supported by the finding that a single prolonged in vivo exposure session produces permanent cure in specific phobia (Öst, 1989).

Why is in vivo exposure so often more effective than imaginal exposure? One explanation for the attenuated effectiveness of imaginal exposure is that at least some patients fail to engage in processing the scripts. It is easier to ignore input arising from a verbal script than it is to ignore input arising from veridical fear stimuli. Indeed, studying agoraphobics, Zander and McNally (1988) found that scripts representing feared stimuli, fear responses, and catastrophic consequences provoked self-reported fear without increasing physiological arousal.

In addition, an imagery script provides a verbal representation of the object of fear, which is designed to activate the cognitive representation of this object. Thus, imaginal exposure merely entails the activation of one representation by another, whereas in vivo exposure entails the activation of a cognitive representation by the object of the representation itself. Accordingly, imaginal scripts inevitably provide impoverished informational input, and are therefore less evocative than real-life exposure.

Another important variable influencing effectiveness of exposure is duration. Prolonged exposure produces better outcome than does brief exposure, regardless of diagnosis (Chaplin & Levine, 1981; Rabavilas, Boulougouris, & Stefanis, 1976; Stern & Marks, 1973). During exposure sessions, most patients exhibit decreases in autonomic responding and reported fear, and the magnitude of these changes predicts successful outcome. Habituation takes time. Changes in S-R associations typically require habituation of feared responses, and this process unfolds gradually. Accordingly, long-duration exposure is most likely to permit habituation, and thereby to abolish these dysfunctional associations.

If emotional processing is construed as the modification of a fear structure through the incorporation of corrective information, an obvious prerequisite is sensory encoding of the information presented. Accordingly, variables that promote attention to fear-relevant information ought to foster activation of the fear structure and promote its subsequent modification. But excessively high levels of fear during exposure will disrupt attention and impair encoding of information, including the information designed to alter pathological elements in the structure. These considerations imply that moderate levels of arousal should yield optimal outcome. Consistent with this hypothesis, Borkovec and Sides (1979) found that moderate arousal during imaginal exposure, achieved by relaxation procedures, was associated with vividness of imagery, initial heart responses, and habituation of fear. Grayson, Foa, and Steketee (1986) further confirmed the importance of attention to fear-relevant information. Treating obsessive–compulsives, they found that no heart rate habituation occurred during exposure with distraction instructions, whereas it did with exposure with attention instructions.

MECHANISMS OF EMOTIONAL PROCESSING

We have adopted the view that fear is represented as a propositional structure in memory, that serves as a program for fear behavior. We have also suggested that pathological fear includes dysfunctional associations among elements. It follows that the target of therapy for pathological fear is to change the pathological components in the structure. Such change, which Foa and Kozak (1986) called "emotional processing," requires the incorporation of information that is incompatible with the pathological elements of the structure. In this section, we discuss processes through which this is accomplished.

Dissociation of Stimulus from Response Elements

Pathological fear structures are partly characterized by S-R associations in which the responses preparatory to escape or avoidance are unwarranted by the context. Exposure promotes within-session physiological habituation of preparatory responses, such as heart rate. Attenuation of these responses in the fear context constitutes information incompatible with that represented in the pathological structure; it thereby weakens the preexisting links between stimulus and response elements. Regardless of the physiological mechanisms that underlie within-session habituation, the process of habituation itself constitutes information that changes the fear structure. This information is available for encoding in response propositions that are inconsistent with the pathological ones represented in the structure. For example, successful habituation of fear to dogs in a dog phobic constitutes information that dogs no longer activate a physiology mobilized for flight.

A common misconception in anxiety-disordered individuals is that their fear will spiral upward indefinitely unless they escape the context that provoked it. An additional misconception is that anxiety itself may have catastrophic consequences if it spirals out of control (e.g., loss of control). Habituation disconfirms both mistaken assumptions. It shows patients that anxiety declines rather than spirals upward, despite their continued engagement with the provocative context. It also shows them that catastrophes they believe will arise from mounting anxiety do not materialize. Even at the peak of anxiety during exposure, before habituation begins to occur, no harm ensues.

Modification of Meaning

In addition to abolishing dysfunctional S-R associations via short-term physiological habituation, harmless confrontation with a feared situation also changes both propositional and nonpropositional aspects of meaning. "Propositional meaning" refers to information that can be represented in language, such as "Dogs are dangerous." "Nonpropositional meaning" refers to information embedded in S-S associations such as "dog–bite." Whereas propositional meanings are always encoded linguistically, nonpropositional meanings need to be transformed into linguistic code, and need not always be capable of such transformations.

One aspect of meaning concerns representations of probability of harm, which can be coded either propositionally or nonpropositionally. Many anxious patients exaggerate the likelihood of aversive consequences' materializing under certain conditions. For example, panic patients overestimate the likelihood that physiological arousal will lead to physical collapse (McNally & Foa, 1987), and obsessive–compulsive checkers often overestimate the likelihood that unchecked doors and locks are indeed open for burglars.

Probability of harm can also be encoded nonpropositionally in S-S associations (i.e., nonlinguistically), with stronger associations reflecting higher probabilities. Regardless of whether they characterize probabilities verbally, many patients act as if inflated probabilities of harm govern their behavior. Reduction in probability of harm can occur through either nonlinguistic (i.e., nonpropositional) or linguistic (i.e., propositional) procedures. Exposure to feared stimuli in the absence of feared consequences reduces the strength of S-S associations, and thereby reduces the probability of harm represented in the structure. For example, patients whose fear structure was once characterized by inflated probabilities of the co-occurrence of dogs and bites will no longer have this information in the structure after exposure to friendly dogs.

A propositional way of modifying representations of probability is via their replacement with incompatible information represented linguistically. For example, the instruction that AIDS cannot be contracted through handshakes changes the perceived probability of AIDS, given handshaking. Changing probabilities via weakening of S-S associations requires neither conscious awareness nor language, whereas modification of propositional representation of probabilities may require both.

In addition to altering probability representations, exposure also diminishes the negativity of valence representations in the fear structure. Like probability representations, valence representations can be altered either nonpropositionally or propositionally. Changes in valence can occur for both feared contexts (akin to Pavlovian conditioned stimuli [CSs]) and feared consequences (akin to Pavlovian unconditioned stimuli [USs]).

We first explicate how exposure diminishes the negative valence of CSs, before addressing how changes in US valence can occur. Exposure attenuates the negative valence of CSs through severing S-S relations. For example, dogs acquire negative valence by virtue of their predictive relation to a feared consequence, and lose negative valence once this association no longer holds. That is, negative valence is diminished via nonpropositional procedures that sever S-S associations. For example, harmless exposure to dogs abolishes the S-S association between dogs and biting, thereby not only altering the representation of probability of harm, but also altering the representation of valence associated with dogs ("Dogs are unlikely to bite," "Dogs are not bad"). Accordingly, although probability of harm and valence are conceptually distinct, in practice they often covary with changes in strength of S-S associations with regard to the valence of the CS.

Exposure cannot diminish the negative valence of feared consequences when they are functionally similar to Pavlovian first-order USs, but can do so when they are akin to second-order USs. For example, exposure to harmless dogs reduces the negative valence of dogs (CSs), but not that of dog bites themselves (USs). On the other hand, exposing social phobics to feared criticism may attenuate the negative valence of criticism (a second-order US). In other words, feared consequences that lack biological significance (e.g., criticism) may be amenable to negative valence reduction, whereas those having biological significance (e.g., bites) are not.

The valence of a feared consequence can change in two ways. First, once experienced, the consequence may not possess many of the aversive properties that the patient envisions it will have (e.g., criticism from a boss does not invariably lead to job loss). In this sense, exposure disconfirms certain expected implications and properties of the consequence, and thereby diminishes its negative valence. Second, reduction of anxiety associated with the consequences may attenuate its negative valence. Habituation of anxiety through repeated contact with feared consequences during exposure treatment may itself diminish the negative valence of these consequences. The social phobic whose anxiety in response to repeated criticism diminishes may evaluate criticism as not so terrible. Reduction in the negative valence of second-order feared consequences can also be achieved through propositional procedures, as in rational–emotive therapy (Ellis, 1962) and cognitive restructuring (Beck, 1976). These interventions employ language to reduce the perceived "badness" of feared consequences, but often incorporate exposure to these consequences in the context of "behavioral experiments" (Salkovskis, 1991).

The foregoing discussion concerns the attenuation of negative valence of feared consequences themselves. Exposure therapy may also involve reducing the negative valence associated with the activation of the representation of these consequences. Feared consequences akin to first-order USs are often objectively highly aversive, and therapy does not entail persuading patients that they are not. No therapist, for example, endeavors to convince rape victims that rape is benign. Yet many patients become excessively distressed by merely thinking about objectively aversive consequences. Exposure therapy is designed not to reduce the valence of the consequence per se, but to reduce the valence associated with the activation of its corresponding cognitive representation. Thus, imaginal exposure often diminishes the negative valence associated with the activation of a representation of a feared consequence, without diminishing the negative valence of the consequence itself. For example, an obsessional patient may habituate to repeated imaginings of murdering her daughter, but this does not alter the negative valence of homicide. That is, the negative valence associated with the thought itself has diminished through imaginal exposure, even though the valence of the represented event (i.e., murdering the daughter) has not.

SOME RECONSIDERATIONS

The foregoing discussion about the mechanisms by which exposure reduces fear prompts several questions. We elaborate here on three of these. First, are fear structures ever changed? Or does exposure entail the formation of new structures? As noted at the beginning of this chapter, exposure therapists originally construed the process of fear reduction as either replacement or erasure of associations. Wolpe (1958) held that successful therapy involves the replacement of pathological S-R associations with nonpathological ones. Associations between feared stimuli and fear responses were thought to be replaced by new associations between these stimuli and responses incompatible with anxiety. By contrast, others held that associations are not replaced, but rather erased through the process of extinction (e.g., Stampfl & Levis, 1967).

In this tradition, Foa and Kozak (1986) proposed that fear reduction results from weakening of associations among elements in the fear structure, as well as through the replacement of pathological elements with nonpathological ones. Research by Bouton (Bouton, 1988; Bouton & Swartzentruber, 1991) among others, however, strongly implies that fear reduction does not involve the weakening of associations per se, but rather involves the formation of new associations. Accordingly, successful exposure therapy may not involve the abolition of existing pathological associations, but rather the establishment of new, nonpathological ones. That is, fear reduction implies new learning, not unlearning. Cast within the framework of Foa and Kozak (1986), Bouton's work implies that after therapy fear structures remain intact, but new structures that override the influence of pathological ones are established via exposure. More specifically, the old pathological and the new nonpathological structures share stimulus representation, but differ in that these representations are associated with different response and meaning elements.

Bouton's research indicates that fear memories are not erased, but can be reinstated under certain contextual cues. Similar phenomena happen clinically. Patients often report reinstatement of fear under certain contexts, such as dysphoric moods and environmental stress. For example, an obsessive–compulsive washer who feared bodily secretions prior to successful treatment will most often access the new, normal structure, and will not exhibit rituals and avoidance. Nevertheless, the patient will not forget fearing these secretions, and under some circumstances may reexperience activation of the entire pathological structure as evinced in relapse.

Bouton's work implies that therapy ought to achieve several aims. It ought to establish new, nonpathological structures, and to increase the accessibility of their subsequent activation in contexts that formerly activated pathological structures. Finally, because therapy cannot abolish pathological structures, it must arrange for their inhibition in contexts that once provoked their activation. Exposure therapists have been remarkably effective in establishing nonpathological structures, but have been less consistently successful in fostering the accessibility of nonpathological structures and in securing the inhibition of pathological ones. Research ought to focus on developing procedures that promote accessibility of new structures and promote inhibition of old ones.

Two assumptions underlie exposure therapy. First, "anxiety" and "fear" have traditionally been regarded as interchangeable terms for the same emotional phenomenon. Second, anxiety disorders have been traditionally viewed as largely problems of pathological fear; accordingly, treatment of anxiety disorders has been largely a matter of reducing pathological fear rather than other emotions. These assumptions seem more valid for some anxiety disorders than for others. Specific phobia entails pathological fear, whereas complex anxiety disorders involve other pathological emotions in addition to fear. Patients with PTSD suffer not only from fear and anxiety, but also from guilt, anger, shame, and sadness. OCD washers experience excessive disgust as much as excessive fear when encountering contaminants, and most OCD patients are also plagued by excessive guilt.

The idea that complex anxiety disorders include pathological emotions other than fear probably has considerable therapeutic implications. Exposure therapy rests on the fundamental assumption that repeated confrontation to distressing stimuli will engender habituation. This is indeed true for fear, but perhaps false for other negative emotions, such as guilt. Unlike fear, guilt is a nonprimitive, complex emotion whose mechanisms are probably different from those of fear. Hence therapeutic procedures effective for fear may be ineffective, or even harmful, for guilt and other complex negative emotions. Consistent with this proposal, Pitman et al. (1991) found that imaginal exposure to traumatic events in Vietnam veterans with PTSD failed to engender habituation when the events concerned atrocities the veterans had committed during the war. In these cases, the most disturbing emotion was guilt, not fear. That is, an exposure therapy found to be highly effective for fear reduction in victims of assault (Foa, Rothbaum, Riggs, & Murdock, 1991) worsened symptoms associated with guilt in combat veterans. Unlike fear, guilt is a complex emotion involving cognitive representation of the self, as well as dysfunctional representations of feared stimuli and fear responses. Accordingly, the involvement of higher-order constructs may render habituation relatively ineffective. Cognitive therapies may be more effective in addressing pathological guilt.

Like guilt, disgust and aversion may fail to habituate during repeated exposure, but perhaps for different reasons. Indeed, aversions (e.g., distress at touching cotton or hearing a fingernail scratch on a chalkboard) are even less complex than fear, but fail to habituate to repeated exposure. Moreover, these stimuli involve nothing but simple auditory and tactile input and thus lack the biological significance of a genuine US (e.g., a pain-producing stimulus). But like fundamental USs, they resist habituation. Aversions demonstrate that exposure can fail not only with complex emotions such as guilt, but also with phenomena simpler than fear. Exposure therapy may be helpful with complex anxiety disorders only to the extent that fear is involved. Its effectiveness will be limited to the extent that other emotions contribute to the clinical picture. For example, an OCD patient whose rituals are motivated more by disgust than by fear may profit less from exposure therapy than an OCD patient who ritualizes to avoid sickness. Further research is warranted to determine the scope and limitations of exposure therapy with other negative emotions other than fear.

Foa and Kozak (1986) suggested that therapy involves replacement of nonrealistic pathological structures with realistic nonpathological ones. Implicit in this formulation is the assumption that mental health involves an accurate match between the world and a person's representation of it. However, social psychologists (e.g., Taylor & Brown, 1988) have shown that psychological adjustment seems to require positive biases. That is, happy people may view themselves and the world in unrealistically positive ways. Accordingly, successful therapy may entail the addition of new (partly) unrealistic but positive structures that compete with the old unrealistic pathological one, rather than the addition of new realistic structures.

REFERENCES

Barlow, D. H. (1988). *Anxiety and its disorders: The nature and treatment of anxiety and panic.* New York: Guilford Press.

Beck, A. T. (1976). *Cognitive therapy and the emotional disorders.* New York: International Universities Press.

Borkovec, T. D. (1985). The role of cognitive and somatic cues in anxiety and anxiety disorders: Worry and relaxation-induced anxiety. In A. H. Tuma & J. D. Maser (Eds.), *Anxiety and the anxiety disorders* (pp. 463–478). Hillsdale, NJ: Erlbaum.

Borkovec, T. D., & Sides, J. K. (1979). The contribution of relaxation and expectancy to fear reduction via graded imaginal exposure to feared stimuli. *Behaviour Research and Therapy, 17,* 529–540.

Bouton, M. E. (1988). Context and ambiguity in the extinction of emotional learning: Implications for exposure therapy. *Behaviour Research and Therapy, 26,* 137–149.

Bouton, M. E., & Swartzentruber, D. (1991). Sources of relapse after extinction in Pavlovian and instrumental learning. *Clinical Psychology Review, 11,* 123–140.

Chaplin, E. W., & Levine, B. A. (1981). The effects of total exposure duration and interrupted versus continuous exposure in flooding therapy. *Behavior Therapy, 12,* 360–368.

Ellis, A. (1962). *Reason and emotion in psychotherapy.* New York: Lyle Stuart Press.

Foa, E. B., & Kozak, M. J. (1986). Emotional processing of fear: Exposure to corrective information. *Psychological Bulletin, 99,* 20–35.

Foa, E. B., Riggs, D. S., Massie, E. D., & Yarczower, M. (in press). The impact of fear activation and anger on the efficacy of exposure treatment for PTSD. *Behavior Therapy.*

Foa, E. E., Rothbaum, B. O., Riggs, D. S., & Murdock, T. B. (1991). Treatment of posttraumatic stress disorder in rape victims: A comparison between cognitive-behavioral procedures and counseling. *Journal of Consulting and Clinical Psychology, 59,* 715–723.

Grayson, J. B., Foa, E. B., & Steketee, G. S. (1986). Exposure *in vivo* of obsessive–compulsives under distracting and attention-focusing conditions: Replication and extension. *Behaviour Research and Therapy, 24,* 475–479.

Kamin, L. J. (1969). Predictability, surprise, attention, and conditioning. In B. A. Campbell & R. M. Church (Eds.), *Punishment and aversive behavior* (pp. 279–296). New York: Appleton-Century-Crofts.

Kazdin, A. E., & Wilcoxin, L. A. (1976). Systematic desensitization and nonspecific treatment effects: A methodological evaluation. *Psychological Bulletin, 83,* 729–758.

Kozak, M. J., Foa, E. B., & Steketee, G. (1988). Process and outcome of exposure treatment with obsessive–compulsives: Psychophysiological indicators of emotional processing. *Behavior Therapy, 19,* 157–169.

Lang, P. J. (1977). Imagery in therapy: An information processing analysis of fear. *Behavior Therapy, 8,* 862–886.

Lang, P. J. (1979). A bio-informational theory of emotional imagery. *Psychophysiology, 16,* 495–512.

Lang, P. J., Kozak, M. J., Miller, G. A., Levin, D. N., & McLean, A., Jr. (1980). Emotional imagery: Conceptual structure and pattern of somatovisceral response. *Psychophysiology, 17,* 179–192.

Marks, I. M. (1987). *Fears, phobias, and rituals.* New York: Oxford University Press.

McNally, R. J., & Foa, E. B. (1987). Cognition and agoraphobia: Bias in the interpretation of threat. *Cognitive Therapy and Research, 11,* 567–581.

McNally, R. J., & Louro, C. E. (1992). Fear of flying in agoraphobia and simple phobia: Distinguishing features. *Journal of Anxiety Disorders, 6,* 319–324.

Öst, L.-G. (1989). One-session treatment for specific phobias. *Behaviour Research and Therapy, 27,* 1–7.

Pitman, R. K., Altman, B., Greenwald, E., Longpre, R. E., Macklin, M. L., Poire, R. E., & Steketee, G. S. (1991). Psychiatric complications during flooding therapy for posttraumatic stress disorder. *Journal of Clinical Psychiatry, 52,* 17–20.

Pylyshyn, Z. W. (1973). What the mind's eye tells the mind's brain: A critique of mental imagery. *Psychological Bulletin, 80,* 1–24.

Rabavilas, A. D., Boulougouris, J. C., & Stefanis, C. (1976). Duration of flooding sessions in the treatment of obsessive–compulsive patients. *Behaviour Research and Therapy, 14,* 349–355.

Rachman, S. (1976). The passing of the two-stage theory of fear and avoidance: Fresh possibilities. *Behaviour Research and Therapy, 14,* 125–131.

Rachman, S. (1977). The conditioning theory of fear-acquisition: A critical examination. *Behaviour Research and Therapy, 15,* 375–387.

Rachman, S. (1980). Emotional processing. *Behaviour Research and Therapy, 18,* 51–60.

Rescorla, R. A., & Wagner, A. R. (1972). A theory of Pavlovian conditioning: Variations in the effectiveness of reinforcement and nonreinforcement. In A. H. Black & W. F. Prokasy (Eds.), *Classical conditioning II: Current research and theory* (pp. 64–99). New York: Appleton-Century-Crofts.

Salkovskis, P. M. (1991). The importance of behaviour in the maintenance of panic and anxiety: A cognitive account. *Behavioural Psychotherapy, 19,* 6–19.

Schwartz, S. G., & Kaloupek, D. G. (1987). Acute exercise combined with imaginal exposure as a technique for anxiety reduction. *Canadian Journal of Behavioural Science, 19,* 151–166.

Stampfl, T. G., & Levis, D. J. (1967). Essentials of implosive therapy: A learning-theory-based psychodynamic behavioral therapy. *Journal of Abnormal Psychology, 72,* 496–503.

Stern, R., & Marks, I. (1973). Brief and prolonged flooding: A comparison in agoraphobic patients. *Archives of General Psychiatry, 28,* 270–276.

Taylor, S. E., & Brown, J. D. (1988). Illusion and well-being: A social psychological perspective on mental health. *Psychological Bulletin, 103,* 193–210.

Watson, J. P., Gaind, R., & Marks, I. M. (1972). Physiological habituation to continuous phobic stimulation. *Behaviour Research and Therapy, 10,* 269–278.

Wolpe, J. (1958). *Psychotherapy by reciprocal inhibition.* Stanford, CA: Stanford University Press.

Zander, J. R., & McNally, R. J. (1988). Bio-informational processing agoraphobia. *Behaviour Research and Therapy, 26,* 421–429.

13

Therapeutic Changes in Phobic Behavior Are Mediated by Changes in Perceived Self-Efficacy

S. LLOYD WILLIAMS

THE PRESENT CHAPTER reviews theory and evidence in support of the theory that phobic behavior is caused by low perceptions of self-efficacy, and that therapeutic changes in phobia are mediated by changes in perceived self-efficacy. The focus here is on current psychological causation of phobic behavior, rather than on the historical development or etiology of phobia.

PHOBIA

Phobia is a most striking and puzzling condition—a prototypical example of the "neurotic paradox" of self-defeating behavior, in which people are disabled despite perceiving every incentive to function normally, having the requisite basic cognitive/motoric abilities, and being well aware that their disability is senseless.

Phobias often cost people their livelihood and their ability to engage in their favorite social and recreational activities. These disabilities, in turn, can be humiliating and damaging to their sense of well-being and self-esteem.

The present chapter is concerned with phobic behavioral disability and with the evidence regarding the influence of self-efficacy on it. Behavior is the single most important dimension of psychological functioning that theories and treatments must address, because behavioral limitations and disabilities are the most serious material hardships and sources of suffering that phobic individuals endure.

THE FAILURE OF ANXIETY THEORY

Traditional phobia theories emphasized anxiety as the main determinant of phobic behavior (e.g., Wolpe, 1958; Mowrer, 1960). The terms "fear" and "anxiety," here considered synonyms, refer to subjective distress and/or autonomic arousal. The anxiety theory of phobia has always suffered from serious explanatory weaknesses (Bandura, 1969; Mineka, 1979; Rachman, 1976; Seligman & Johnston, 1973; Williams, 1987, 1988). In the first place, the term "anxiety" has tended to be a catch-all label for dissimilar phenomena, so that simply measuring "it" can be unclear. Some analyses of anxiety, such as the "three systems" approach, went so far as to include phobic behavior in the very definition of anxiety (Lang, 1971). This renders into circular nonsense the proposition that anxiety *causes* phobic behavior, since a thing cannot cause itself. The proliferation of meanings has resulted in part from to the long-standing failure of any particular index of anxiety to strongly predict avoidant behavior (Williams, 1987, 1988).

Perhaps the most usual ways of defining anxiety are either as a feeling of fear rated on a subjective intensity scale, or as autonomic arousal. But anxiety's various indices are only weakly correlated with one another, and only weakly correlated with phobic behavior (Bandura, 1969, 1978, 1988; Lang, 1971; Mineka, 1979; Rachman, 1976). People can be very anxious but still perform an activity, as in the case of terrified but frequent fliers; and people can be *not* very anxious but still avoid something, as in the case of bridge-phobic people who calmly drive far out of their way to stay clear of large bridges. Moreover, treatment effects bear no clear relation to anxiety arousal. Whether anxiety is minimized, evoked, or ignored during treatment makes little difference, and numerous studies show that the anxiety people experience during treatment correlates weakly with how much they benefit from treatment (Mathews, Gelder, & Johnston, 1981; Williams, 1987, 1990a).

A variation on anxiety theory—namely, that panic anxiety is the primary determinant of agoraphobic behavior—is equally dubious, since the correlation between the severity or frequency of panic attacks and severity of agoraphobia tends to be low (Craske & Barlow, 1988). Many persons with severe agoraphobia have not panicked for months or years, and many panickers are not particularly agoraphobic. Panic may well play a role in the historical etiology of agoraphobic fears, but it is largely unrelated to the phobias once they develop.

Since correlation is a necessary condition for causation, the weak correlations show that the fearful feelings, panic attacks, and autonomic distress cannot be the major determinants of phobic behavior. There is no doubt that fear arousal can accompany phobia, and that phobia theories must explain anxiety and phobia treatments must remedy it. But anxiety is better conceived of as part of the problem to be solved than as the mechanism of therapeutic behavior change. I discuss below the issue of *anticipated* future anxiety and panic, which is a cognitive factor that has a somewhat stronger relationship with agoraphobic behavior than does fear per se. However, we will see that even anticipated fear is eclipsed in behavioral predictiveness by people's perceptions of self-efficacy.

THE FAILURE
OF STIMULUS-ORIENTED THEORIES

With the growing realization that anxiety has little power to explain phobic behavior or its change during treatment, some theorists proposed that therapeutic changes occur because of "exposure" to fearsome stimuli (Marks, 1978). This view emphasizes the amount of time the person remains in proximity to scary stimuli, and posits that this time factor accounts for change. The exposure view gained a wide following, and now disparate phobia treatments are known widely as "exposure" therapies.

The exposure notion and associated terminology are unfortunate, however, because they encourage neglect of inner psychological processes (Rosenthal & Bandura, 1978; Williams, 1987, 1988, 1990). Of course, learning in any domain requires spending time in commerce with domain-relevant material, but beyond this obvious truism the exposure concept says little. Exposure encounters serious difficulties in explaining why a given amount and kind of treatment will benefit one person very much but another person not at all. Indeed, the exposure concept has not been plainly operationally defined, so as to permit empirical tests of the relationship between amount of "exposure,'" and amount of therapeutic benefit. Some have even incorporated treatment benefit into the very definition of exposure, thereby rendering it circular and devoid of meaning. Understanding the mechanisms of phobia, and developing more effective treatments for it, require operationally specifying its underlying psychological processes, rather than trying to externalize the locus of psychological causation. In self-efficacy theory, phobic behavior derives largely from conscious cognitive self-appraisal processes within the phobic individual.

SELF-EFFICACY THEORY

Self-efficacy theory is a subpostulate of social-cognitive theory, which emphasizes the central importance to human functioning of higher cognitive capabilities such as symbolic representation, vicarious learning, forethought, self-reflection, and self-direction (Bandura, 1986; Cervone & Williams, 1992). Self-efficacy theory posits in particular that psychological treatment procedures benefit people largely by increasing their perceptions of self-efficacy (Bandura, 1977)—that is, their largely domain-specific judgments that they can manage particular kinds of activities and control their own cognitive and emotional reactions (Bandura, 1988). In this view, people's belief that they cannot cope with potential threats, either cognitively or behaviorally, is what makes them anxious, avoidant, and beset with disturbing thoughts (Bandura, 1986, 1988).

Perceived threat is a function of the relationship between appraisals of possible danger and of one's capacities to deal with it. If people believe they can prevent, control, or manage a potential difficulty, they will not see it as highly threatening, and they will have little reason to fear and avoid it. What matter in treatment, therefore, are not the amount and quality of stimulus exposure or anxiety extinction, but the quality and amount of information people gain about their ability to manage challenging activities. In self-efficacy theory, reductions in anxiety and increases in coping capabilities are not directly causally related, but are each effects of increased self-efficacy.

Self-efficacy theory embodies predictions regarding the factors that affect self-efficacy judgments, the effects of self-efficacy judgments on other psychological responses, and the principles of effective psychological treatment. The present chapter emphasizes the influence of self-efficacy judgments on coping behavior, while only briefly discussing the sources of self-efficacy and self-efficacy-based treatment of phobia. Readers interested in more detailed discussions of these other aspects of self-efficacy theory can consult Bandura (1986, 1988), Cervone and Williams (1992), and Williams (1990, 1992, in press).

RESEARCH ON SELF-EFFICACY: INITIAL FINDINGS

Establishing that an internal psychological factor influences behavior requires at a minimum showing that the factor (in this case, self-efficacy) does indeed correlate strongly with the effect to be explained (in this case phobic disability). This is by no means a trivial test, because many proposed causes of phobia, such as anxiety arousal, in fact do *not* correlate well with phobic behavior (Williams, 1987, 1988). In the standard methodology, phobic people rate their self-efficacy for doing a graduated series of phobia-related tasks, then attempt the tasks, and then rate their self-efficacy a second time; after this they complete a treatment program, and the sequence of measures is repeated (Williams, 1985). The multiple measurement of self-efficacy allows investigators to disentangle the effects of treatment from the effects of behavioral testing. Behavioral approach tests such as those used in self-efficacy research are highly reliable, valid, and meaningful measures of phobic disability (Williams, 1985).

The results of diverse studies with diverse phobic conditions show that regardless of whether treatment is vicarious, imaginal, or performance-based, a close correspondence exists between subjects' level of self-efficacy and their level of actual functional capability (Arnow, Taylor, Agras, & Telch, 1985; Bandura & Adams, 1977; Bandura, Adams, & Beyer, 1977; Bandura, Adams, Hardy, & Howells, 1980; Bandura, Reese, & Adams, 1982; Bandura, Taylor, Williams, Mefford, & Barchas, 1985; Biran & Wilson, 1981; Bourque & Ladouceur, 1980; Emmelkamp & Felten, 1985; Ladouceur, 1983; Southworth & Kirsch, 1988; Telch, Agras, Taylor, Roth, & Galen, 1985; Williams, Dooseman, & Kleifield, 1984; Williams, Kinney, & Falbo, 1989; Williams & Rappoport, 1983; Williams, Turner, & Peer, 1985; Williams & Watson, 1985). Both before and after treatment, the correlations between self-efficacy and subsequent behavior generally fall in the range of .90 to .50, with a median of about .75.

The causal potency of self-efficacy judgments has not gone unchallenged, however. Indeed, more than simple correlational data alone are required to conclude that an internal psychological factor causes behavior. In the following section I consider some of the relevant issues and data. Readers interested in a more extensive discussion of related issues and controversies can consult other sources—for example, Bandura (1978, 1982, 1984, 1988), Rachman (1978), and Williams (1992, in press).

SELF-EFFICACY AS A CAUSE OF BEHAVIOR

Self-Efficacy Influences Coping Behavior

A substantial body of evidence verfies the causal role of self-efficacy beliefs in diverse domains of human functioning (Bandura, 1986, in press). The findings also clarify the cognitive, motivational, affective, and choice processes by which self-efficacy perceptions influence psychological functioning. Efficacy beliefs affect the choices people make, how much effort they mobilize, how long they persevere, their recovery from setbacks, and their vulnerability to stress and depressions. The limited space available here does not permit exploring the broad sweep of this research; I will focus primarily on the domain of phobic dysfunction, in which the findings strongly support the causal role of self-efficacy beliefs.

Phobic people's perceptions of self-efficacy strongly predict subsequent phobia-related behavior even after vicarious or imaginal treatments that involve no actual coping with phobic threats, and that therefore provide no behavioral basis for judging self-efficacy (Bandura & Adams, 1977; Bandura et al., 1977, 1980, 1982). For example, severely snake-phobic subjects who all view an identical therapeutic film typically show widely varying amounts of behavioral benefit, ranging from almost none to virtually complete mastery of the phobia. The individual degrees of behavioral change are accurately predicted by changes in self-efficacy measured prior to subjects' having any posttreatment opportunity to enact phobia-related tasks (Bandura et al., 1977). Self-efficacy perceptions have been systematically manipulated to differential levels by modeling alone, and then related to performance accomplishments (Bandura et al., 1982). The causal contribution of self-efficacy was replicated regardless of whether an intergroup or intrasubject experimental design was used. In all such research, the changes in overt behavior came *after* the experimentalally induced changes in self-efficacy.

Second, cognitive causation is shown by the capacity of self-efficacy to predict generalized behavioral changes (Williams et al., 1989). When agoraphobics are given performance-based treatment for one phobia (e.g., driving), while a distinct and dissimilar phobia (e.g., grocery shopping) is left untreated, generalized improvements occurring in the untreated phobias are more accurately predicted by improvements in self-efficacy for the untreated phobias than by the person's previous behavior with respect to the untreated phobic areas (Williams et al., 1989) I review this generalization study in more detail later, including its finding that self-efficacy judgments also surpassed a variety of alternative cognitive factors in predicting generalized behavioral changes.

Third, even when only phobias that have been directly treated with performance-based approaches are considered, posttreatment coping behavior tends to be more accurately predicted by changes in self-efficacy than by the level of performance achieved during treatment. This is because previous behavior does not perfectly determine self-efficacy judgments. People who achieve a given performance level during treatment will in some cases subsequently think they can do less than they did during treatment, and in other cases that they can do more. When such discrepancies between self-efficacy and previous behavior occur, self-efficacy tends to be the more accurate predictor of coping behavior (e.g., Bandura et al., 1977, 1980; Williams et al., 1984, 1989).

These findings show clearly that self-efficacy changes cause behavioral changes.

Subjects Do Not Try to Match Their Behavior to Their Efficacy Ratings

Some commentators have expressed concern that the superior predictive accuracy of self-efficacy judgments indicats only that subjects feel social pressure to match their performances on behavioral tests to their earlier efficacy judgments. This interpretation is implausible and is invalidated by direct empirical evidence.

First, the phobia research procedure minimizes social pressure and subjects' concern about the efficacy ratings per se. Subjects complete the scales in relative or complete privacy. In any case, the efficacy ratings are not very salient because in many studies they are embedded among numerous other rating forms, all of which may have been completed long before behavioral testing. Moreover, subjects are asked to judge what they believe they are capable of doing, using a confidence scale with many intermediate values reflecting uncertainty; they are decidedly *not* asked to "predict" what they "will" do. When efficacy measures and experimenter surveillance are deliberately made salient, the ratings are found to be *less* rather than more congruent with behavior, because subjects tend to underestimate conservatively underestimate what they can do so as not to appear smugly overconfident (Telch, Bandura, Vinciguerra, Agras, & Stout, 1982).

Second, the psychological context of treatment research with phobic subjects renders the efficacy-matching hypothesis highly inplausible. The subjects have come for treatment of what they see as a serious personal problem. They are asked in the tests to do as much as they can. They are every bit as interested as the experimenter, if not much more so, in just what their disabilities and capabilities are. They are confronted with real phobic threats, which cause considerable distress. To suppose that under these circumstances people would be preoccupied with matching their behavior to some marks they made on a piece of paper embedded among other pieces of paper many minutes, hours, or days ago strains the utmost limits of credulity.

Third, data showing directly that self-efficacy ratings do not have reactive effects upon behavior are found in the pattern of discrepancies between the ratings and subsequent coping behavior. If people were motivated to match behavior to rating, they would infrequently do more than they judged, because once their performance reached the level of their self-efficacy rating, they would simply stop so as to produce an exact match. In fact, however, analyses of many hundreds of behavioral tests with diverse severe phobias reveal the opposite asymmetry, in which coping behavior tends more often to *surpass* than to fall short of the preceding efficacy judgment (Williams & Bauchiess, 1993). This hardly suggests a motivation to produce efficacy–behavior matches (see also Bandura, 1982; Gauthier & Ladouceur, 1981).

Self-Efficacy Is Not Merely "Willingness"

It has been suggested that when subjects rate self-efficacy scales, they are indicating their "willingness," not their perceived ability (Kirsch, 1982, 1990). The "will" to do something is the same essentially as the intention to do it. In self-efficacy theory, such intention is rooted in two beliefs: (1) that one can carry out the act (positive self-efficacy judgment), and (2) that the act will produce positive outcomes (positive outcome expectations). In Kirsch's view, willingness is a function solely of perceived outcomes. Below I will review a large body of data showing that perceived outcomes have little capacity to predict phobic behavior independently of self-efficacy judgments. The willingness view also overlooks the growing body of evidence that judgments of coping ability influence both intentions and coping behaviors (e.g., Ajzen & Madden, 1986; Bandura, in press). Kirsch's analysis suggests that despite rating their self-efficacy as zero for some tasks, phobic individuals really *can* do anything they want; they lack incentives and desire, not ability. Characterizing people with serious behavioral restrictions as willfully misbehaving just does not square with reality. Phobias are fascinating precisely because seemingly sensible people who possess the requisite rudimentary cognitive and motoric skills, who are aware that their fears are senselessness, and who have and perceive every reason to function normally nevertheless *cannot* do so.

People with phobias and compulsions pay frightfully high costs for their disabilities — not only in major financial reversals, but in poor social and recreational functioning and in lowered self-esteem. People who have abandoned fulfilling and lucrative careers, or have endured other severe personal hardships because of a phobia or compulsion, will be surprised to hear that they are simply unwilling to act sensibly. Heartbroken agoraphobics who cannot attend their children's weddings are not just being obstinate or holding out for the right price. Phobic disability is genuine disability.

Kirsch's (1982) finding that mildly fearful undergraduates who were selected according to minimal self-report criteria of timidity, and whose behavioral inhibitions were never actually tested, expressed increased willingness to approach a snake when offered strong make-believe incentives says little about genuine phobic behavior or self-efficacy. Kirsh (1982) interprets his finding that incentives altered undergraduates' self-efficacy ratings as evidence that the subjects were "invoking a linguistic habit" (p. 133) of confusing their confidence in what they could do with their willingness to do it. It is not clear how (or that) these linguistically normal, educated English speakers misunderstood the commonplace distinction between "confidence" that they "can do" (the literal terms that label self-efficacy scales) and their "willingness to do." Perhaps these subjects were simply bored and therefore inattentive to the instructions.

Genuinely phobic people whose lives are severely restricted and who are otherwise tormented by their problem, have and perceive strong incentives to function normallly. Their self-perceived disabilities will not be much affected by additional incentives. It is not inducements that they lack, but the belief that they can cope with what they fear. The following section presents strong evidence that self-efficacy perceptions affect coping behavior independently of outcome expectations.

A Self-Efficacy Judgment Is Not an Outcome Expectation

Social-cognitive theory points out that self-efficacy judgments and outcome expectations constitute two conceptually distinct and partially independent sources of motivation and behavior (Bandura, 1977, 1986; Cervone & Scott, in press). The difference between efficacy judgments and outcome expectatations is generally straightforward. "Self-efficacy" refers to one's self-perceived ability to execute a given course of action, regardless of what may result from that action. Thus, for example, my belief that I can walk four blocks along a busy street is a perception of self-efficacy. "Outcome expectations," in contrast, refer to one's beliefs about what consequences one will experience as a result of a course of action. For example, my belief that I will faint, die, or experience panic if I walk four blocks along the street is an outcome expectation. I can judge myself quite able to do something that I believe will result in undesirable outcomes (e.g., park illegally in Manhattan); and I can judge myself quite *un*able to do something that I believe will result in desirable outcomes (e.g., write beautiful poetry).

In social-cognitive theory, environmental consequences influence behavior largely by creating and altering expectations about action–outcome relationships. It is clear that outcome expectations can affect behavior independently of self-efficacy judgments. People are obviously more likely to do what they expect to be enjoyable and rewarding than what they expect to be aversive and harmful, other factors being equal. But self-efficacy perceptions can also strongly influence behavior independently of outcome expectations. However marvelous the outcomes of an action might seem, people will not attempt it or persist at it if they profoundly believe they cannot execute it. Two people may both expect that if they cross over a large bridge they will enjoy increased vocational and recreational opportunities, but if only one of them believes he or she can do it, they may well differ in actually crossing the bridge. On the other hand, if people see no reason to cross a bridge, then despite maximum bridge-crossing self-efficacy they will not attempt to do so. Resolute action requires both positive outcome expectations and positive self-efficacy judgments.

But the conceptual independence of self-efficacy perceptions and outcome expectations does not mean that they never influence each other. On the contrary, self-efficacy judgments often determine outcome expectations, because outcomes often depend on preceding actions. Inept social approach fosters rejection, whereas adept approach fosters welcoming acceptance. Self-efficacy is not the sole determinant of expected outcomes; however, in the many circumstances where adroit actions produce desirable outcomes but inept actions produce undesirable outcomes, then the outcome one expects must logically be influenced by how well one thinks one can execute the antecedent behavior. In the following subsection I discuss a sizable body of evidence showing that self-efficacy perceptions and outcome expectations are empirically quite distinct.

Self-Efficacy Is Not Reducible to Outcome Expectations

Some commentators have suggested that self-efficacy owes its capacity to predict behavior to its correlation with another cognitive or emotional factor, and that this "third variable" is what actually causes maladaptive behavior and low self-efficacy. This view requires specifying the alternative factor, of course, because it would be gratuitous merely to speculate that an unspecified other variable *might* be at work. In the view of some, the third variable is conditioned anxiety but we have already seen that anxiety arousal is not a viable explanation of phobic behavior.

A more cognitively oriented proposal is that phobic people's expectation of negative outcomes is the third variable driving phobic behavior. Two broad classes of negative outcome expectations have been proposed; these might be called "perceived danger" and "anticipated anxiety." These variables and the research that has directly compared them with self-efficacy judgments are now discussed.

Perceived Danger

In Beck's (Beck, 1976; Beck & Emery with Greenberg, 1985) cognitive theory, phobic disability and distress invariably derive from a belief that phobia-related activities or objects will cause the person physical or psychosocial harm. For example, height phobics fear falling, social phobics fear humiliation and rejection, agoraphobics fear loss of control or death, and so on.

Beck (1976) argues further that although phobic people are by definition aware of the irrationality of their fears, "the phobic individual is usually better able to appraise realistically the actual danger of his feared situations from a distance" (Beck et al., 1985, p. 117). From afar, a phobic man may rate the probability of harm as being near zero, but "as he approaches the situation, the odds change. He goes to 10 percent, to 50 percent, and finally in the situation, he may believe 100 percent that harm will occur" (Beck, 1976, p. 176). This proposition encounters some difficulty in explaining why much phobic avoidance takes place when the individual is far removed in time and space from feared settings. Social phobics decline party invitations from the safety of their living rooms, and bridge phobics plan circuitous routes to ensure that they are never confronted with a large bridge. Despite this difficulty in Beck's theory, it remains possible that danger perceptions contribute to phobic behavior independently of self-efficacy perceptions. My colleagues and I have examined this possibility in a series of studies with height phobics and agoraphobics.

We measured danger perceptions in four studies, using Beck's (1976) procedure of having subjects indicate the likelihood of a harmful consequence occurring if they were to perform each task. Specifically, in two studies with height phobics (Williams & Watson, 1985; Williams et al., 1985), we asked subjects to rate the likelihood that they would fall if they were to ascend to a balcony at each level of a tall building and look down. In two studies in which agoraphobic subjects were behaviorally tested for a variety of phobic areas, subjects were first asked to specify what harmful event they thought could occur if they were to engage in the target test activity (Williams, 1991; Williams et al., 1989). They then rated the likelihood of that event occurring for each task of the behavioral test. If they thought no harmful event could occur, perceived danger was scored as zero. Self-efficacy was also assessed for each test task.

Self-efficacy was consistently the far stronger predictor of behavioral approach. Partial correlation analyses were performed to determine whether either variable predicted approach behavior independently of the other; the results for three of the studies are presented in Table 13.1.[1] Self-efficacy consistently remained a very strong predictor of behavior when perceived danger was held constant, whereas perceived danger consistently lost its capacity to predict behavior when self-efficacy was held constant. The lack of relationship between thoughts of danger and phobic behavior appears to derive in part from phobic people's awareness of the irrationality of their phobias. They often really believe that the activity is not dangerous. It is not unusual for clients (whether severe agoraphobics or height phobics), even when in the phobic situation and experiencing a high level of fear, to state that they know they will not die, go crazy, or the like (Williams & Watson, 1985; Williams et al., 1985). So although phobic individuals may at times perceive danger, they extent to which they do

TABLE 13.1. Partial Correlations between Self-Efficacy and Behavior
(Perceived Danger Held Constant) and between Perceived Danger and Behavior
(Self-Efficacy Held Constant), by Study and Assessment Phase

Study/test phase	n	Self-efficacy predicts behavior (perceived danger held constant)	Perceived danger predicts behavior (self-efficacy held constant)
Williams & Watson (1985)			
Pretreatment	15	.62**	.19
Posttreatment	15	.75***	−.38
Williams et al. (1985)			
Pretreatment	38	.45**	−.05
Posttreatment	38	.91***	.34[a]
Follow-up	38	.90***	−.10
Williams (1991)[b]			
Pretreatment	37	.35*	−.20
Posttreatment	37	.82***	−.08
Follow-up	26	.84***	−.02

[a]Significant in the direction contrary to expectation, $p < .05$.
[b]The n's for this study refer to the number of phobias rather than the number of subjects (26), because multiple phobias were evaluated within some subjects, and the analyses' logic required correlating at the level of phobias.
*$p < .05$. **$p < .01$. ***$p < .001$.

so is highly variable and can be minimal even in people with quite severely disabling phobia.

Anticipated Anxiety

Another kind of anticipated consequence that has been emphasized in explaining phobic behavior, especially agoraphobic behavior, is the expectation that engaging in phobia-related activities will produce aversive feelings of fear and distress (e.g., Chambless & Gracely, 1989). I have pointed out earlier that actual anxiety and panic per se do not have a strong influence on phobic behavior; however, the hypothesis here is that regardless of actual anxiety or panic, the belief that coping behavior will produce intense fear is sufficient to inhibit coping attempts. Of course, even before the evidence is considered, there is the problem of identifying the source of anticipated fear — that is, why someone should expect to be fearful in the first place.

A number of studies have measured "anticipated anxiety" as the level of anxiety phobic subjects expect to experience during each task in a hierarchy of phobia-related approach tasks (Arnow et al., 1985; Kirsch, Tennen, Wickless, Saccone, & Cody, 1983; Telch et al., 1985; Williams, 1991; Williams et al., 1984, 1985, 1989; Williams & Rappoport, 1983).

Correlational analyses showed that both anticipated anxiety and self-efficacy were strong predictors of approach behavior, with self-efficacy consistently being more accurate. Partial correlation analyses, in which anticipated anxiety and self-efficacy were each correlated with behavior when the other was held constant, are shown in Table 13.2. The first column indicates that across studies and assessment phases, self-efficacy remained strongly correlated with approach behavior when anticipated anxiety was held constant, whereas the second column shows that anticipated anxiety lost much or all of its capacity to predict behavior when self-efficacy was held constant.

Anticipated Panic

A closely related but distinct kind of outcome expectation is "anticipated panic," the judged likelihood that a panic attack would occur if one were to engage in phobia-related tasks. Note that this clearly differs from anticipated anxiety, because it is a prediction of the *likelihood* of panic, rather than the *level* of anxiety. Anticipated panic was measured in the Williams (1991) study, as well as in the generalization study to be described later. The pattern of results closely resembles that for anticipated anxiety. In the Williams (1991) data, 37 phobic areas were measured in a series of 26 agoraphobic subjects. The results showed that when the perceived likelihood of panicking was held constant, self-efficacy still strongly predicted approach behavior at pretreatment ($r = .64$), posttreatment ($r = .81$), and follow-up ($r = .86$) (all p's $< .001$). In contrast, with self-efficacy held constant, anticipated panic did not significantly predict behavior at any of the three phases (r's $= .07$, $-.05$, and $.07$, respectively, all nonsignificant).

These data certainly support the view that perceptions of self-efficacy are primary, and that self-efficacy theory cannot be dismissed by simply assuming the primacy of some other kind of cognitive process. The results from the generalization research, described next, further support the conclusion that perceptions of self-efficacy play a central role in phobic disability.

SELF-EFFICACY MEDIATES GENERALIZATION OF BEHAVIORAL CHANGE

The causal status of self-efficacy judgments is shown clearly in a study on generalization of behavioral changes in agoraphobia (Williams et al., 1989). Generalization is well suited to testing the predictive power of self-efficacy, because it involves changes in phobic areas with which a person has had no direct learning experiences during treatment (or, in stimulus terms, without any direct exposure to phobia-relevant stimuli).

TABLE 13.2. Partial Correlations between Self-Efficacy and Behavior (Anticipated Anxiety Held Constant) and between Anticipated Anxiety and Behavior (Self-Efficacy Held Constant) by Study and Testing Phase

Study/test phase	n	Self-efficacy predicts behavior (anticipated anxiety held constant)	Anticipated anxiety predicts behavior (self-efficacy held constant)
Williams & Rappoport (1983)			
Pretreatment 1	20	.40*	−.12
Pretreatment 2	20	.59**	−.28
Posttreatment	20	.45*	.13
Follow-up	18	.45*	.06
Williams et al. (1984)			
Pretreatment	32	.22	−.36*
Posttreatment	32	.59**	−.21
Williams et al. (1985)			
Pretreatment	38	.25	−.36*
Posttreatment	38	.72***	.05
Follow-up	38	66***	−.12
Arnow et al. (1985)			
Pretreatment	24	.77***	.17
Posttreatment	24	.43*	−.08
Follow-up	22	.88***	−.06
Kirsch et al. (1983)			
Pretreatment		.54***	−.34*
Posttreatment		.48**	−.48**
Telch et al. (1985)			
Pretreatment	29	−.28	−.56***
Posttreatment	29	.48**	.15
Follow-up	25	.42*	−.05
Williams (1991)[a]			
Pretreatment	37	.35*	−.20
Posttreatment	37	.82***	−.08
Follow-up	26	.84***	−.02

[a]The n's in this study refer to the number of phobias rather than the number of subjects (26), because multiple phobias were evaluated within some subjects, and the analyses' logic required correlating at the level of phobias.
*p < .05. **p < .01. ***p < .001.

In traditional learning theory, generalization is analyzed in terms of stimulus similarity, with transfer expected to occur in proportion to the number of stimulus features shared by the learning situation and the transfer situation. This approach is problematic because of the great difficulties in quantifying the amount of stimulus overlap between distinct complex situations, as well as in quantifying how much the treatment has exposed the person to the shared stimuli.

Cognitive theories offer a more promising approach, in which transfer is determined by changes in people's cognitive appraisal of the transfer tasks. Thus, for example, Beck's (1976) theory would predict transfer according to changes in people's perceptions of danger, whereas self-efficacy theory would predict generalization according to the changes in people's self-efficacy for coping with the transfer tasks.

Our strategy was to select subjects who showed marked behavioral disability in several phobic areas; to give them performance-based treatment for only some of their phobias (e.g., driving and shopping); and then, in a midtreatment assessment, to measure the resulting behavioral changes in the untreated ("transfer") phobias (e.g., heights and walking). Measures of subjects' perceived self-efficacy, perceived danger, anticipated anxiety, anticipated panic, subjective anxiety, and previous behavior were used to compare possible mechanisms of generalization. After the midtreatment assessment, subjects completed a second treatment phase for some previously untreated phobias, and then completed posttreatment and follow-up assessments. Control subjects completed the measures twice without intervening treatment. Subjects were prohibited from tackling phobia-related activities on their own during the study, and their diary records showed full compliance with this instruction.

First, the results showed that the treated phobias improved significantly more than the transfer phobias, and that the transfer phobias improved significantly more than the control phobias. Thus, there were significant generalized changes in behavior, and on all the cognitive measures as well.

Second, generalization effects varied markedly between subjects and, perhaps even more interestingly, within subjects. That is, individuals whose treated phobias improved a great deal might simultaneously experience both large and small changes in their various transfer phobias. The degree of generalized change was highly idiosyncratic and variable within and between subjects, and could not be predicted simply from stimulus features shared by treated and transfer activities. Predicting the highly variable and idiosyncratic generalized behavioral changes at the midtest and posttest thus constituted a major challenge for each proposed cognitive mediator. It was also of interest to predict the changes in the treated phobias, and in all the phobias between the pretest and follow-up.

The capacity of self-efficacy to predict behavior with the alternative factors held constant, and the capacity of the alternative factors to predict behavior with self-efficacy held constant, are presented in Table 13.3. These results are entirely consistent with the findings reported earlier. Self-efficacy remained significantly predictive of behavioral outcome at all phases, and for both the treated and the transfer phobias, with outcome expectations and prior behavior held constant. In contrast, the alternative factors lost most or all of their predictive capacity with self-efficacy held constant. Previous behavior did not independently predict subsequent

TABLE 13.3. Partial Correlations between Self-Efficacy and Behavior
(Alternate Factors Held Constant) and between Alternate Factors and Behavior
(Self-Efficacy Held Constant) in Generalization Study by Williams et al. (1989)

Alternate factor		Treated phobias		Transfer phobias		
	Pre	Mid	Post	Mid	Post	Follow-up
Self-efficacy predicts behavior (alternate factors held constant)						
Perceived danger	.71***	.79***	.56***	.75***	.75***	.87***
Anticipated anxiety	.45***	.65***	.47**	.53***	.36	.71***
Anticipated panic	.71***	.63***	.41*	.51***	.41*	.75***
Previous behavior	—	.67***	.40*	.59***	.58**	.74***
df	99	35	25	61	16	78
Alternate factors predict behavior (self-efficacy held constant)						
Perceived danger	.02	−.21	−.20	.09	.11	−.02
Anticipated anxiety	−.13	−.15	.02	−.15	−.16	−.03
Anticipated panic	−.10	−.17	−.04	−.20*	−.40*	.05
Previous behavior	—	.49***	.33*	.19	.39	.54***
df	99	35	25	61	16	78

Note. All tests were one-tailed. Pre, pretreatment assessment; Mid, midtreatment assessment; Post, posttreatment assessment. The *df* are based on the number of phobias rather than the number of subjects (26), because multiple phobias were evaluated within some subjects, and the analyses' logic required correlating at the level of phobias. There were many fewer phobias at posttreatment than at midtreatment, because the analysis at posttreatment considered only those phobias that remained severe at the midtreatment assessment phase.
*p < .05. **p < .01. ***p < .001.

behavior in the transfer phobias, and did so in the treated phobias only weakly. The findings thus support the proposition that perceptions of self-efficacy are the primary mediators of both direct and generalized therapeutic changes in phobia.

SELF-EFFICACY AND PERCEIVED CONTROL

It is worth noting in passing the growing convergence of theory and evidence on the power of perceived control to ameliorate defensiveness and stress reactions. Perceived self-efficacy is intimately related to perceived control, because having control means being able to exercise it effectively. Without the self-efficacy belief that one can enact a controlling response, the perception of control does not exist. People who believe they can moderate noxious stimulation will be less anxious than others who cannot do so, even when both groups experience the identical aversive events (Miller, 1979; Seligman, 1975). Moreover, perceived control has benefits even if a person makes no controlling responses (Miller, 1979; Mineka

& Kelly, 1989; Sanderson, Rapee, & Barlow, 1989). The growing emphasis on perceived control in theories of anxiety-related problems (e.g., Barlow, 1988; Foa, Zinbarg, & Rothbaum, 1992) is thus quite consistent with self-efficacy theory.

SOURCES OF SELF-EFFICACY

Self-efficacy theory is embedded in an extensively researched theory of human agency that specifies the social cognitive origins of efficacy beliefs, the processes through which they operate, their diverse effects and how to change them (Bandura, 1986, in press). Self-efficacy perceptions are products of cognitive processing in which individuals access, interpret, and integrate information from diverse sources. There are six principal sources of self-efficacy information: performance accomplishments, vicarious experiences, imaginal experiences, verbal persuasion, physiological arousal, and subjective emotional states.[2]

Performance Accomplishments

Performance accomplishments are the most potent single source of efficacy information, because they convey vivid and self-relevant information based on firsthand experiences of success or failure. Self-efficacy and accomplishments are linked reciprocally: Successes tend to increase efficacy perceptions, which in turn promote further success. However, the effect of attainments on efficacy judgments is not automatic. Sometimes people will judge themselves unable to do again what they have just performed, and at other times they will believe they can do what they have not yet performed (Bandura et al., 1982).

Vicarious Experiences

People base self-efficacy judgments partly on vicarious experiences—the observed actions of others. Vicarious sources are less trustworthy than direct personal experiences because their personal relevance is more open to question, so they are generally less potent means of enhancing self-efficacy (Bandura et al., 1977, 1980; 1982; Bandura & Adams, 1977).

Imaginal Experiences

In imagery-based learning, such as systematic desensitization therapy (Wolpe, 1958), implosion (Stampfl & Levis, 1967), and covert modeling

(Kazdin, 1984), clients imagine themselves or others succeeding in coping actions. A vast body of research reveals that imagined success experiences do clearly benefit many anxious individuals (Bandura, 1969; Kazdin, 1984; Leitenberg, 1976). Nonetheless, imaginal treatments for phobia are substantially less effective than performance-based treatments, because imagining oneself doing something is just not as convincing as actually doing it (Leitenberg, 1976; Williams, 1990).

Verbal Persuasion

People can sometimes be led to a stronger belief in their own capabilities through persuasory dialogue. Because talking about coping is highly indirect experience, it should be less potent than direct coping successes in improving self-efficacy; indeed, verbal cognitive therapies for phobia have generally not been found to be particularly effective, compared with performance-based treatments (Biran & Wilson, 1981; Emmelkamp, Kuipers, & Eggeraat, 1978; Emmelkamp & Mersch, 1982; Ladouceur, 1983; Williams & Rappoport, 1983).

Physiological Arousal

Physiological responses provide another source of efficacy information, but a relatively weak one, because people know from long experience that their viscera tell them relatively little about what they can manage. People are notoriously poor at estimating their autonomic arousal (e.g., Ehlers & Breuer, 1992), and this makes it a treacherous guide. Even if people could accurately perceive their viscera, they would be badly misled because of the empirically poor relationship between physiological arousal and coping capabilities (Bandura, 1978; Lang, 1978; Williams, 1987).

Emotional States

People judge their self-efficacy partly by their subjective states of feeling and mood, which are not simply a function of physiological arousal, and indeed are often quite unrelated to it (e.g., Morrow & Labrum, 1978). Although high anxiety may have some dampening effects on self-efficacy and coping effectiveness, people know that they sometimes do well despite feeling scared, as is often the case with stage actors, dissertation defenders, or panicky agoraphobics (Bandura, 1988; Williams, 1987). And people also know that they can be quite incompetent despite being calm. For these reasons, emotional arousal has only a modest impact on self-efficacy judgments.

SELF-EFFICACY–BASED PSYCHOLOGICAL TREATMENT

Limitations of Exposure Therapy

Self-efficacy theory generally prescribes performance-based mastery experiences as central elements in treatment programs, because such experiences constitute the most potent source of information for building a strong sense of efficacy (Bandura, 1977; Williams, 1990). As mentioned earlier, conceptions of phobia treatment often emphasize the concept of exposure to phobic stimuli (Marks, 1978); this likens treatment to a classical extinction procedure. The exposure principle not only has the serious conceptual failings mentioned earlier in this chapter (Williams, 1987, 1988, 1990), but it gives therapists little guidance as to optimal procedures to follow, beyond a generalized suggestion to bring clients somehow into some kind of prolonged contact with phobic stimuli.

The exposure view does not recognize the active quality of clients' attempts at mastery, gives stimulus proximity and duration of time precedence over performance accomplishments, neglects how therapists might help clients tackle difficult tasks, and neglects the proficiency with which clients perform phobia-related activities in therapy.

Guided Mastery Therapy

In treatment based on self-efficacy theory, or "guided mastery therapy" (Williams, 1990), the emphasis is not on mere stimulus exposure; rather, it is on the quality and amount of information people gain from treatment experiences about what they can manage, and the sense of personal coping effectiveness they thereby develop. Time and fear arousal are incidental, since what counts is rapid mastery, regardless of initial fear levels. During therapeutic performance, people are not passively absorbing stimuli, but actively mastering a challenge.

Therapists, too, can play an active role. The guided mastery therapist uses several classes of techniques to foster success and ensure that clients develop a robust and generalized sense of mastery.

First, the therapist assists people in tackling tasks that otherwise would be too difficult. For example, the therapist may accompany a freeway-phobic woman the first few times she attempts to drive the freeway, then may follow her in another car, increasing the distance behind her until she can drive the freeway unaided. The point of the assistance is to create an interim increase in self-efficacy, which will enable the person to take on yet more challenging tasks; this should result in an ascending spiral of therapeutic change.

Second, the mastery therapist helps clients to increase the quality and flexibility of their performance by guiding them in doing therapeutic tasks more proficiently, without embedded ritualistic defensive maneuvers and self-restrictions. For example, the therapist can encourage the freeway-phobic woman to turn off the radio rather than have it blaring, and to change lanes and pass slower cars instead of just keeping to the slow lane. Such defensive maneuvers and self-restrictions, which are very common but much neglected in accounts of agoraphobia therapy, tend to limit clients' sense of self-efficacy by vividly reminding them of their incompetence, and by leading them to attribute successes to the defensive activities rather than to their own growing capabilities (Kinney, 1992; Williams, 1985).

Third, when people are progressing well, the therapist guides them to do the tasks increasingly independently—fading out the therapist and "safe" persons, as well as reducing and then removing other performance aids. The therapist arranges for varied independent success experiences so that clients' self-efficacy will be unconditional.

Research on Guided Mastery

The most exacting and direct test of the power of guided mastery is to compare it to the same or a longer duration of "pure" stimulus exposure. Eight studies with phobic individuals have compared one group receiving a varied repertoire of guided mastery aids during therapeutic performance to another group receiving strong encouragement to remain fully exposed to the same frightening stimuli, but few specific mastery aids (Bandura, Jeffrey, & Wright, 1974; Bourque & Ladouceur, 1980; O'Brien & Kelley, 1980; Öst, Salkovskis, & Hellstrom, 1991; Williams et al., 1984, 1985; Williams & Zane, 1989; Zane & Williams, 1993). Six of the eight studies (all but the Bourque & Ladouceur, 1980, and Zane & Williams, 1993 studies) found therapist-guided mastery to be substantially superior to mere exposure.

Theories of psychological mechanisms must be judged in part by their capacity to generate effective psychological treatments. These findings provide additional support for self-efficacy theory, illustrating that it can be a highly useful guide for increasing the power of treatment interventions.

CONCLUSIONS

Self-efficacy theory has demonstrated its power to account for behavioral change brought about by diverse treatments for diverse phobias. Perceptions of self-efficacy are causal determinants of behavior in their own right. Their accuracy in predicting behavior cannot easily be explained in terms

364   *III. TREATMENT*

of other cognitive, emotional, or stimulus factors. Moreover, self-efficacy
theory helps promote more effective means of reducing phobic disability
and distress. The evidence to date thus strongly encourages continued systematic efforts to investigate the role played by self-efficacy perceptions
in anxiety disorders.

ACKNOWLEDGMENT

Preparation of this chapter, and much of my research reported in it, were supported by U.S. Public Health Service Grant No. R29-MH43285.

NOTES

1. The Williams et al. (1989) study of generalization had a somewhat more
involved design, and so is presented in subsequent section ("Self-Efficacy Mediates Generalization of Behavioral Change"). Its findings were quite consistent with
those reported here.
2. Bandura (1977, 1986) cites only performance accomplishment, vicarious
experiences, physiological arousal, and verbal persuasion as sources. He includes
systematic desensitization and subjective emotion under physiological arousal, but
this seems misleading. Since subjective emotion is so poorly correlated with physiological arousal (e.g., Morrow & Labrum, 1978), it seems ill advised to include
subjective emotion in the physiological category. In systematic desensitization, treatment may be keyed to subjective anxiety, and in any case the operative procedural
ingredient in systematic desensitization as in covert modeling (Kazdin, 1974) and
implosion (Stampfl & Levis, 1967) appears to be simply the act of imagining oneself coping with the phobic object (Leitenberg, 1976). Such imaginal self-modeling
could be called "vicarious experience," but "imaginal experience" seems more
straightforward.

REFERENCES

Ajzen, I., & Madden, T. J. (1986). Prediction of goal-directed behavior: Atti-
tudes, intentions, and perceived behavioral control. *Journal of Experimental
Social Psychology, 22,* 453–474.
Arnow, B. A., Taylor, C. B., Agras, W. S., & Telch, M. J. (1985). Enhancing
agoraphobia treatment outcome by changing couple communication pat-
terns. *Behavior Therapy, 16,* 452–467.
Bandura, A. (1969). *Principles of behavior modification.* New York: Holt, Rine-
hart & Winston.
Bandura, A. (1977). Self-efficacy: Toward a unifying theory of behavioral change.
Psychological Review, 84, 191–215.
Bandura, A. (1978). Reflections on self-efficacy. *Advances in Behaviour Research
and Therapy, 1,* 237–269.

Bandura, A. (1982). The assessment and predictive generality of self-percepts of efficacy. *Journal of Behavior Therapy and Experimental Psychiatry, 13,* 195–199.

Bandura, A. (1984). Recycling misconceptions of perceived self-efficacy. *Cognitive Therapy and Research, 8,* 231–255.

Bandura, A. (1986). *Social foundations of thought and action: A social cognitive theory.* Englewood Cliffs, NJ: Prentice-Hall.

Bandura, A. (1988). Self-efficacy conception of anxiety. *Anxiety Research, 1,* 77–98.

Bandura, A. (in press). *Self efficacy: The exercise of control.* New York: Freeman.

Bandura, A., & Adams, N. E. (1977). Analysis of self-efficacy theory of behavioral change. *Cognitive Therapy and Research, 1,* 287–308.

Bandura, A., Adams, N. E., & Beyer, J. (1977). Cognitive processes mediating behavior change. *Journal of Personality and Social Psychology, 35,* 125–139.

Bandura, A., Adams, N. E., Hardy, A., & Howells, G. (1980). Tests of the generality of self-efficacy theory. *Cognitive Therapy and Research, 4,* 39–66.

Bandura, A., Jeffrey, R. W., & Wright, C. L. (1974). Efficacy of participant modeling as a function of response induction aids. *Journal of Abnormal Psychology, 83,* 56–64.

Bandura, A., Reese, L., & Adams, N. E. (1982). Microanalysis of action and fear arousal as a function of differential levels of perceived self-efficacy. *Journal of Personality and Social Psychology, 43,* 5–21.

Bandura, A., Taylor, C. B., Williams, S. L., Mefford, I. N., & Barchas, J. D. (1985). Catecholamine secretion as a function of perceived self-efficacy. *Journal of Consulting and Clinical Psychology, 53,* 406–414.

Barlow, D. H. (1988). *Anxiety and its disorders: The nature and treatment of anxiety and panic.* New York: Guilford Press.

Beck, A. T. (1976). *Cognitive therapy and the emotional disorders.* New York: International Universities Press.

Beck, A. T., & Emery, G., with Greenberg, R. L. (1985). *Anxiety disorders and phobias: A cognitive perspective.* New York: Basic Books.

Biran, M., & Wilson, G. T. (1981). Treatment of phobic disorders using cognitive and exposure methods: A self-efficacy analysis. *Journal of Consulting and Clinical Psychology, 49,* 886–899.

Bourque, P., & Ladouceur, R. (1980). An investigation of various performance-based treatments with agoraphobics. *Behaviour Research and Therapy, 18,* 161–170.

Cervone, D., & Scott, W. D. (in press). Self-efficacy theory of behavioral change: Foundations, conceptual issues, and therapeutic implications. In W. O'Donohue & L. Krasner (Eds.), *Theories in behavior therapy.* Washington, DC: American Psychological Association.

Cervone, D., & Williams, S. L. (1992). Social cognitive theory and personality. In G.-V. Capara & G. L. Van Heck (Eds.), *Modern personality psychology: Critical reviews and new directions* (pp. 200–252). New York: Harvester-Wheatsheaf.

Chambless, D. L., & Gracely, E. J. (1989). Fear of fear and the anxiety disorders. *Cognitive Therapy and Research, 13,* 9–20.

Craske, M. G., & Barlow, D. H. (1988). A review of the relationship between panic and avoidance. *Clinical Psychology Review, 8,* 667–685.

Ehlers, A., & Breuer, P. (1992). Increased cardiac awareness in panic disorder. *Journal of Abnormal Psychology, 101,* 371–382.

Emmelkamp, P. M. G., & Felten, M. (1985). The process of exposure *in vivo:* Cognitive and physiological changes during treatment of acrophobia. *Behaviour Research and Therapy, 23,* 219–223.

Emmelkamp, P. M. G., Kuipers, C. M., & Eggeraat, J. B. (1978). Cognitive modification versus prolonged exposure *in vivo:* A comparison with agoraphobics as subjects. *Behaviour Research and Therapy, 16,* 33–41.

Emmelkamp, P. M. G., & Mersch, P. P. (1982). Cognition and exposure *in vivo* in the treatment of agoraphobics: Short-term and delayed effects. *Cognitive Therapy and Research, 6,* 77–88.

Foa, E. B., Zinbarg, R., & Rothbaum, B. O. (1992). Uncontrollability and unpredictability in post-traumatic stress disorder: An animal model. *Psychological Bulletin, 112,* 218–238.

Gauthier, J., & Ladouceur, R. (1981). The influence of self-efficacy reports on performance. *Behavior Therapy, 12,* 436–439.

Kazdin, A. E. (1984). Covert modeling. *Advances in Cognitive-Behavioral Research and Therapy, 3,* 103–129.

Kinney, P. J. (1992). *The role of attributions in self-efficacy and behavioral changes following performance-based treatment of phobia.* Unpublished doctoral dissertation, Lehigh University.

Kirsch, I. (1982). Efficacy expectations or response predictions: The meaning of efficacy ratings as a function of task characteristics. *Journal of Personality and Social Psychology, 42,* 132–136.

Kirsch, I. (1990). *Changing expectations: A key to effective psychotherapy.* Pacific Grove, CA: Brooks/Cole.

Kirsch, I., Tennen, H., Wickless, C., Saccone, A. J., & Cody, S. (1983). The role of expectancy in fear reduction. *Behavior Therapy, 14,* 520–533.

Ladouceur, R. (1983). Participant modeling with or without cognitive treatment of phobias. *Journal of Consulting and Clinical Psychology, 51,* 942–944.

Lang, P. J. (1971). The application of psychophysiological methods to the study of psychotherapy and behavior modification. In A. E. Bergin & S. L. Garfield (Eds.), *Handbook of psychotherapy and behavior change.* New York: Wiley.

Lang, P. J. (1978). Anxiety: Toward a psychophysiological definition. In H. S. Akiskal & W. L. Webb (Eds.), *Psychiatric diagnosis: Exploration of biological predictors* (pp. 365–389). New York: Spectrum.

Leitenberg, H. (1976). Behavioral approaches to the treatment of neuroses. In H. Leitenberg (Ed.), *Handbook of behavior modification and behavior therapy* (pp. 124–167). Englewood Cliffs, NJ: Prentice-Hall.

Marks, I. (1978). Behavioral psychotherapy of adult neurosis. In S. L. Garfield & A. E. Bergin (Eds.), *Handbook of psychotherapy and behavior change* (pp. 493–547). New York: Wiley.

Mathews, A. M., Gelder, M. G., & Johnston, D. W. (1981). *Agoraphobia: Nature and treatment.* New York: Guilford Press.

Miller, S. M. (1979). Controllability and human stress: Method, evidence and theory. *Behaviour Research and Therapy, 17,* 287–304.

Mineka, S. (1979). The role of fear in theories of avoidance learning, flooding, and extinction. *Psychological Bulletin, 86,* 985–1010.

Mineka, S., & Kelly, K. A. (1989). The relationship between anxiety, lack of control and loss of control. In A. Steptoe & A. Appels (Eds.), *Stress, personal control and health* (pp. 163–191). New York: Wiley.

Morrow, G. R., & Labrum, A. H. (1978). The relationship between psychological and physiological measures of anxiety. *Psychological Medicine, 8,* 95–101.

Mowrer, O. H. (1960). *Learning theory and behavior.* New York: Wiley.

O'Brien, T., & Kelley, J. (1980). A comparison of self-directed and therapist-directed practice for fear reduction. *Behaviour Research and Therapy, 18,* 573–579.

Öst, L., Salkovskis, P. M., & Hellstrom, K. (1991). One-session therapist-directed exposure vs. self-exposure in the treatment of spider phobia. *Behavior Therapy, 22,* 407–422.

Rachman, S. (1976). The passing of the two-stage theory of fear and avoidance: Fresh possibilities. *Behaviour Research and Therapy, 14,* 125–131.

Rachman, S. (Ed.). (1978). Perceived self-efficacy: Analyses of Bandura's theory of behavioural change [Special issue]. *Advances in Behaviour Research and Therapy, 1*(3).

Rosenthal, T. L., & Bandura, A. (1978). Psychological modeling: Theory and practice. In S. L. Garfield & A. E. Bergin (Eds.), *Handbook of psychotherapy and behavior change* (2nd ed., pp. 621–658). New York: Wiley.

Sanderson, W. C., Rapee, R. M., & Barlow, D. H. (1989). The influence of an illusion of control on panic attacks induced via inhalation of 5.5% carbon dioxide-enriched air. *Archives of General Psychiatry, 46,* 157–162.

Seligman, M. E. P. (1975). *Helplessness: On depression, development, and death.* San Francisco: W. H. Freeman.

Seligman, M. E. P., & Johnston, J. C. (1973). A cognitive theory of avoidance learning. In F. J. McGuigan & D. B. Lumsden (Eds.), *Contemporary approaches to conditioning and learning* (pp. 69–110). Washington, DC: V. H. Winston.

Southworth, S., & Kirsch, I. (1988). The role of expectancy in exposure-generated fear reduction in agoraphobia. *Behaviour Research and Therapy, 26,* 113–120.

Stampfl, T. G., & Levis, D. J. (1967). Essentials of implosive therapy. *Journal of Abnormal Psychology, 72,* 496–503.

Telch, M. J., Agras, W. S., Taylor, C. B., Roth, W. T., & Gallen, C. C. (1985). Combined pharmacological and behavioral treatment for agoraphobia. *Behaviour Research and Therapy, 23,* 325–335.

Telch, M. J., Bandura, A., Vinciguerra, P., Agras, A., & Stout. A. L. (1982). Social demand for consistency and congruence between self-efficacy and performance. *Behavior Therapy, 13,* 694–701.

Williams, S. L. (1985). On the nature and measurement of agoraphobia. *Progress in Behavior Modification, 19,* 109–144.

Williams, S. L. (1987). On anxiety and phobia. *Journal of Anxiety Disorders, 1,* 161–180.

Williams, S. L. (1988). Addressing misconceptions about phobia, anxiety, and self-efficacy: A reply to Marks. *Journal of Anxiety Disorders, 2,* 277–289.

Williams, S. L. (1990). Guided mastery treatment of agoraphobia: Beyond stimulus exposure. *Progress in Behavior Modification, 26,* 89–121.

Williams, S. L. (1991). [Cognitive processes in agoraphobia] Unpublished raw data.

Williams, S. L. (1992). Perceived self-efficacy and phobic disability. In R. Schwarzer (Ed.), *Self-efficacy: Thought control of action* (pp.149–176). New York: Hemisphere.

Williams, S. L. (in press). Role of self-efficacy in anxiety and phobic disorders. In J. Maddux (Ed.), *Self-efficacy, adaptation, and adjustment.* New York: Plenum Press.

Williams, S. L., & Bauchiess, R. (1993). *Agoraphobics overestimate their disability and anxiety proneness: Implications for the maintenance and treatment of agoraphobia.* Unpublished manuscript, Lehigh University.

Williams, S. L., Dooseman, G., & Kleifield, E. (1984). Comparative effectiveness of guided mastery and exposure treatments for intractable phobias. *Journal of Consulting and Clinical Psychology, 52,* 505–518.

Williams, S. L., Kinney, P. J., & Falbo, J. (1989). Generalization of therapeutic changes in agoraphobia: The role of perceived self-efficacy. *Journal of Consulting and Clinical Psychology, 57,* 436–442.

Williams, S. L., & Rappoport, A. (1983). Cognitive treatment in the natural environment for agoraphobics. *Behavior Therapy, 14,* 299–313.

Williams, S. L., Turner, S. M., & Peer, D. F. (1985). Guided mastery and performance desensitization treatments for severe acrophobia. *Journal of Consulting and Clinical Psychology, 53,* 237-247.

Williams, S. L., & Watson, N. (1985). Perceived danger and perceived self-efficacy as cognitive determinants of acrophobic behavior. *Behavior Therapy, 16,* 237–247.

Williams, S. L., & Zane, G. (1988). Guided mastery and stimulus exposure treatments for severe performance anxiety in agoraphobics. *Behaviour Research and Therapy, 27,* 237–247.

Wolpe, J. (1958). *Psychotherapy by reciprocal inhibition.* Stanford, CA: Stanford University Press.

Zane, G., & Williams, S. L. (1993). Performance-related anxiety in agoraphobia: Treatment procedures and cognitive mechanisms of change. *Behavior Therapy, 24,* 625–643.

The Limitations of Self Efficacy Theory in Explaining Therapeutic Changes in Phobic Behavior

RICHARD J. MCNALLY
EDNA B. FOA

WILLIAMS HAS LUCIDLY DESCRIBED the self-efficacy theory of phobia reduction in Chapter 13. We agree that a satisfactory account of treatment for pathological fear should elucidate the mechanisms underlying therapeutic change, and that a descriptive theory that includes merely parametric variables is inadequte. However, we differ strongly from Williams on level of analysis and in matters of detail. This commentary concerns points of disagreement.

SELF-EFFICACY VERSUS EXPOSURE

Williams commits a conceptual error by comparing self-efficacy theory with exposure "theory." Self-efficacy is indeed a theory of behavior change, "exposure" is not. "Exposure" denotes a set of therapeutic procedure whose effects themselves require a theoretical explanation. The inability of exposure to explain treatment effectiveness arises not because it is a false theory, as Williams implies, but because it is not a theory at all. Some proponents of exposure treatment mistakenly attribute a status of an explanatory theory to the techniques themselves. The relative merits of self-efficacy theory are best tested against other theories of behavior change that explain *why*, not only *how*, behavioral treatments for phobia work (e.g., Foa & Kozak, 1986).

CONSCIOUS AND NONCONSCIOUS
COGNITIVE DETERMINANTS OF PHOBIA

The theoretical account that Williams provides for why treatment for phobia works rests on the assumption that the phobic patient is capable of verbalizing all the cognitive determinants of phobic behavior. Although we do not deny the importance of conscious cognitive processes, many dysfunctions associated with phobic disorders are not accessible to introspection. Indeed, a major research emphasis during the past decade has concerned the application of experimental psychology methods that elucidate automatic, nonconscious information-processing biases that figure in the maintenance, and perhaps the etiology, of phobic and other anxiety disorders (for reviews, see Mathews & MacLeod, 1994; McNally, 1994). These studies imply that disordered cognition in phobia is not confined to inaccurate estimates of perceived self-efficacy, or to other conscious forms of cognitive disturbance. Some theorists even suggest that the crucial mechanisms in emotional disorders are largely unavailable to conscious processing. Accordingly, a theory that relies totally on conscious processes is bound to be inaccurate or at best insufficient.

IS BEHAVIORAL AVOIDANCE
ALWAYS THE PRIMARY PROBLEM?

Williams rightly emphasizes the disabilities stemming from behavioral avoidance. But motoric avoidance behavior is not invariably the most problematic aspect of anxiety disorders. For example, many socially phobic individuals do not avoid anxiety-evoking situations, but endure them with great distress. Moreover, avoidance behavior is not especially prominent in generalized anxiety disorder, "pure" obsessional disorder, or panic disorder without agoraphobia. The relevance of self-efficacy theory for these nonavoidant anxiety disorders has yet to be fully explored.

HOW DOES SELF-EFFICACY ACCOUNT
FOR DIFFERENTIAL EFFECTS OF TREATMENT
ON PHOBIC ANXIETY AND AVOIDANCE BEHAVIOR?

Several studies revealed that after exposure treatment for agoraphobia, avoidance greatly diminished while panic attacks remained (e.g., Arnow, Taylor, Agras, & Telch, 1985). Conversely, after cognitive-behavioral therapy with panic-disordered individuals who had mild agoraphobia, panic attacks greatly diminished while avoidance not infrequently persisted

(Barlow, Craske, Cerny, & Klosko, 1989). Along similar lines, how does self-efficacy theory explain why exposure to contaminants reduces obsessional anxiety in "washers" but does not reduce rituals (e.g., active avoidance behavior), whereas response prevention ameliorates rituals but not obsessional anxiety (Foa, Steketee, & Milby, 1980)?

DO SELF-EFFICACY SCALES REFLECT PERCEIVED ABILITY OR WILLINGNESS?

Williams misunderstands Kirsch's (1982, 1985) argument that self-efficacy scales measure willingness to perform feared tasks, not perceived ability to perform them. Kirsch does not claim that phobic individuals are "willfully misbehaving" (Williams, Chapter 13) by exhibiting behavioral avoidance, nor does he hold that phobics "simply do not wish to act sensibly" (Williams, Chapter 13). He does not morally condemn patients, nor does he underestimate their disability. Instead, Kirsch holds that behavioral self-efficacy scales make sense only if one interprets them as tapping willingness to engage in avoided activities. For example, if we ask obsessive–compulsive washers whether they "can" reach down and pick up trash off the street, low estimates of perceived self-efficacy do not reflect doubts about their capability of executing the requisite motor movements (e.g., bending over, grasping the trash with their fingers). Rather, their low estimates of perceived self-efficacy can only reflect an unwillingness to engage in feared activities.

Unlike Williams, other self-efficacy theorists, such as Telch and his colleagues (e.g., Telch, Brouillard, Telch, Agras, & Taylor, 1989; Valentiner, Telch, Petruzzi, & Bolte, in press), have persuasively argued that self-efficacy ought to be framed in terms of the patient's perceived ability to cope with the consequences of encountering phobic threats, rather than in terms the ability (willingness?) to engage in certain motor behaviors. For example, it makes more sense to evaluate an agoraphobic's perceived self-efficacy for coping with panic and its consequences than to evaluate his or her perceived self-efficacy for walking through a crowded shopping mall. An efficacy assessment for coping with panic taps perceived skill, not willingness, whereas an efficacy assessment for walking through a mall taps willingness, not perceived skill.

SUMMARY

In summary, self-efficacy theory's limitations stem from its sole focus on one aspect of anxiety disorders (i.e., avoidance behavior), its disregard

for the nonconsciouos processes that are probably involved in the maintenance of these disorders, and the conceptual confusion between willingness to engage in a give behavior and perceived ability to cope with
the feared consequences of that behavior.

REFERENCES

Arnow, B. A., Taylor, C. B., Agras, W. S., & Telch, M. J. (1985). Enhancing
agoraphobia treatment outcome by changing couple communication patterns. *Behavior Therapy, 16,* 452–467.

Barlow, D. H., Craske, M. G., Cerny, J. A., & Klosko, J. S. (1989). Behavioral
treatment of panic disorder. *Behavior Therapy, 20,* 261–282.

Foa, E. B., & Kozak, M. J. (1986). Emotional processing of fear: Exposure to
corrective information. *Psychological Bulletin, 99,* 20–35.

Foa, E. B., Steketee, G., & Milby, J. B. (1980). Differential effects of exposure
and response prevention in obsessive–compulsive washers. *Journal of Consulting and Clinical Psychology, 48,* 71–79.

Kirsch, I. (1982). Efficacy expectations or response predictions: The meaning of
efficacy ratings as a function of task characteristics. *Journal of Personality
and Social Psychology, 42,* 132–136.

Kirsch, I. (1985). Self-efficacy and expectancy: Old wine with new labels. *Journal of Personality and Social Psychology, 49,* 824–830.

Mathews, A., & MacLeod, C. (1994). Cognitive approaches to emotion and emotional disorders. *Annual Review of Psychology, 45,* 25–50.

McNally, R. J. (1994). *Panic disorder: A critical analysis.* New York: Guilford
Press.

Telch, M. J., Brouillard, M., Telch, C. F., Agras, W. S., & Taylor, C. B. (1989).
Role of cognitive appraisal in panic-related avoidance. *Behaviour Research
and Therapy, 27,* 373–383.

Valentiner, D. P., Telch, M. J., Petruzzi, D. C., & Bolte, M. C. (in press). Cog-
nitive mechanisms in claustrophobia: An examination of Reiss and
McNally's expectancy model and Bandura's self-efficacy theory. *Cognitive
Therapy and Research.*

Overcoming Phobia: Unconscious Bioinformational Deconditioning or Conscious Cognitive Reappraisal?

S. LLOYD WILLIAMS

ARE PHOBIC PEOPLE AVOIDANCE MACHINES, driven mainly by an unconscious conditioned bioinformational fear program, as Foa and McNally propose in Chapter 12? Or are they reflective thinking individuals, whose phobias spring largely from self-beliefs about their vulnerabilities and limitations, as I propose in Chapter 13? Foa and McNally hold that conscious thought is neither the main contributing cause of phobia nor the main factor in its treatment; rather, they contend that phobic behavior is caused by an underlying bioinformational "fear structure," and that therapeutic change in phobia results from a kind of neoclassical deconditioning of anxiety. Their analysis is seriously flawed. It yields weak predictors of, and treatments for, phobic behavior.

The bioinformational model's fear structure presents a mechanical view of people. It consists of declarative and procedural stimulus, response, and meaning propositions represented in multiple levels of brain code in a network of memory nodes. This network processes information via spreading activation across nodes and levels, extending to inhibitory and excitatory somatovisceral afferents and efferents, with associated prototypes, emotional images, schemas, templates, and diverse other contents (Lang, 1985). This polymorphous "mechanism" seems an overview of the entire human mental faculty. But broad allusions to variegated collections of poorly defined phenomena, caused by all kinds of processes, portray a cause so extremely complicated and hard to measure that it has little

value. And the few meaningful predictions this model yields are discon-
firmed by a vast quantity of evidence.

Testing causal mechanisms requires identifying the measures we must
gather from phobic people during treatment in order to determine whether
changes in the mechanism predict changes in how people manage phobia-
related tasks after treatment. Changes in the self-efficacy mechanism are
measured directly, using simple, straightforward self-efficacy questionnaires. Foa and McNally do not say how to measure the fear structure
or its multifarious unconscious components. Instead, they propose to measure plain old anxiety. They thereby leap from the frying pan of an un-
testable mechanism into the fire of a long-invalidated mechanism.

Their unswerving loyalty to anxiety theory, despite its dismal record
of empirical failure, is striking. Whether anxiety is offered as a causal
mechanism in its own right, or as a stand-in for bioinformational processing, it can be confidently ruled out as the major determinant of change
in phobia.

One difficulty is that "anxiety" is a house divided against itself. The
various physiological and subjective fear responses diverge routinely from
one another (Lang, 1985; Williams, 1987), and so yield contradictory
predictions of benefit. Indeed, why the discordant responses should be
called aspects of the same underlying "anxiety" entity is far from clear
(Williams, 1987).

Foa and McNally specifically predict that the people who benefit most
will, when initially confronting phobic threats, become highly anxious
(both physiologically and subjectively) but not too anxious. They do not
specify at what levels each of the various anxiety responses start or stop
being therapeutic, but in any case the prediction is empirically false.
Response to treatment typically bears little relation to anxiety levels (Williams, 1987). For example, among 299 agoraphobics tested and treated
for 426 areas of disability in my research program, initial subjective anxiety predicted behavioral change very poorly, $r(424) = .13$, and continued
to do so after those with maximum initial anxiety were excluded, $r(359)$
$= .11$. The respective figures for self-efficacy change predicting behavior
change were .64 and .63; thus self-efficacy explained over 20 times the
variance explained by initial anxiety!

Foa and McNally further state that people whose anxiety declines
most during each treatment session, and from one session to the next,
will benefit most. To say that decline in anxiety "predicts" treatment benefit
is to say that treatment benefit predicts treatment benefit. Some predictor! If benefit refers to improved behavior, then improvement will not be
predicted accurately by decline in anxiety (Williams, 1987, 1988, Chapter 13). In my data, decline in anxiety from pretreatment to posttreatment predicted increase in coping behavior very weakly, $r(424) = -.22$
(and if one excludes those with initial maximum anxiety, $r[359] = -.16$).

Nor is the Foa and McNally analysis of much value for conducting therapy. They hold that "emotional processing" requires activating the fear structure by giving the client information that matches it, and then altering it by giving the client information incompatible with its "pathological elements." They do not say how the therapist is to know what information is in the unconscious fear structure in the first place; how to measure the degree of match between it and potential therapeutic information; how much match is needed to activate it; most importantly, how much and *what kind* of unmatch is needed to alter it; or what the therapist must actually do to bring about the required matches and unmatches. Self-efficacy theory specifies all that is needed to make detailed therapeutic use of the self-efficacy mechanism (Williams, 1990). What is required is not matching or unmatching unconscious fear structures, but rather giving people opportunities for gaining a sense of confidence about coping with previously avoided activities.

Foa and McNally acknowledge that traditional conditioning theories have failed, but then they propound those same failed theories—at times using the old conditioning language, at times using fancy modern "information-processing" language. Similarly, they rely heavily on the concepts of stimulus exposure and habituation, which make people into passive receivers of conditioned stimuli, and which liken treatment to mechanical Pavlovian extinction. I have described elsewhere how this kind of exposure/deconditioning analysis gives dysfunctional guidance for conducting phobia treatment (Williams, 1987, 1990).

Why should we adopt the cumbersome tedious terminology of conditioning when we have available the much more potent, parsimonious, apprehensible, and measurable mechanisms of conscious thought? Parsimony is conceptual simplicity and directness, not the reflexive rejection of awareness. In self-efficacy theory, people undergoing treatment are behaviorally active in trying to master phobia-related tasks, and cognitively active in reappraising their growing coping abilities and diminishing vulnerability. Among many other advantages, the self-efficacy analysis empowers therapists and clients to actively accelerate the process of cognitive and behavioral change (Williams, 1990), rather than passively relying on the prolonged passage of time to bring about "habituation."

Foa and McNally's heavy use of conditioning and stimulus exposure terminology springs from an apparent ambivalence, if not antipathy, toward conscious causation. Foa and McNally state that *after* fear habituation takes place, positive cognitive changes occur. But they do not explain what causes the habituation in the first place. They posit that the structures that generate fear are not accessible to introspection. Yet they emphasize phobic people's dysfunctional beliefs, pathological meanings, and danger estimations. So, are such cognitions causal factors in their own right, or merely inert by-products of the fear structure and epiphenomena of conditioning processes? One cannot have it both ways.

Theories of phobia must take cognition seriously. Reflective thinking, and the persons who engage in it, cannot be dismissed without paying a heavy price in lost scientific and therapeutic power. People with phobias are conscious beings whose thoughts strongly affect their well-being, for good or ill. Because self-efficacy theory takes that reality into account, it will continue to be more successful than bioinformational deconditioning in explaining and treating phobia.

REFERENCES

Lang, P. J. (1985). The cognitive psychophysiology of emotion: fear and anxiety. In A. H. Tuma & J. D. Maser (Eds.), *Anxiety and the anxiety disorders* (pp. 131–170). Hillsdale, NJ: Erlbaum.

Williams, S. L. (1987). On anxiety and phobia. *Journal of Anxiety Disorders, 1,* 161–180.

Williams, S. L. (1988). Addressing misconceptions about phobia, anxiety, and self-efficacy: A reply to Marks. *Journal of Anxiety Disorders, 2,* 277–289.

Williams, S. L. (1990). Guided mastery treatment of agoraphobia: Beyond stimulus exposure. *Progress in Behavior Modification, 26,* 89–121.

Index